LIFETIME Physical Fitness

A Personal Choice

LIFETIME Physical Fitness
A Personal Choice

Melvin H. Williams
Old Dominion University

uucb
Wm. C. Brown Publishers   Dubuque, Iowa

Book Team

Edward G. Jaffe *Senior Editor*
Lynne M. Meyers *Associate Editor*
Lisa Bogle *Designer*
Beverly ODell-Potter *Production Editor*
Carol M. Schiessl *Photo Research Editor*
Mavis M. Oeth *Permissions Manager*
Aileene Lockhart *Consulting Editor*, Texas Woman's University

Wm. C. Brown *Chairman of the Board*
Mark C. Falb *President and Chief Executive Officer*

wcb

Wm. C. Brown Publishers, College Division

Lawrence E. Cremer *President*
James L. Romig *Vice-President, Product Development*
David A. Corona *Vice-President, Production and Design*
E. F. Jogerst *Vice-President, Cost Analyst*
Bob McLaughlin *National Sales Manager*
Marcia H. Stout *Marketing Manager*
Craig S. Marty *Director of Marketing Research*
Marilyn A. Phelps *Manager of Design*
Eugenia M. Collins *Production Editorial Manager*
Mary M. Heller *Photo Research Manager*

Cover Photo by John Kelly/The Image Bank
Photographs by author except as indicated.
Illustrations by Ruth Krabach and Fine Line Illustrations, Inc.

Library of Congress Catalog Card Number: 84–071677

ISBN 0–697–00147–01

2–00147–01

Printed in the United States of America
10 9 8 7 6 5 4 3 2 1

Contents

Preface

The United States is in the midst of a health and fitness boom, with millions of Americans initiating aerobic exercise programs, shifting to a more natural healthful diet, breaking the smoking habit, decreasing alcohol consumption, and using various stress reduction techniques, all in order to look and feel better. This trend is a positive one, for these life-style changes may help to prevent many of the degenerative diseases that plague our modern society. These healthful changes characterize a Positive Health Life-style in which proper exercise and sound nutrition are two of the key elements.

The health and fitness boom originated among individuals in their thirties and forties, but increasing numbers of college-aged students appear to be adopting a Positive Health Life-style. This textbook is designed to provide contemporary information about the beneficial effects of a Positive Health Life-style and how to implement and live such a life-style. It is designed primarily to be used in conjunction with a physical activity course in colleges and universities such as "Health through Exercise," but the presentation of the material is also suitable for students to use on an individual basis. The basic premise of this book is that, with proper knowledge and guidance, the student can design and implement his or her own Positive Health Life-style.

The book is organized into eleven chapters. Most chapters contain Laboratory Inventories that help to assess the individual's current health life-style and provide guidelines for modification if necessary. Key concepts and key terms are highlighted at the beginning of each chapter, and numerous figures and tables are also included to help explain the major concepts. Contemporary research studies that support the chapter content are documented at the end of each chapter.

Chapter 1 is designed to establish the basis for adopting a Positive Health Life-style, while chapter 2 emphasizes the major degenerative diseases in our society today and how a Positive Health Life-style may affect them. Chapter 3 presents an overview of human energy systems and the basic principles of designing and implementing an individualized exercise program.

The heart of the textbook is found in chapters 4 through 9, where specific guidelines for adopting a Positive Health Life-style are offered. Chapter 4 covers aerobic exercise; chapter 5 provides the basis for sound nutrition; chapter 6 deals with methods to lose body weight, while chapter 7 documents how to gain muscle weight; chapter 8 provides guidelines for improved flexibility and prevention of low back pain, while chapter 9 is concerned with stress reduction techniques. Chapter 10 briefly discusses some issues relevant to females, while chapter 11 stresses a Positive Health Life-style as a lifelong program.

Other features include a glossary of terms used and six appendices including the Recommended Dietary Allowances, the six Food Exchange Lists, salt, fat, and cholesterol content of common foods, and the Calories expended through a variety of exercises.

This text is designed to get the individual to think about the possible consequences of his or her current life-style. But more importantly, it provides a mechanism for change by actively involving the student in a number of Laboratory Inventories designed to help implement a Positive Health Life-style.

I would like to acknowledge Mr. Ed Jaffe, editor for Wm. C. Brown Publishers, who encouraged me to write this textbook in the first place and who has been extremely supportive in its development over the past year. Special thanks also goes to Sue Hedrick for her excellent work in the preparation of the final manuscript.

The contributions of the following reviewers to the development of this text are gratefully acknowledged: Norman William Johanson, City College of the City University of New York; Ralph Honderd, Calvin College; Scott K. Powers, Louisiana State University; Bruce Drummond, California State University at Sacramento; Normand Gionet, University of Moncton; and Candace J. Norton, Georgia Department of Education.

Melvin H. Williams

LIFETIME Physical Fitness

A Personal Choice

Your Personal Health Profile 1

Key Terms

chronic diseases
disuse phenomena
life expectancy
life span
personal choice

physical fitness
Positive Health Life-style
prudent health behavior
rectangular society
risk factor

Key Concepts

Aging is inevitable, and the catabolic effects of the aging process also appear to be inevitable, although many may be lessened by following a Positive Health Life-style.

The most prominent theory of aging suggests that the genes begin to make errors in protein synthesis in the cells, which may eventually lead to cellular dysfunction.

Although the average life span in the United States should be about eighty-five years, it is actually only seventy-four years which indicates the average death is eleven years premature.

Most premature deaths in the United States today are due to chronic diseases (such as coronary heart disease), many of which are preventable to some degree.

A Positive Health Life-style is not solely concerned with the prevention of chronic disease, but also incorporates a striving to achieve the healthiest body possible, within our natural limitations.

Health life-style assessment inventories are educational tools designed to analyze your current health life-style and to offer you a general idea of those areas in your life that may pose a health risk.

Several key risk factors are associated with the onset of chronic disease: physical inactivity; excess body weight; a diet high in fat, cholesterol, and salt; high blood pressure; excessive stress; smoking habits; and excessive alcohol intake.

The major thrust of personal preventive medicine is to encourage personal choices of positive health behaviors that will help counteract the key risk factors mentioned above.

The development of a Positive Health Life-style should be encouraged as early in life as possible, but the benefits attributed to adopting such a life-style may be achieved at almost any age.

Two major components of a Positive Health Life-style are a properly planned exercise program and a sound nutrition program.

Introduction

Have you ever thought about getting old? Have you ever contemplated how many years you would live? Have you ever wondered if you will be able to take care of yourself during your old age? Have you ever wondered if there is anything you could do to increase both the quantity and quality of your life? As a young college student, you probably do not spend a great deal of time worrying about such questions as these, but they may have crossed your mind at one time or another. For those of you who are older than the typical college age (eighteen to twenty-four), these questions may have become increasingly important.

The major thrust of this book is to develop a particular set of health behaviors that may help to increase the quantity of your life and, at the same time, improve the quality. Many young adults exercise or diet, not to prevent the onset of coronary heart disease in their later years, but to improve their appearance and to feel good about themselves now. With the selection of proper health-related behaviors, both short-term and long-term benefits may be achieved concomitantly. Most of this book deals with the implementation of such health behaviors so that they constitute a life-style that we label a *Positive Health Life-style*.

The Aging Process

We all begin to age from the first day of conception, and our first twenty years or so are characterized by a dominance of anabolic processes in which the skeleton, muscles, nerves, and other bodily systems grow and develop. In general, this anabolic phase is completed in the late teens or early twenties. Following this anabolic phase are the maintenance and catabolic phases, wherein the body systems are maintained at an optimal functioning level, then begin to deteriorate as the body gets older. Some of these catabolic changes in the aging process are readily observable, while others are not as easily detected (fig. 1.1). We can note rather easily such symptoms as gray hair, impaired hearing and vision, increased body weight, stiff joints, and wrinkled skin; however, clogged arteries, less efficient lungs and heart, and diminished function of certain glands may not be readily noticed.

At the present time, aging is inevitable, and the catabolic effects that accompany the aging process also appear to be inevitable. In an affluent society that places a high value on a youthful appearance, certain technological and medical advances have been made to counteract some of these adverse catabolic effects. We can obtain an almost invisible device to improve hearing and soft contact lenses to correct vision or undergo plastic surgery to replace lost hair, smooth facial wrinkles, and remove excess body fat. Some of these applications may not be necessary, for although not all of the effects of aging are preventable, some of them can be diminished. There appears to be little we can do to deter the gradual erosion of proper vision, so glasses or contact lenses become a necessity. Hearing losses may or may not be preventable, depending on whether hearing loss is a natural occurrence of the aging process or is brought about by exposure to continuous periods of loud noise during younger years (such as from using stereo headsets). On the other hand, in most individuals, body weight may be controlled by a proper nutrition and exercise program so no excess body fat accumulates.

Figure 1.1 Physiological Changes Associated with the Aging Process. A number of physiological changes occur during the natural aging process. Some of the changes, such as decreased visual ability, are not too preventable. However, others, such as decreased cardiovascular functions, may be prevented to some degree by a Positive Health Life-style.

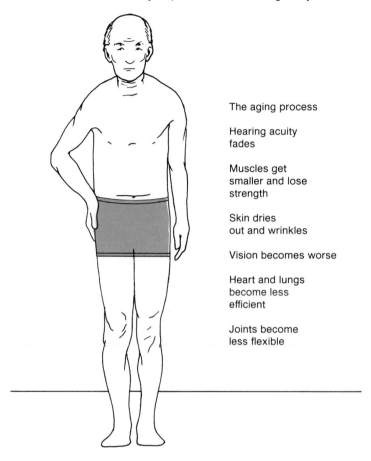

The aging process

Hearing acuity fades

Muscles get smaller and lose strength

Skin dries out and wrinkles

Vision becomes worse

Heart and lungs become less efficient

Joints become less flexible

Many of the effects of aging are not primarily life-threatening. You are not likely to die from poor vision or hearing, but a decreased capacity to see or hear may lead to a greater probability of an accident—an indirect relationship to an actual cause of death. Conversely, clogged arteries, cancer, decreased heart efficiency, and altered organ (kidney or pancreas) functions, may be immediately life-threatening. How preventable are these conditions? We shall return to this question after a brief look at the aging process.

Theories of Aging

Why do we age? Aging is a very complex process that results from the interaction of a wide variety of factors. Thus a number of different theories have been advanced in attempts to explain why we grow older, and why aging produces its catabolic effects on the body. The most prominent theories center around genetic control. One genetic

Figure 1.2 Genetic Error Theory of Aging. The genetic error theory of aging proposes that defective DNA and RNA produce a defective or inadequate amount of protein within a particular cell and thus contribute to the aging of that cell and the related body tissues.

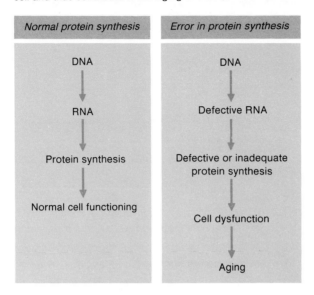

theory suggests that aging is an inherited factor—that a genetic clock or tape is present at conception, and cell function ceases when that clock or tape runs out. The second genetic theory (fig. 1.2) is that aging results when the genes that control the synthesis of every protein in the body begin to make random errors that eventually disrupt normal cellular functioning. Every cell in the body has a genetic control mechanism, designed to make that cell perform its major function—be it to form muscle proteins, produce an enzyme that may be used in energy-producing processes, or manufacture a hormone such as insulin. In simple terms, the genetic material, DNA, activates several types of RNA that control these cellular functions. Thus, the cumulative effect of random errors eventually disrupts this process and may result in cellular dysfunction. Fries and Crapo, in their excellent book on the aging process, *Vitality and Aging,* suggest that the second theory has the most supporting evidence.

Longevity

How long can you expect to live? According to Fries and Crapo, the **life span** (the biological limit to the length of life) of humans has been constant for at least 100,000 years and no change is anticipated in the near future. In their proposed rectangular society (discussed in figure 1.3), Fries and Crapo note that the median length of life is eighty-five years—one-half of all Americans can live to be eighty-five. They see a maximal age of one hundred, with the possibility of some individuals passing that barrier. However, life span must be differentiated from life expectancy. **Life expectancy** represents the number of years of life expected for a given individual or population. Life expectancy and life span do not necessarily coincide. For example, although the

Figure 1.3 Ideal Survival Curve Resulting from the Elimination of Premature Disease in the United States. By 1980, over 80 percent of the area between the curve for 1900 and the ideal curve was reduced. To interpret this figure, simply select an age, and move vertically until you intersect one of the three curves; then move horizontally to the Percent Surviving scale. For example, in 1900 less than 50 percent of the American population survived to age sixty, whereas over 80 percent survived in 1980. The ideal curve indicates a survival rate of nearly 95 percent. (Data from the National Bureau of Health Statistics).
Source: From *Vitality and Aging,* by J. Fries and L. Crapo. Copyright © 1981 by W. H. Freeman and Company. All rights reserved.

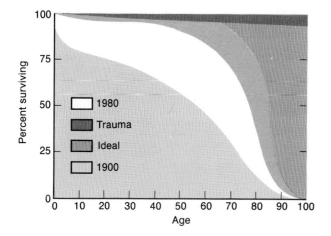

average life span may be eighty-five, the average life expectancy in the United States for men is about seventy-one years and for women is about seventy-six years. Thus, Americans are not attaining their full potential life span. Why?

The United States is becoming a **rectangular society.** Figure 1.3 helps explain this concept. Note that as the time frame progresses from 1900 to 1980, the curve becomes more rectangular in shape. The general interpretation of this curve is that more and more people are living longer, but the maximal life span is the same. Life span is fixed, but life expectancy is increasing. In 1900, only about 50 percent of the population survived to age sixty, whereas in 1980, about 83 percent were still living. This increase in life expectancy has resulted from the elimination of premature death rather than from extension of the natural life span, primarily due to the complete elimination or reduced mortality from such infectious diseases as tuberculosis, diphtheria, influenza, pneumonia, kidney disease, and diseases of early infancy. The 1980 curve can be improved so that it may begin to approach the ideal (nearly rectangular) curve. In order to do this, the **chronic diseases** (diseases that develop over a long period of time), such as atherosclerosis and other arterial diseases, cancer, diabetes, arthritis, emphysema, and cirrhosis—which account for nearly 80 percent of all premature deaths and over 90 percent of all disabilities—must be reduced. In 1900, the average individual died thirty-eight years prematurely, in 1950 seventeen years prematurely, and in 1980 twelve years prematurely. Thus, reducing the mortality rate from some of these chronic diseases could possibly add eleven to twelve years to the average American's life span. Note, also, that trauma, or accidents, are contributing factors to premature deaths. Although it is not reflected in the curves for 1900 and 1980, accidental deaths have increased to the point where they, too, are a major cause of premature death.

Table 1.1
Developmental Stages of Several Chronic Diseases

Age	Stage	Atherosclerosis	Diabetes	Cirrhosis
20 or younger	Start	Elevated cholesterol	Obesity	Drinker
30	Discernable	Small plaques in arteries	Abnormal glucose tolerance	Fatty liver
40	Subclinical	Larger plaques in arteries	Elevated blood glucose	Enlarged liver
50	Threshold	Leg pain on exercise	Sugar in urine	Bleeding in upper intestines
60	Severe	Pain in chest	Drug requirement	Fluid accumulated in abdomen
70	End	Stroke, heart attack	Blindness, nerve damage	Hepatic coma

Premature Death

Other than premature deaths in the young, caused by trauma (primarily automobile accidents), most premature deaths are concentrated in the years over sixty and are due to the chronic diseases noted previously. Although we may think of these as diseases of old age, their beginnings may start at age twenty or even as early as ages seven or eight. Table 1.1 represents some possible progressions of several of the chronic diseases prevalent in American society today.

If you want to live to obtain the greatest quantity of life—to approach that ideal rectangular curve—then your greatest opportunity is to reduce the possibility of contracting those chronic diseases that are somewhat preventable. Along with increased quantity of life, we would all like increased quality as well—to be full of vim, vigor, and vitality throughout our lives, including old age. Many of the chronic diseases have their beginnings in the early phases of life. Therefore, preventive measures should be initiated early in order to help counteract the disabling effects or premature death caused by such diseases. The earlier a healthy life-style is developed, the better, but life-style modification may have some positive benefits at almost any age. The remainder of this chapter deals with this concept, the development of a life-style conducive to maximizing both the quantity and quality of life.

The Positive Health Life-style

A **Positive Health Life-style** is not concerned solely with preventing the onset of chronic disease. It also includes a striving to achieve the healthiest body possible within our natural limitations. Per Olaf Astrand, a world-renowned authority on exercise and health, has stated that, in order to attain optimal function and optimal health, we must intellectually learn and understand how the human body functions, and how to treat it well. We need to develop a life-style that, according to current medical evidence,

Figure 1.4 Both a sound mind and body are important to optimal health.

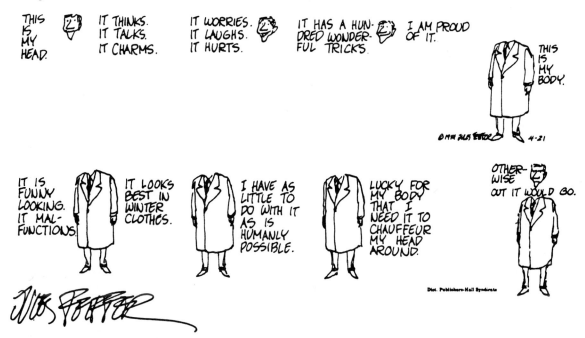

provides us with the greatest statistical probability of remaining healthy. This is not to say that adopting a Positive Health Life-style is going to guarantee protection against all chronic diseases, but it may delay the onset of such diseases or reduce the severity of disabling symptoms.

Mind-Body Interrelationships

A Positive Health Life-style is based on a model that views the individual as a whole, such that there is a unity between the mind and body, and disease processes or disturbances in one can cause disease in the other. Figure 1.5 illustrates this concept of the interrelationships between the mind and the body, and some possible contributing factors to physical/emotional diseases. This partial list of contributing factors to physical and emotional diseases involves a number of life-style practices over which we do have some degree of control. Before we proceed with an expanded discussion of this topic, let's try to analyze your current health life-style.

Health Life-style Assessment Inventory

There are a large number of health assessment inventories available. Some are very simple and can be completed in less than a minute, giving you a general measurement of your health life-style. On the other extreme are those that may take an hour or so to complete and can give you an estimate of your probability of developing a particular

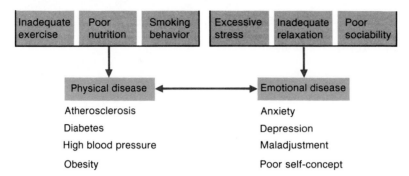

Figure 1.5 Mind-Body Interrelationships. Physical disease may lead to emotional disease, and vice versa. Contributing risk factors to each type of disease may be modified by Positive Health Behaviors, i.e., elimination of the risk factors.

chronic disease or even forecast how many years you will live. Since no validity studies of these more extensive inventories are yet available, we cannot verify their accuracy and will not duplicate them here. Those who are interested in such an analysis may contact several of the companies or agencies that administer them. A listing can be found in the pamphlet, *Health Risk Appraisals: An Inventory,* which may be obtained by writing to the National Health Information Clearinghouse, P.O. Box 1133, Washington, DC 20013. The major point to keep in mind concerning any of these inventories is that, although they may be effective health education tools, they are not to be used for diagnosis or even for general screening purposes.

The Health Life-style Assessment Inventory (Laboratory Inventory 1.1) is designed to assess your current health life-style and to give you a general idea of those areas in your life that may need to be modified in order to achieve a Positive Health Life-style. It is not designed to provide a specific assessment of your health risks in any given area or to predict the development of any specific chronic disease. It also does not take into account your family history of diseases that may exert a significant influence on your future health. A number of chronic diseases appear to be related to genetic predisposition and, thus, tend to run in some families. Moreover, with the exception of body weight and blood pressure, it does not look at your personal health history. You may have or have had diabetes, asthma, allergies, rheumatic heart disease, or other disorders that may influence your health life-style. With these limitations in mind, please complete the Health Life-style Assessment Inventory at the end of this chapter before reading any further. It will take a little effort on your part to evaluate your behavior in several of the areas listed.

Preventive Medicine and Personal Choice

Risk Factors

After completion of the Health Life-style Assessment Inventory you should have some idea of your personal health behaviors that may pose some risk relative to your future health—those life-style components for which you checked either the poor or dangerous categories. The life-style components listed in the inventory, among others, are often called **risk factors.** A risk factor is a health behavior or a personal characteristic that has been associated with a particular disease. A cause-and-effect relationship does not necessarily have to be present in order to label a particular factor as a risk to health, but some form of statistical relationship should be evident, such as that obtained from epidemiological studies. For example, obesity is a risk factor associated with the development of diabetes in adulthood. Individuals who become obese have a higher statistical probability of developing diabetes than those who remain relatively lean. However, no exact cause (obesity) and effect (diabetes) relationship has yet been determined, although some theories are available. In other cases, a direct cause-and-effect relationship can be observed, such as that between excessive alcohol consumption and cirrhosis of the liver. The following list indicates only one of the disease states or complications associated with the dangerous category for each of the major risk factors in the Health Life-style Assessment Inventory.

1. Excessive body weight—Diabetes
2. Low occupational exercise—Obesity
3. Low levels of planned exercise—Coronary heart disease
4. Poor basic diet—Malnutrition
5. High fat and cholesterol diet—Atherosclerosis
6. High salt diet—High blood pressure
7. High blood pressure—Stroke
8. Excessive stress—Ulcers
9. Tobacco smoking—Lung cancer
10. Excessive alcohol consumption—Cirrhosis of the liver
11. Poor driving habits—Accidents
12. Poor physical exam habits—Cancer

Treatment versus Prevention

Most of us have been exposed to individuals who have developed a chronic disease, and we may also be aware of the excellent treatment they have received from our technologically sophisticated medical community. Physicians and hospitals today are equipped with a wide array of diagnostic tools, advanced surgical techniques, medicines, and drugs to treat some of the major chronic diseases. In many cases, what may have been a fatal disease in the past now has a favorable prognosis for partial or complete recovery. Medical advances have been phenomenal during the first fifty to sixty years of this century, and have been instrumental in eradicating many of the previous causes of premature death—tuberculosis, polio, diphtheria, etc. Moreover, medical advances in the past twenty years have been even more phenomenal, and are helping to treat the major chronic diseases that are now the major threats to our health. However, the research and development of these modern medical techniques for treating chronic and other diseases has been extremely costly, with medical care costs expanding at an extremely rapid rate during the past decade.

This rapid rise in medical care costs, coupled with an increasing tendency towards national health care legislation, are two factors that have helped to begin to change the focus of medical care from treatment to prevention. Dr. Richard E. Palmer, of the

American Medical Association, has noted that the medical system affects only about 10 percent of the usual factors that influence an individual's state of health. The remaining 90 percent are determined by factors over which doctors have little or no control. In other words, 90 percent of the health problems in the United States are preventable to one degree or another. Palmer stressed the point of personal health decisions as the key to preventive health behavior. Although the concept of preventive medicine has been around for a long time, its value and need now appear to be taking on added significance in American society, among both the medical community and the general public. Schools of medicine are now developing departments of preventive medicine; some hospitals are developing wellness clinics for healthy people who want to learn how to stay healthy. A fitness boom has also spread across the country, beginning as a ripple in the early 1970s and coming to full bloom in the 1980s, without any indication of abating. The medical community and many of the general public appear to be genuinely concerned with means to preserve an optimal state of physical and mental health and to prevent the onset of chronic disease.

Personal Preventive Medicine

What can you do in order to develop a Positive Health Life-style? The ultimate goal is to develop a set of permanent health behaviors that, based upon current scientific evidence, should provide you with the greatest opportunity to attain and/or maintain a state of optimal health. A model often used to explain the development of a set of behaviors involves a sequence of acquisition of knowledge, formation of an attitude or set of values, and development of a particular behavior (fig. 1.6). For example, you may acquire the knowledge that eggs are very high in cholesterol, and that high levels of some forms of cholesterol in the blood are associated with the development of atherosclerosis and coronary heart disease. This knowledge, plus other information you possess about coronary heart disease, may help you to shape a personal attitude that eggs are bad for your health. This attitude may then be reflected in your actual behavior with the result that you will not eat eggs. On the other hand, you may have learned that eggs are an inexpensive, excellent source of complete protein, and are high in nutrient value. This knowledge may help you acquire an attitude that eggs are good for your nutritional health, and your behavior may reflect this attitude with the result that you eat a lot of eggs. Thus, one of the keys to shaping your health behavior patterns is the knowledge you receive. Unfortunately, we often have incomplete or controversial information relative to the impact of certain health behaviors upon the development of optimal health or the prevention of chronic diseases. In the previous example, it is true that eggs are high in cholesterol, but it is also true that they are an excellent source of nutrients. Moreover, although it is known that high levels of some forms of cholesterol in the blood are associated with atherosclerosis, the amount of dietary cholesterol needed to raise these blood cholesterol levels in the average individual is still questionable. Eating eggs may or may not have an impact upon the development of atherosclerosis, but the generally prevailing medical attitude is to restrict the amount of high cholesterol foods, including eggs, in the diet. Based upon the available scientific evidence, this appears to be a **prudent health behavior.** Thus, although

Figure 1.6 Development of Different Health Behaviors. Knowledge influences attitude development, which leads to actual behavior.

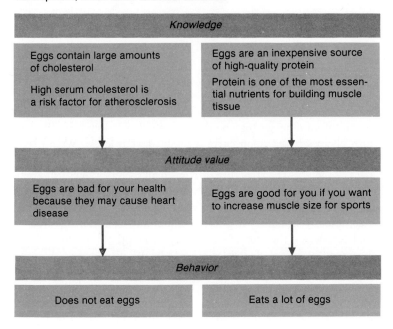

we do not, in many cases, possess absolute proof that a recommended health behavior will prevent the development of certain chronic diseases, the available scientific information does provide us with a base for making a prudent choice in light of the knowledge at hand.

What are some recommended prudent behaviors that may have a positive effect on our health? Several surveys using healthy individuals have been conducted to determine whether there are any behaviors that appear to help attain or maintain a state of good health. A synthesis of these reports suggests the following behaviors:

1. Exercise—Get at least 20 minutes per day of regular, moderate, aerobic exercise.
2. Nutrition—Eat a good breakfast and two other well-balanced meals per day, and avoid unnecessary snacking.
3. Body weight—Maintain an optimal body weight through a sound exercise and diet program.
4. Rest—Get about 7 to 8 hours of restful sleep each night, and use relaxation techniques when necessary.
5. Alcohol—If you do drink, use alcohol in moderation.
6. Smoking—If you do not smoke, do not begin; and stop smoking if you currently do smoke.
7. Personal environment—Avoid toxins and pollutants when possible.
8. Personal injury—Be safety-conscious; when driving, use seat belts, and avoid excessive speed or use of alcohol or drugs.

9. Stress—Use socially acceptable, yet effective techniques to deal with daily problems.
10. Self-worth—Develop a feeling of personal value, a feeling that you are in control of your personal environment, a feeling that you are able to make a personal choice.

Personal Choice

The concept of **personal choice** in relationship to health behaviors is an important one. An estimated 90 percent of all illnesses may be preventable if individuals would make sound personal health choices based upon current medical knowledge. We all relish our freedom of choice and do not like to see it constrained when it is within the legal and ethical boundaries of society. The structure of American society allows us to make almost all our own personal decisions that may be relevant to our health. If we so desire, we can smoke, drink excessively, refuse to wear seat belts, eat whatever foods we want, and live a completely sedentary life-style without any exercise. The freedom to make such personal decisions is the crux of our society, although the wisdom of these decisions can be questioned. Personal choices relative to health often pose a dilemma. As one example, a teenager may know the facts relative to smoking cigarettes and health but may be pressured by peer approval into believing it is the socially accepted thing to do.

A multitude of factors, both inherited and environmental, influence the development of health-related behaviors, and it is beyond the scope of this text to discuss all these factors as they may impact upon any given individual. However, the decision to adopt a particular health-related behavior is usually one of personal choice. There are healthy choices and there are unhealthy choices. In discussing the ethics of personal choice, Fries and Crapo drew a revealing analogy. They suggest that to knowingly indulge in a behavior that has a statistical probability of shortening life is similar to attempting suicide. Thus, for those individuals who are interested in preserving both the quality and quantity of life, personal health choices should reflect those behaviors that are associated with a statistical probability of increased vitality and longevity (such as the ten behavioral patterns listed in the last section).

Benefits of a Positive Health Life-style

Many individuals do not adopt a Positive Health Life-style because it does require some personal restraint and effort. For example, they might not buckle seat belts because it takes a little effort. Moreover, Americans, in general, expect immediate results and benefits from such personal restraints and efforts. Unfortunately, many of the physiological benefits of sound positive health behaviors are not readily observable. Without medical technology, we cannot see the fall in blood lipids, the changes in blood cholesterol, the increased vitality of the lungs and liver, the alteration in hormones to reduce the stress on the heart, and other such physiological changes that may help to prevent the development of certain chronic diseases. However, there are some clues that a Positive Health Life-style program is working. We can see our body weight begin

Table 1.2
Modifiable Aspects of Aging by Personal Choice
of a Positive Health Behavior

Aging Factor	Positive Health Behavior Required
Body weight	Exercise, diet
Cardiovascular functioning	Exercise, diet, nonsmoking
Dental decay	Diet, proper cleaning
Glucose tolerance	Weight control, exercise, diet
Intelligence tests	Training, practice
Memory	Training, practice
Osteoporosis	Weight-bearing exercise, diet
Physical endurance	Exercise, weight control
Physical strength	Exercise
Pulmonary reserve	Exercise, nonsmoking
Reaction time	Training, practice
Serum lipids and cholesterol	Diet, weight control, exercise
Skin aging	Sun avoidance
Social ability	Practice
Systolic blood pressure	Weight control, salt limitation, exercise

Source: From *Vitality and Aging,* by J. Fries and L. Crapo. Copyright © 1981 by W. H. Freeman and Company. All rights reserved.

to change, feel our breathing improve, experience less coughing in the morning, measure our slower heart rate, suffer less physical and mental fatigue, and develop a feeling of self-worth.

Although we cannot alter the true aging process at the present time, it appears that the development of positive health behaviors may help to prevent some of the adverse effects that may be due to factors other than the true aging process. One such factor may involve **disuse phenomena,** which, simply translated, means that if we don't use something, we lose it. Physical abilities, intellectual capacity, memory, and social skills may deteriorate if they are not continually utilized. Thus, disuse may add to the deterioration that usually occurs in these processes as a natural consequence of the true aging process.

Numerous research studies have indicated that a proper exercise program and other positive health behaviors can aid in slowing down many physiological aging processes. Table 1.2 presents some of the factors associated with aging that may be ameliorated by personal choice of a positive health behavior.

Exercise, Nutrition, and Health

Total health involves a balanced relationship between the mind and the body. To be healthy, you should possess an optimal level of both emotional and physical fitness. Both types of fitness are interrelated and very complex, but our concern in this book is primarily with physical fitness and the associated benefits for mental health.

Table 1.3
Physical Fitness Categories and Components

Health-Related Fitness Components	Motor Skill-Related Fitness Components
1. Cardiovascular-respiratory function	1. Strength and power
2. Body composition	2. Local muscular endurance
3. Abdominal muscle strength and flexibility in low back-hamstring area	3. Agility and balance
	4. Speed

Physical Fitness

What is **physical fitness** and how do you know if you have an optimal level of it? The concept and definition of physical fitness have been undergoing some important changes in the past decade, and there now appears to be some consensus on its definition—particularly as it relates to health. However, the level of physical fitness necessary for optimal health has not been as clearly defined, although some guidelines are available to let us know where we stand on certain individual physical fitness components.

The development of physical fitness is an important concern of the American Alliance for Health, Physical Education, Recreation and Dance (AAHPERD), which has categorized fitness components into two different categories, health-related and motor skill-related (table 1.3). Motor skill-related physical fitness components, although important for participation in athletics, do not appear to emphasize health-related benefits. On the other hand, the health-related fitness components appear to be related to the development of cardiovascular-respiratory health, maintenance of an optimal body weight, and prevention of low back injury and pain. Thus physical fitness needs to be defined in relationship to its components. For the purpose of this textbook, the definition of physical fitness refers to physical fitness as it is related to functional health, not motor skill ability. The exercise programs recommended in this textbook are, in general, designed to contribute to the development of health-related physical fitness.

Key Positive Health Behavior—Exercise

Exercise and physical fitness appear to be key elements in the preventive health movement, for physical inactivity may be one of the most significant, readily modifiable, personal factors contributing to the poor health status of many Americans. The United States Public Health Service notes that habitual inactivity is thought to contribute to hypertension, chronic fatigue and resulting physical inefficiency, premature aging, poor musculature, and lack of flexibility. Such factors are the major causes of low back pain and injury, mental tension, obesity, and coronary heart disease. By contrast, the American Heart Association, in their recent *Statement on Exercise,* reports that regular exercise can lower serum lipid levels, reduce the clinical manifestations of heart disease, improve the efficiency of the heart and circulation, and reduce blood pressure levels in individuals with hypertension.

Several reviews indicate that physicians have begun to recognize the beneficial effects of exercise in a wide variety of disease states. They believe that exercise is a neglected medicine. Bortz even goes as far to state that there is no product in the *Physician's Desk Reference* that offers such an array of benefits in such a diverse set of pathological conditions as does exercise. Leach notes that physicians should write exercise prescriptions and attempt to persuade their patients to view them in the same light as a prescription for a drug. The viewpoint is also advanced that an active exercise program may help to retard many of the adverse effects commonly attributed to aging and, thus, such a program should be a part of daily living patterns at all age levels.

The Surgeon General of the United States recently issued a report entitled *Promoting Health/Preventing Disease: Objectives for the Nation*. This report lists fifteen priority areas in which attempts will be made to improve the health knowledge and behavior of the American population by 1990. Nine of these priority areas, such as family planning, immunization, and toxic agent control, are beyond the scope of this book. However, six will be addressed, including high blood pressure control, smoking, alcohol, nutrition, control of stress, and physical fitness and exercise. Exercise as a mechanism to promote health and prevent disease is a major component of the Surgeon General's report. The following are a few of the major objectives that, hopefully, will be realized by 1990.

1. Ninety percent of children and adolescents between the ages of ten and seventeen will participate regularly in cardiovascular fitness programs that can be carried into adulthood.
2. Sixty percent of adults aged eighteen to sixty-five will participate in vigorous physical exercise.
3. Fifty percent of adults over age sixty-five will participate in appropriate physical activity of an aerobic nature.
4. Seventy percent of all adults should be able to identify the intensity, duration, and frequency of exercise thought to be necessary for cardiovascular health.

The role that exercise may play in the prevention of some chronic diseases and the other risk factors associated with the aging process are discussed throughout this book. A well-designed exercise program appears to be a key factor in diminishing many of the adverse processes of aging.

Key Positive Health Behavior—Nutrition

A program of sound nutritional practices is also a key component in a Positive Health Life-style. *Nutrition* represents the sum total of all the processes whereby food is ingested, digested, absorbed, and metabolized in order to promote growth and maintenance or repair of body tissues. In order to have proper nutrition, the body must obtain a sufficient number of Calories and essential nutrients from the foods consumed on a daily basis.

A *diet* represents the foods we eat in order to obtain Calories and nutrients, and is said to be *balanced* when it meets our nutritional needs. Diets may be modified to meet certain health needs, such as a low-sodium, low-cholesterol, or low-Calorie diet. For the purpose of this book, the terms nutrition and diet are used interchangeably.

One of the most important objectives of sound nutrition is to regulate caloric intake in order to attain and maintain an optimal body weight. Excessive body weight has been associated with a wide variety of chronic diseases, including high blood pressure, diabetes, and arthritis. Thus proper body weight control is a major objective of the Positive Health Life-style, and a balanced program of both nutrition and exercise may help achieve this objective by regulating caloric balance.

Modification of the diet may have some implications for other health conditions as well. For example, a sodium-free diet may be helpful in the treatment of high blood pressure; a low-saturated-fat and low-cholesterol diet may be recommended to reduce or help prevent atherosclerosis; and an increased intake of natural fiber may ameliorate bowel dysfunctions. The dietary recommendations of a United States Senate committee on nutrition, designed to help improve the health of the American population, include such changes as decreased intake of salt, simple sugars, saturated fat and cholesterol, and an increase in fruits and vegetables containing natural fiber.

Adopting a nutritional program that stresses the consumption of a balanced diet of natural foods and limits the intake of highly processed foods is a move towards a Positive Health Life-style. Combined with a proper exercise program, you will have made two very important decisions that may significantly improve the quality and quantity of your life.

General Guidelines

1. Body weight: Consult the average height-weight charts in tables 6.3 and 6.4. Assess your body frame size using table 6.5.

2. Exercise, occupational: Consult appendix E to find the approximate MET rating of your current occupation. If you are a full-time academic student, doing a lot of desk work with some walking, you may be classified as sedentary. Although a completely sedentary occupation is listed under the dangerous category, you need not change jobs to improve your life-style, but you should be aware of the possible dangers of complete inactivity and compensate by developing a planned exercise program, as in the next category.

3. Exercise, planned: Consult appendix E to find the approximate MET rating of your planned exercise program. These exercises should be done continuously for 20 minutes per day, at least 3 to 4 days per week, and, optimally, 6 to 7 days per week.

4. Diet, basic: Consult appendix B to find foods that are contained in the Food Exchange Lists that include the Milk List, the Meat List, the Bread List, the Fruit List, the Vegetable List, and the Fat List.

5. Diet, saturated fats and cholesterol: Consult tables 5.3 and 5.4, respectively, to find foods that are high in saturated fats and cholesterol. In general, animal products such as whole milk, red meats, luncheon meats, and eggs are high in saturated fats and/or cholesterol.

6. Diet, salt: Consult table 5.14 to locate foods high in salt and sodium. Table salt is an obvious example, as are high salt foods such as pretzels, potato chips, and peanuts (unless unsalted). Less obvious examples are canned foods, many processed foods, and some breakfast cereals. Check the list of ingredients on the foods you buy; if salt is listed near the front of the list, it is a high-sodium food.

7. Blood pressure: The only way you can know this value is to have it checked while you are in a resting state. You may be able to have this done by your class instructor, the student health service, your physician, or one of the commercial instruments now available in certain public places such as shopping malls and airports.

8. Stress: This is often a difficult category to assess, as we are all under some type of stress at one time or other during the day. In general, if you are generally relaxed and are exposed to acute periods of stress that do not persist, you should score yourself to the left of center on the inventory. If you are chronically stressed, and experience symptoms of stress such as an upset stomach, depression, tension headaches, and the like, then you should score yourself to the right of center.

9. Tobacco smoking: This category is self-explanatory.

10. Alcohol consumption: A drink is considered to be one 12-ounce bottle of beer or ale, one 4-ounce glass of wine, or one 1.5-ounce shot of bar whiskey or the equivalent.

11. Driving habits: The 20,000 mile criteria applies, whether you are a driver or a passenger in an automobile. The use of seat belts and shoulder harness is self-explanatory, as is the determination of whether or not you drive under the influence of alcohol or other drugs (including prescription drugs or over-the-counter drugs) which may impair your judgment, cause drowsiness, or delay reaction times.

12. Women only: This category includes several tests that may help to detect the early stages of cancer.

13. Based upon your own feelings about your own physical health, check the appropriate box.

14. Based upon your own feelings about your own emotional health, check the appropriate box.

Health Life-style Assessment Inventory

	Excellent	Good	Fair	Poor	Dangerous
1. Body Weight	☐ Lean: about 5 pounds below standard weight range	☐ Standard weight range	☐ Slightly overweight: about 10–25 pounds above standard weight range	☐ Considerably overweight: about 25–50 pounds above standard weight range	☐ Grossly overweight: more than 50 pounds above standard weight range
2. Exercise, Occupational	☐ Intensive: 6–8 METS	☐ Moderate: 4–5 METS	☐ Mild: 3–4 METS	☐ Sedentary: 2–3 METS	☐ Completely sedentary: 1–2 METS
3. Exercise, Planned	☐ 10 METS or above for at least 20 continuous minutes/day	☐ 7–9 METS for at least 20 continuous minutes/day	☐ 4–6 METS for at least 20 continuous minutes/day	☐ 2–3 METS for at least 20 continuous minutes/day	☐ No planned exercise program
4. Diet, Basic	☐ Wide variety from The Food Exchange Lists 7 days/week	☐ Wide variety from The Food Exchange Lists 5 days/week	☐ Wide variety from The Food Exchange Lists 3 days/week	☐ Wide variety from The Food Exchange Lists 1 day/week	☐ Wide variety from The Food Exchange Lists 0 days/week
5. Diet, Saturated Fats and Cholesterol	☐ Diet excludes animal foods high in saturated fat and cholesterol	☐ Eat animal foods high in saturated fat and cholesterol sparingly	☐ Eat animal foods high in saturated fat and cholesterol at 1 meal/day	☐ Eat animal foods high in saturated fat and cholesterol at 2 meals/day	☐ Eat animal foods high in saturated fat and cholesterol at 3 meals/day
6. Diet, Salt	☐ Diet excludes salt and foods high in sodium	☐ Eat some high-sodium foods sparingly; do not add salt to meals	☐ Eat some high-sodium foods daily; do not add salt to meals	☐ Eat some high-sodium foods daily; lightly salt meals	☐ Eat a lot of high-sodium foods; heavily salt all meals daily
7. Blood Pressure	☐ 100 upper reading	☐ 120 upper reading	☐ 140 upper reading	☐ 160 upper reading	☐ 180 upper reading
8. Stress	☐ Generally relaxed; able to relieve stress by exercise or relaxation techniques	☐ Generally relaxed, but feel short periods of stress that cannot be relieved immediately	☐ Moderate degree of stress; occasionally feel average tension at job or home	☐ Above average stress at job and/or home	☐ Unusual stress at job and/or home; need drugs to relieve tension

Health Life-style Assessment Inventory (*continued*)

	Excellent	Good	Fair	Poor	Dangerous
9. Tobacco Smoking	☐ Never smoked or stopped smoking	☐ Smoke cigar or pipe	☐ Smoke less than 10 cigarettes/day	☐ Smoke 10–19 cigarettes/day	☐ Smoke more than 20 cigarettes/day
10. Alcohol Consumption	☐ 0–7 drinks/week; judgment never impaired	☐ 7–14 drinks/week; judgment never impaired	☐ 15–21 drinks/week; judgment rarely impaired	☐ 22–35 drinks/week; judgment occasionally impaired	☐ 35 or more drinks/week; judgment frequently impaired
11. Driving Habits	☐ Less than 20,000 miles/year; always wear seat belts; never drive under influence of alcohol or drugs	☐ Greater than 20,000 miles/year; always use seat belts; never drive under influence of alcohol or drugs	☐ Less than 20,000 miles/year; rarely use seat belts; never drive under influence of alcohol or drugs	☐ Greater than 20,000 miles/year; rarely use seat belts; occasionally drive under influence of alcohol or drugs	☐ Greater than 20,000 miles/year; never use seat belts; often drive under influence of alcohol or drugs
12. Women Only	☐ Pap smear every year; monthly self-examination of breasts, with periodic check by physician	☐ Pap smear every 2 years; monthly self-examination of breasts, but no periodic check by physician	☐ Pap smear every 3 years; self-examination of breasts every 6 months	☐ Pap smear every 4 years; self-examination of breasts every year	☐ Pap smear every 5 years or never; no breast self-examination
13. Your own rating of your physical health	☐	☐	☐	☐	☐
14. Your own rating of your emotional health	☐	☐	☐	☐	☐

References

American Alliance for Health, Physical Education, Recreation and Dance. *Lifetime Health Related Physical Fitness.* Reston, VA: AAHPERD, 1980.

American Heart Association. "Statement on Exercise." *Circulation* 64:1302 A (1981).

Anonymous. "How Healthy Are You—Really?" *Changing Times* 36:32–37 (August 1982).

Astrand, P. O. "Optimal Function and Health." *Bibliotheca Cardiologica* 36:11–18 (1976).

Bortz, W. "Effect of Exercise on Aging—Effect of Aging on Exercise." *Journal of the American Geriatric Society* 28:49–51 (1980).

Bucher, C. "National Adult Physical Fitness Survey: Some Implications." *Journal of Health, Physical Fitness and Recreation* 45:25 (1974).

deVries, H. "Physiological Effects of an Exercise Training Regimen upon Men Aged 52–88." *Journal of Gerontology* 25:325–36 (1970).

Fentem, P. "Exercise: A Prescription for Health? Self Medication: The Benefits of Exercise." *British Journal of Sports Medicine* 12:223–36 (1979).

Fries, J., and Crapo, L. *Vitality and Aging.* San Francisco: W. H. Freeman, 1981.

Leach, R. E. "Rx Exercise: Effects and Side Effects." *Hospital Practice* 16:72A–72W (1981).

Pollock, M. "Exercise—A Preventive Prescription." *Journal of School Health* 49:215–19 (1979).

Sharman, J. "Exercise—The Neglected 'Medicine'." *Alabama Journal of Medical Science* 16:56–58 (1979).

Strasser, A. "The Exercise Fad: A Risk/Benefit Analysis." *Occupational Health and Safety* 50:6–12 (1981).

United States Department of Health and Human Services. *Health Risk Appraisals: An Inventory.* Washington, DC: National Health Information Clearinghouse, 1981.

———. *Promoting Health/Preventing Disease: Objectives for the Nation.* Washington, DC: U.S. Government Printing Office, 1980.

2 Prevention of Chronic Diseases through a Positive Health Life-style

Key Terms

alcohol
arteriosclerosis
arthritis
atherosclerosis
blood pressure
body image
coronary arteries
coronary heart disease (CHD)
coronary occlusion
coronary thrombosis
diabetes mellitus

ECG
high blood pressure
high density lipoproteins (HDL)
hypertension
hypoglycemia
insulin
lipids
lipoproteins
low back pain syndrome
low density lipoproteins (LDL)
myocardial infarct

obesity
osteoarthritis
osteoporosis
peripheral vascular disease
plaque
rheumatoid arthritis
stroke
substance abuse
type A personality
very low density lipoproteins (VLDL)

Key Concepts

The major chronic disease of the cardiovascular-respiratory system is coronary heart disease (CHD), which is characterized by atherosclerosis in the arteries of the heart.

Primary risk factors associated with the development of CHD are high blood pressure, high blood lipids, and cigarette smoking. Heredity, obesity, diabetes, stressful life-style, improper diet, and lack of physical activity are some of the secondary risk factors.

High blood pressure (hypertension) is a major disease, afflicting nearly one out of every six Americans, but, because it displays few obvious symptoms, it often remains undetected; blood pressure should be checked regularly.

A stroke may be caused by diseased blood vessels in the brain. This condition is associated with the same risk factors as CHD and high blood pressure.

Peripheral vascular disease is arteriosclerosis in blood vessels other than those of the heart or brain.

Obesity is one of the major health problems in the United States. Although it is simply defined as an excess storage of Calories, many different factors may be the cause of the caloric imbalance.

Diabetes, a major disease in the United States, is a condition in which the body cannot properly metabolize carbohydrates.

The lower part of the back, particularly the lumbar-sacral area, when subjected to excessive stresses, may develop a low back pain syndrome.

Osteoporosis (softening of the bone) is usually a disease of older adults, but preventive measures should be initiated in young adulthood.

Arthritis is a disease of the cartilage in the joints and, although the cause and cure are not known, the severity of its effects may be lessened by a proper exercise program.

Abuse of substances such as alcohol and tobacco may have significant adverse effects on health.

A Positive Health Life-style may help to prevent and treat many of the major chronic diseases found in the United States today.

Table 2.1
Major Health Problems that May Be Prevented or Ameliorated by a Positive Health Life-style

Cardiovascular-Respiratory Diseases

Coronary heart disease	Stroke
Hypertension—High blood pressure	Peripheral vascular disease

Metabolic Disorders

Obesity
Diabetes

Musculoskeletal Problems

Low back pain
Osteoporosis
Arthritis

Substance Abuse Problems

Alcohol-related health problems
Cigarette-related health problems

Introduction

As mentioned in chapter 1, the average American's life expectancy could be increased appreciably—by approximately eleven years—if accidental deaths could be considerably reduced, and the major chronic diseases, such as coronary heart disease and cancer, could be eliminated. Moreover, the quality of life could also be improved if we could minimize or eliminate the disabling mental and physical effects of these chronic diseases. Many of the chronic diseases that limit both the quantity and quality of life begin to develop in our early years, and may be associated with various risk factors in our particular life-styles.

The purpose of this chapter is to discuss the etiology, or developmental process, of certain chronic diseases, and how identifiable risk factors may contribute to the developmental process. The preventive effects of a Positive Health Life-style, which basically represents a reduction or elimination of those risk factors that can be modified, are incorporated in the discussion. Since this book is primarily centered around the beneficial effects of exercise and nutrition, their preventive roles are stressed whenever relevant.

The major chronic diseases with which we are concerned may be grouped under four major headings. First, cardiovascular-respiratory (CVR) diseases disrupt normal functioning of the heart, blood vessels, and lungs. The major CVR disease is coronary heart disease (CHD). Second, metabolic disorders may be numerous, but we are concerned primarily with obesity (an imbalance in energy metabolism), and diabetes (a disturbance of carbohydrate metabolism). Third, musculoskeletal problems, such as low back pain, although not usually life-threatening, may be a source of constant discomfort, impairing the quality of life. And fourth, other major health problems (including cirrhosis of the liver and automobile accidents resulting from excessive consumption of alcohol, and lung cancer from cigarette smoking) are associated with use of substances toxic to the body. An overview of the major health problems that may possibly be prevented or ameliorated by a Positive Health Life-style is presented in table 2.1.

Figure 2.1 The Cardiovascular-Respiratory Systems. The cardiovascular and respiratory systems function to deliver oxygen (O_2) to all body cells and remove carbon dioxide (CO_2) which is a metabolic waste product. Oxygen is taken into the lungs from the atmospheric air, and in the alveoli (small air sacs) it is diffused into the blood. This oxygenated blood travels to the left side of the heart, where it is eventually pumped to the body tissues (such as muscle tissue) via the arterial blood vessels. The tissues use the oxygen for their energy needs, producing carbon dioxide in the process. The carbon dioxide is then returned in the blood to the right side of the heart, where the blood is pumped to the lungs, and the carbon dioxide is expelled from the body. **Source:** Courtesy Ward's Natural Science, Inc., Rochester, New York.

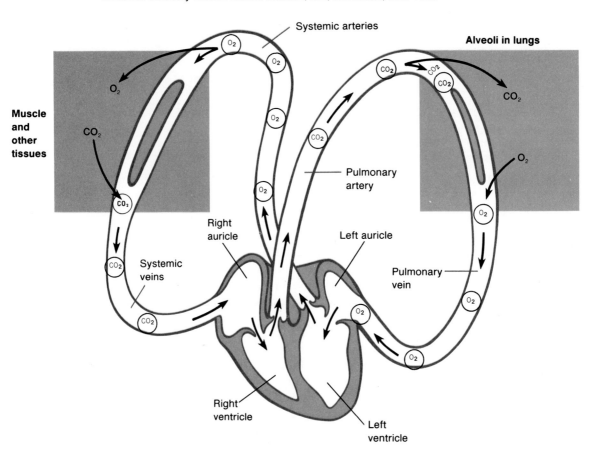

Cardiovascular-Respiratory Diseases

Oxygen is the element most vital to life. The most important function of the cardiovascular and respiratory systems is to maintain a constant supply of oxygen to all body tissues, according to their needs. Figure 2.1 depicts the interrelationships between the cardiovascular and respiratory systems relative to gaseous exchange of oxygen (O_2) and carbon dioxide (CO_2).

The respiratory system takes in oxygen from the atmospheric air and conveys it to the alveoli (small air sacs in the lungs, surrounded by a capillary network). In the alveoli, oxygen is picked up and dissolved in the blood, and carbon dioxide is eliminated from the blood. The bronchi and bronchioli are air pathways that may cause respiratory distress if they become constricted or narrowed for any reason.

The cardiovascular system serves as a plumbing system, functioning to transport the oxygen in the blood throughout the body. The heart serves as a muscular pump to provide the force or pressure for ejecting the blood into the blood vessels, which serve as the channels to transport the blood to all living body cells. There are several different types of blood vessels in the body. The major classifications include arteries, capillaries, and veins. The arteries transport blood away from the heart; the capillaries permeate the various tissues and release oxygen and other nutrients to the cells; the veins transport the blood back to the heart.

The major health problems associated with the cardiovascular system arise in the blood vessels, primarily the arteries, and, more specifically, the arteries in the heart. The heart is a large muscle with four blood-filled chambers, but the heart itself cannot extract much oxygen directly from the blood in its chambers. Like other organs in the body, it has its own internal network of arteries, capillaries, and veins. The arteries that supply blood to the heart muscle are called **coronary arteries**—mainly the left coronary, right coronary, and circumflex (fig. 2.2). In order to function efficiently, the coronary arteries and all other arteries throughout the body must maintain a normal interior diameter. When the normal opening of an artery is narrowed or closed, cardiovascular problems develop.

Coronary Heart Disease (CHD)

Coronary heart disease (CHD) is one of several major diseases of the cardiovascular system. It is also known as coronary artery disease because obstruction of the blood flow in the coronary arteries is responsible for the pathological effects of the disease. The major manifestation of coronary heart disease is a heart attack, which results from a sudden stoppage of blood flow to parts of the heart muscle. Other terms often used for heart attack include **coronary thrombosis,** which is a blockage of a blood vessel by a clot (thrombus), **coronary occlusion,** which simply means blockage, and **myocardial infarct,** which is defined as death of some heart cells that do not get enough oxygen due to the blocked coronary artery.

Nearly one out of every two deaths in the United States is due to diseases of the heart and blood vessels. Each year, approximately one million Americans die from some form of cardiovascular disease, including CHD, stroke, hypertensive disease, rheumatic heart disease, and congenital heart disease. Of these million deaths, about two-thirds are attributed to CHD. Although the total percentage of deaths due to CHD has been declining in recent years, it is still an epidemic and the number one cause of death among Americans.

Arteriosclerosis

Arteriosclerosis is a term applied to a number of different pathological conditions wherein the arterial walls thicken and lose their elasticity. It is often defined as hardening of the arteries. **Atherosclerosis,** one form of arteriosclerosis, is characterized by deposits of fat, cholesterol, cellular debris, calcium, and fibrin on the inner linings of

Figure 2.2 The Coronary Arteries. The heart muscle itself receives its blood supply from the coronary arteries. The main coronary arteries are the left coronary artery, one of its branches named the *circumflex,* and the right coronary artery. Atherosclerosis of these arteries leads to coronary heart disease.
Source: From Fox, Stuart Ira, *Human Physiology.* © 1984, Wm. C. Brown Publishers, Dubuque, Iowa. All Rights Reserved. Reprinted by Permission.

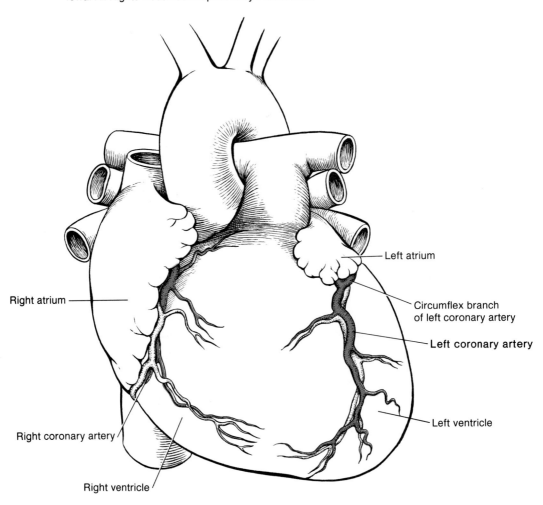

the arterial wall. These deposits, known as **plaque,** result in a narrowing of the blood channel, making it easier for blood clots to form, eventually resulting in complete blockage of blood flow to vital tissues such as the heart or the brain. Figure 2.3 illustrates the gradual, progressive narrowing of the arterial channel. Figure 2.4 presents a schematic of the content of arterial plaque.

Atherosclerosis is a slow, progressive disease, beginning in childhood and usually manifesting itself later in life. Severe coronary atherosclerosis is the cause of almost all heart attacks. Because of its prevalence in industrialized society, scientists throughout the world have been conducting intensive research efforts in attempts to identify the

Figure 2.3 Atherosclerosis. The developmental process of atherosclerosis is illustrated from top to bottom. Deposits of cholesterol, fat, and other debris accumulate in the inner lining of the artery, leading to a decrease or cessation of blood flow to the tissues. Atherosclerosis in the heart is a major cause of coronary heart disease.

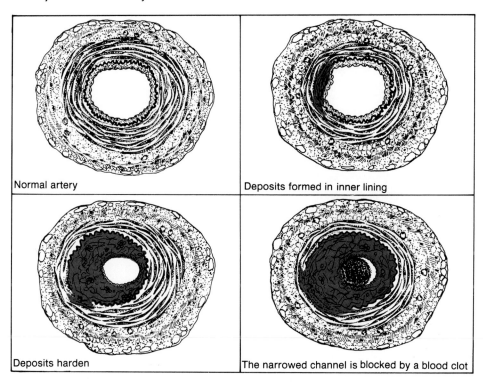

cause, or causes, of atherosclerosis and coronary heart disease. Although the actual cause has not yet been completely identified, considerable evidence has accumulated that helps us to identify those risk factors that may predispose an individual to atherosclerosis and CHD.

Risk Factors

Research into the etiology, or origin, of CHD has utilized several approaches. One approach involves epidemiological techniques whereby certain populations of people are studied in order to isolate risk factors. For example, a number of epidemiological studies have compared physically active and inactive individuals and found that physical activity may help to prevent the development of CHD. Other research techniques involve experimental studies with both animals and humans, designed to determine the effect of some factor such as a high-cholesterol diet or jogging on the development of atherosclerosis or the level of blood cholesterol. The results of epidemiological and experimental research have helped to document a number of the risk factors associated with CHD. This research has also shown that the greater the number and severity of risk factors present, the greater is the predisposition to CHD. Many of these risk factors are presented in the Health Life-style Assessment Inventory in chapter 1.

Figure 2.4 An Enlargement of Atherosclerotic Plaque. Cholesterol, fats, dead cells, and other debris collect within or beneath the inner lining of an artery. There is often an ulceration (opening) in the inner layer of the arterial wall through which the cholesterol and other plaque constituents enter.

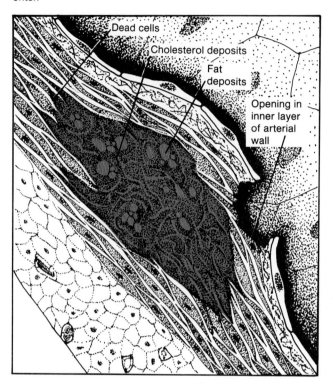

Table 2.2 highlights risk factors that have been identified from epidemiological or experimental studies. Primary risk factors are those that are directly related to the development of CHD, while secondary risk factors may predispose an individual to a primary risk factor. Although some of the risk factors cannot be changed, many may be modified by adopting a Positive Health Life-style. Let us look briefly at each risk factor and how it is associated with CHD.

High Blood Pressure. Hypertension, or high blood pressure, is a disease by itself and is discussed in more detail later in this chapter. For now, however, we may note that it is probably the major risk factor associated with CHD and stroke.

High Blood Lipids. In atherosclerosis, the plaque that develops in the arterial walls is composed partly of fats and cholesterol. Hence, high levels of blood **lipids** (triglycerides and cholesterol) are associated with increased levels of plaque formation. Most triglycerides and cholesterol are carried in the blood as **lipoproteins,** which are small capsules of triglycerides, cholesterol, phospholipids (another lipid substance), and protein. The protein acts as a carrier for these lipids, hence the name lipoproteins. Various

Figure 2.5 Risk Factors in Coronary Heart Disease. The danger of developing coronary heart disease and experiencing a heart attack increases with the number of risk factors. The three major risk factors are cigarette smoking, high blood serum cholesterol levels, and high blood pressure.
Source: © American Heart Association. Reproduced with permission.

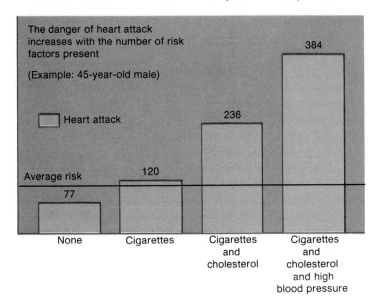

Table 2.2
Risk Factors Associated with Coronary Heart Disease

Risk Factors	Classification	Positive Health Life-style Modification
High blood pressure	Primary	Proper nutrition, exercise
High blood lipids	Primary	Proper nutrition, exercise
Smoking	Primary	Stop smoking
ECG abnormalities	Primary	Exercise
Obesity	Secondary	Low-Calorie diet, exercise
Diabetes	Secondary	Proper nutrition, weight reduction, exercise
Stressful life-style	Secondary	Stress reduction, exercise
Dietary intake	Secondary	Proper nutrition
Sedentary life-style	Secondary	Exercise
Family history	Secondary	Not modifiable
Sex	Secondary	Not modifiable
Race	Secondary	Not modifiable
Age	Secondary	Not modifiable

Figure 2.6 The Major Lipoproteins in the Plasma. Triglyceride (TG) is the major constituent of the very low density lipoproteins (VLDL). The low density lipoproteins (LDL) contain high proportions of cholesterol (C) and phospholipids (PL), while the high density lipoproteins are high in cholesterol and protein (P). It is theorized that the LDL may be a risk factor in the development of atherosclerosis while the HDL may serve a preventive role.
Source: From Wood, Peter, et al, *Annals of the New York Academy of Sciences.* Reprinted by permission of the publisher and the author.

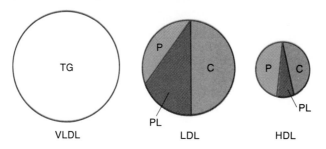

forms of lipoproteins are found in the blood, and are classified according to their density, which depends on their composition (various lipids and protein). In brief, the **very low density lipoproteins (VLDL)** are composed primarily of triglycerides; the **low density lipoproteins (LDL)** contain high amounts of cholesterol; the **high density lipoproteins (HDL)** have a high concentration of protein. Figure 2.6 graphically presents the composition of the major lipoproteins in the blood. Some cholesterol is found in all types of lipoproteins. In recent years much research has been devoted to the role of LDL-cholesterol and HDL-cholesterol in the development of CHD. Individuals with high levels of HDL-cholesterol appear to experience less CHD in comparison to those with high levels of LDL-cholesterol. Total cholesterol is still important, but an analysis should examine the different types of lipoprotein cholesterol. The exact mechanism of how one form of cholesterol may help prevent CHD and another may predispose an individual to CHD has not been elucidated, but one theory suggests that HDL picks up cholesterol from the arterial wall and transports it to the liver for removal from the body, while LDL helps to deposit cholesterol in the arterial wall. High blood triglyceride and cholesterol levels are often treated with drug therapy, but may also be modified by diet and exercise.

Smoking. The degree of CHD risk from cigarette smoking is affected by the number of cigarettes smoked daily (whether or not the smoke is inhaled) and the number of years of smoking. Smoking stresses the cardiovascular system in several ways. Nicotine, a drug present in cigarette smoke, stimulates adrenalin release in the body, which elevates blood pressure by constricting blood vessels and increasing the heart rate. Also, carbon monoxide in the smoke displaces oxygen from hemoglobin and, thus, increases the work load of the heart in delivering oxygen to the tissues. Moreover, certain hydrocarbons in cigarette smoke may act as mutagens (substances that cause a change or transformation) on the cells in the arterial walls, possibly accelerating the atherosclerotic process. However, the American Heart Association has noted that the rate of fatal heart disease in cigarette smokers who stop smoking is nearly as low as for those people who have never smoked.

ECG Abnormalities. The **ECG,** or electrocardiogram, is a record of the electrical activity generated in the heart. An abnormal pattern may be indicative of insufficient blood flow and oxygen to part of the heart muscle. In many cases, resting ECGs may not detect these abnormalities, but exercise stress tests usually can detect the presence of CHD. In most cases, an abnormal ECG response is indicative of CHD. Other types of tests may then be conducted to determine the severity of the disease. A prescribed exercise program may help alleviate some ECG abnormalities.

Obesity. Obesity, in itself, does not appear to have a very high relationship to CHD, but excess weight predisposes individuals toward high blood pressure and high blood lipid levels, both of which are primary risk factors. Obesity is also a factor in the development of adult-onset diabetes, another secondary risk factor. The causes of obesity are complex and are discussed later in this chapter, but a low-Calorie diet and exercise are effective means to lose excess weight in most individuals.

Diabetes. Individuals with diabetes have an increased risk of CHD and stroke. In essence, the high levels of glucose in the blood of diabetics may damage some of the small blood vessels in the heart or brain. Diabetes can be controlled with proper medication, diet, weight reduction, and exercise. An expanded discussion of diabetes is presented later in this chapter.

Stressful Life-style. Psychological stress is prevalent in today's modern society, and may be a factor involved in CHD. Individuals who have a high-strung personality, who are always tense, and who are constantly imposing stressful demands upon themselves have been labeled as having a **type A personality.** Type A coronary-prone behavior patterns, or constant stress, may elicit various hormonal responses in the body, which may predispose an individual to CHD. Elevated blood pressure, due to constricted blood vessels and elevated blood lipids, are two possible effects. Stressful situations in life should be identified and actions taken to eliminate them whenever possible. Proper exercise programs and stress reduction techniques may be helpful in reducing the effects of stress.

Dietary Intake. A number of different types of foods that we consume have been associated with CHD, primarily because they increase blood lipid levels, or contribute to the development of high blood pressure. In brief, the general recommendation today is to consume less saturated fat, cholesterol, refined sugars, and alcohol, because excessive amounts of any of these may increase blood lipid levels. Salt intake should also be restricted because excessive salt may aggravate high blood pressure. In addition, a low-Calorie diet may help reduce excess body weight.

Sedentary Life-style. In general, people who are physically active experience a lower incidence of heart attacks and clinical symptoms such as chest pain and abnormal ECGs. Also, people who do have heart attacks have a greater survival rate if they have been physically active. The best type of exercise involves aerobic activities that engage the cardiovascular system.

Family History.   Although there is little evidence to indicate that either CHD or the atherosclerotic process are directly inherited through the genes, there does appear to be a tendency for CHD to run in certain families. This familial tendency may be related to the fact that other risk factors, such as high blood lipid levels, high blood pressure, diabetes, and obesity tend to be familial also. If your family has a history of CHD before age sixty, you may be exposed to this risk factor. This risk factor may not be modified, since we have no choice in the selection of our parents.

Sex.   Young females experience fewer heart attacks than males. This protection against CHD may be attributed to estrogen, a female sex hormone that may raise blood levels of HDL-cholesterol. Due to hormonal changes, some of this protection decreases after menopause, and the rate of CHD among women increases sharply. However, the rate of CHD never reaches that of men. There is, of course, little that we can do about our sex type, since it is genetically determined.

Race.   In the United States, blacks are almost 50 percent more likely to have high blood pressure than are whites. As noted previously, high blood pressure is a major risk factor in CHD. Unfortunately, the cause of this racial tendency toward high blood pressure is not understood at present. Race is also genetically determined, and, thus, cannot be modified.

Age.   As we get older, our chances of developing CHD increase. Most fatalities from CHD occur after age sixty-five, yet one out of every four deaths does occur under age sixty-five. Although we can do nothing about our chronological age (actual age), we may be able to maintain a younger physiological age by adopting a Positive Health Life-style early in life so that some of the natural consequences of the aging process may possibly be slowed down.

Positive Health Life-style

Many of the risk factors associated with CHD may be beneficially affected by the development of a Positive Health Life-style. Those that may be modified include high blood pressure, high blood lipid levels, cigarette smoking, obesity, stressful life-style, dietary intake, and physical activity.

The risk of CHD decreases when smokers stop their habit. This would appear to be one of the easiest methods to reduce CHD risk. Unfortunately, the smoking habit is so engrained in some people's life-styles that it is extremely difficult to break. Some helpful hints for stopping smoking are presented later in this chapter.

Stress reduction techniques, which are discussed in detail in chapter 9, provide another mechanism whereby a CHD risk factor may be modified. These techniques help to counteract some of the adverse effects of a stressful life-style.

Modification of the diet may have a significant impact upon several risk factors. Reduction of the dietary intake of salt, cholesterol, and saturated fats may significantly reduce high blood pressure and high blood lipid levels, while a low-Calorie diet can prevent or reduce obesity. Dietary modifications to reduce salt, cholesterol, and saturated fats are presented in chapter 5. Weight reduction methods are included in chapter 6.

Figure 2.7 Ranges of Systolic and Diastolic Blood Pressures from Birth to Age One Hundred. Blood pressure levels vary among individuals, as noted by the wide ranges, particularly as one ages. Systolic hypertension occurs at a pressure of 140 mm Hg while diastolic hypertension is rated at 90 mm Hg. Note that advancing age increases the probability of hypertension, but even young adults may have high blood pressure.
Source: Reprinted from *What about Blood Pressure,* Daniel E. James, © 1981 by Carolina Biological Supply Company.

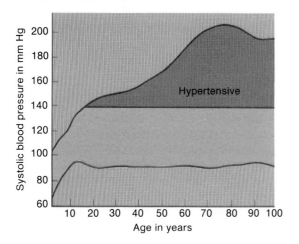
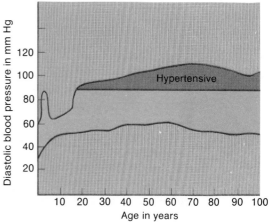

A properly designed exercise program, primarily aerobic, will remove one risk factor—physical inactivity. Additionally, aerobic exercise may have a healthful effect on other risk factors as well. Aerobic exercise may help to reduce high blood pressure, exert a beneficial effect upon blood lipid and cholesterol levels, prevent or reduce obesity, and help to counteract the effects of stress on the body. The mechanisms whereby exercise elicits these effects are presented in later chapters, primarily chapter 4.

High Blood Pressure (Hypertension)

Everybody has blood pressure, for without it we would not be able to sustain body metabolism. Simply speaking, **blood pressure** is the force that the blood exerts against the blood vessel walls. Although pressure is present in all types of blood vessels, the arterial blood pressure is the one most commonly measured and most important to our health. Systolic blood pressure represents that phase during which the heart is pumping blood through the arterial system when the pressure is greatest against the arterial wall. Increases in the amount of blood being pumped from the heart can increase the systolic blood pressure. The diastolic blood pressure represents that phase when the heart is resting (between beats).

A number of factors influence the normal range of blood pressure, including age, body position (such as sitting or standing), time of day, recency of exercise, and intake of drugs (such as caffeine, alcohol, or nicotine). As noted in figure 2.7, there is a rather wide range in blood pressure levels, both systolic and diastolic, from one individual to another. For example, at age twenty the range is about 90–145 for systolic and 50–95 for diastolic. A level of 140 for systolic and 90 for diastolic is considered to be hypertension. Thus, some twenty-year-olds have high blood pressure. You may also note from this figure that, as age increases, the upper ranges of both systolic and diastolic pressures also increase and a greater percentage of individuals become hypertensive. A persistent resting blood pressure of over 140 systolic and/or 90 diastolic is considered high and in need of medical attention.

Two major factors are involved in the regulation of blood pressure. They are the cardiac output (the amount of blood pumped by the heart each minute), and the peripheral vascular resistance (the resistance offered to blood flow by the vessels). Increasing either the cardiac output or the peripheral vascular resistance increases the blood pressure.

High blood pressure, also known as **hypertension** (hyper = high; tension = pressure) is a silent disease. The American Heart Association indicates that over thirty-seven million Americans (about 15 percent of the population) have high blood pressure. It is 50 percent more prevalent among black Americans than whites. However, millions do not know they have it because it has no outstanding symptoms. Some general symptoms include headaches, dizziness, and fatigue, but they can be caused by a multitude of other factors, so they may not be recognized as symptoms of high blood pressure. Although a great deal of research has and is being conducted into the cause of high blood pressure, the exact cause is unknown in about 90 percent of all cases. In these cases the condition is known as *essential hypertension,* for which there is no cure.

High blood pressure is dangerous for two reasons. First, it drastically increases the work load of the heart in pumping the extra blood volume or overcoming the peripheral vascular resistance. As noted previously, high blood pressure is a primary risk factor for coronary heart disease. Second, high blood pressure may directly damage the arteries, due to the constant pressure, and thus be a major contributing factor to stroke. High blood pressure is a disease unto itself, but it is also involved in the etiology of other diseases.

Positive Health Life-style

Since high blood pressure is such a potentially dangerous disease, it is important that it be controlled. In many cases, this means the utilization of drug therapy (antihypertension drugs) under a physician's direction. However, several life-style modifications may also help to reduce blood pressure, possibly decreasing, or in some cases eliminating, the need for drug therapy.

Two rather universally accepted Positive Health Life-style changes to reduce blood pressure are to decrease dietary intake of salt and decrease body fat. Excessive amounts of salt (sodium) in the body hold more water, thereby increasing the blood volume, which then increases the blood pressure. Excessive body fat places extra demands on the heart to pump blood through more blood vessels, again increasing the blood pressure.

Stress reduction techniques have been advocated as a means to reduce blood pressure, but results are not as conclusive as with salt restriction and weight loss. Behavioral techniques involving the relaxation response (see chapter 9) have successfully reduced blood pressure in some highly motivated subjects, but the general success of this technique in lowering high blood pressure is still considered to be questionable.

Regular aerobic exercise has also been recommended as a modality to reduce high blood pressure. Since exercise may be an effective means to lose excess body fat, it may exert a beneficial effect through this avenue. However, the role of exercise as an independent factor in lowering high blood pressure is more controversial. One effect of chronic exercise training may be a lessened blood pressure rise during exercise, which confers a protective effect. A number of other studies also note that exercise training helps to decrease resting systolic blood pressure in those who have high blood pressure, but has no effect on those with normal blood pressure. Although most investigators who have reviewed the relevant research note that the available evidence does not conclusively show that exercise training will benefit the general hypertensive population, they suggest that the present information is sufficient to justify an aerobic exercise program for the treatment of high blood pressure.

One type of exercise, however, is not recommended for hypertensive individuals. Isometric exercise, such as straining to move an immovable object, creates a physiological response and raises the blood pressure rapidly to rather high levels. This increase may be hazardous to someone whose resting blood pressure is already at an elevated level.

Stroke

Stroke, which is also known as apoplexy or a cerebral vascular accident, annually afflicts almost two million Americans and is responsible for nearly 170,000 deaths. A stroke occurs when the blood supply to the brain is inadequate, usually due to a blocking of one of the arteries to the brain by atherosclerosis or by a clot. A stroke may also occur if a cerebral blood vessel ruptures, forming a clot in the brain tissue, or if a tumor blocks normal blood flow. The severity of the stroke may vary from slight loss of memory, slight paralysis, and speaking difficulty to severe paralysis or death, depending on the location and extent of the brain damage.

An individual with atherosclerosis and/or high blood pressure is more likely to have a stroke. Thus, the risk factors associated with the development of both of these diseases may contribute to cerebral vascular accidents.

Positive Health Life-style
A Positive Health Life-style, which reduces the severity of the risk factors associated with coronary heart disease and high blood pressure, is also an effective preventive measure against stroke.

Peripheral Vascular Disease

Peripheral vascular disease (PVD) is similar to coronary heart disease (CHD), but in PVD, the arteriosclerosis is found in blood vessels other than those in the heart. Individuals with PVD experience pain during physical activity due to the inability of the vessels to deliver enough blood to the active tissues. The risk factors for CHD and PVD are similar.

Figure 2.8   Stroke. A stroke, or apoplexy, is caused by inadequate blood flow to parts of the brain. One cause is a cerebral thrombosis, or clot, which decreases blood flow, and hence oxygen, with resultant damage to brain function. The observable effects depend upon the area of the brain and the amount of tissue damaged.

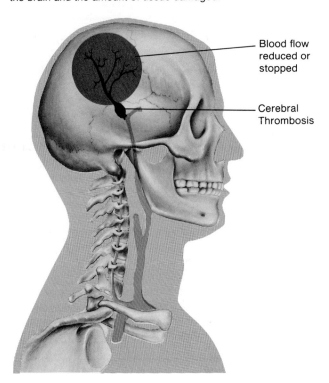

Blood flow
reduced or
stopped

Cerebral
Thrombosis

Positive Health Life-style

Whether or not an exercise and a proper nutrition program may help reduce the severity of PVD once it has developed is uncertain. Research conducted at the Longevity Research Institute supports a beneficial effect of exercise and dietary modification upon the symptoms of PVD. They found that exercise training, in conjunction with a normal American diet, was effective in prolonging walking endurance without symptoms of pain. However, their dietary program (10 percent fat, 10 percent protein, and 80 percent complex carbohydrates and no cholesterol), in conjunction with exercise training, was even more effective. On the other hand, a recent report in the Journal of the American Medical Association reveals no improvement of blood flow in the limbs following a year of daily exercise and a diet similar to the one used at the Longevity Research Institute. Although the atherosclerosis may not be reversed, the onset of the pain symptoms are usually reversed through a combined exercise-nutrition program. This general finding may, in itself, justify the recommendation for an exercise-nutrition program for individuals with PVD. Moreover, such a program may have greater value as a preventive measure. Adoption of the Positive Health Life-style recommended for the prevention of CHD is prudent behavior to also help prevent PVD.

Metabolic Disorders

Metabolism represents the sum total of all the physical and chemical processes in the human body that are concerned with the energy transformations essential to life. Although general metabolism includes all processes involved in the utilization of ingested nutrients, there are also special types, such as carbohydrate metabolism, fat metabolism, and protein metabolism. There are a vast number of different metabolic disorders that are harmful to health, but two of the most prevalent in American society are obesity (unbalanced Calorie metabolism) and diabetes (a disorder of carbohydrate metabolism).

Obesity

Obesity is a condition marked by excessive deposition and storage of fat throughout the body. Overweight is often used as a synonym for obese, but this may depend on the ratio of body fat to lean tissue. Obesity affects both children and adults. Approximately 25 percent of the American population are too fat for optimal health (20–30 percent over their recommended normal weights). Being obese is associated with a host of health problems—both physical and socio-emotional. Obesity is a risk factor associated with the development of high blood pressure and diabetes, both of which are also risk factors for CHD. Obesity has also been associated with kidney disease and cirrhosis of the liver. Thus, mortality rates are higher among the obese than in their normal-weight peers. Obesity may also contribute to the development of psychological disturbances, particularly in adolescents who are conscious of their body images. **Body image** is a term used to describe the feelings an individual has toward his or her body. Body image tends to solidify during adolescence and persists into adulthood. Thus, a youngster who develops a poor body image may experience personality difficulties that can retard proper socio-emotional development. Excess body fat may also exert an adverse effect on the ability to perform physical activities well, so that the obese child may avoid sports and other activities, and possibly be deprived of their socialization value.

Although the ultimate cause of obesity is a simple problem of energy balance—an excessive caloric intake beyond caloric expenditure—the factors contributing to this energy imbalance may be very complex. The current theory of obesity is centered around a multicausal etiology, suggesting that a number of factors may interact to create an energy surplus of fat in the body. There may be a genetic predisposition to obesity, for children of an obese parent have a greater probability of being obese, possibly because they inherit the tendency to develop more fat cells. Endocrine imbalances or metabolic disturbances may lower the body's ability to utilize its energy sources. Damage to the hunger (satiety) centers in the hypothalamus may disrupt feeding reflexes so an individual overeats. Social customs, such as serving large meals of high-Calorie foods, may be a contributing factor. Psychological trauma may foster overeating. Physical inactivity eliminates an important avenue for caloric expenditure. Any one of these causes, or the interaction of several, may affect the ability of an individual to achieve or maintain normal weight.

Positive Health Life-style

Basically, there are two general means to treat or prevent obesity. You must either decrease your energy intake or increase your energy output. In essence, you must initiate a low-Calorie diet, or an exercise program, or both. Just as adding 150 Calories to the daily diet will increase body fat by 15 pounds in one year, so too will decreasing 150 Calories from the daily diet result in an annual loss of 15 pounds. Jogging a mile and a half per day will accomplish the same result. A Positive Health Life-style centered around a low-Calorie nutritious diet and an aerobic exercise program can be a sound means to prevent or treat obesity. Research has indicated that a combination of a nutritious diet and an aerobic exercise program is the best approach to weight control.

Diabetes

Diabetes is one of the most prevalent diseases in the United States, afflicting over five million Americans. It is the third leading cause of death, claiming 300,000 lives annually, due to both the disease itself and its complications, such as heart attack and stroke. Diabetes affects almost all body tissues. Millions of diabetics suffer consequences such as blindness, high blood pressure, and chronic infections. Every minute, another American is diagnosed as diabetic.

Diabetes is a condition in which excessive amounts of urine are excreted from the body daily. It may be caused by such problems as a malfunctioning adrenal or pituitary gland. However, its most common form is **diabetes mellitus,** a disorder in which the body cannot metabolize carbohydrates properly. The main effect is a high level of glucose in the blood. The major problem is associated with **insulin,** a hormone secreted by the pancreas. Insulin is necessary for blood glucose to enter the body cells. Diabetics may have a decreased pancreatic production of insulin, or a deficiency of insulin receptors in the liver, muscle, and fat tissues, so that the insulin, even if it is present in normal amounts, may have no effect on the tissues. In essence, diabetics have impaired carbohydrate, or glucose, metabolism, as the body turns to fat for its major energy sources. The rise in serum lipids then becomes a contributing factor for other diseases, such as CHD.

Diabetes may develop in one of two general ways. Juvenile-onset diabetes usually occurs in children, and may be caused by a virus or other toxic agent that in some way destroys the ability of the pancreas to produce insulin. This is the most severe type of diabetes. Heredity does not appear to play a major role in its development. Maturity-onset diabetes, as the name implies, usually develops later in life. Its onset is more gradual, and the disease is usually milder than the juvenile-onset type. Most maturity-onset diabetics are overweight, and nearly 85 percent of these diabetics have a diabetic parent. The two recently adopted terms used to describe diabetic patients are insulin-dependent and noninsulin-dependent. All juvenile-onset diabetics, and about 20 percent of maturity-onset diabetics, are insulin-dependent (they must take insulin in order to control the disease). Noninsulin-dependent diabetics, who constitute about 80 percent of all diabetics, may be able to control their blood sugar by proper nutrition and exercise, or other drugs.

Figure 2.9 Role of Insulin. Insulin binds to insulin receptors in the cell membrane, which then activates a carrier system (*C*). The carrier system transports glucose through the cell membrane to the interior where it is released for further use. One cause of diabetes is a deficiency of insulin receptors in the body. Another cause is insufficient insulin production by the pancreas.

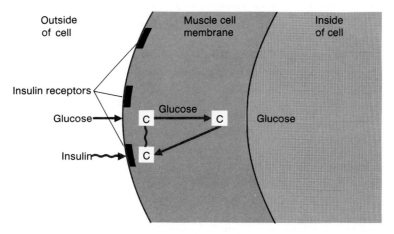

Positive Health Life-style

As with the other diseases discussed previously in this chapter, a Positive Health Life-style can be viewed as both treatment and prevention for diabetes. Medical treatment of diabetes usually centers around four aspects—insulin or other drugs, diet, exercise, and weight control. Of these four factors, the latter three are important components of a Positive Health Life-style.

Insulin-dependent diabetics need medical supervision in order to determine how much insulin they need and how often they should take it. The dosage must be tailored to the life-style of the individual. Exercise may reduce the insulin requirement somewhat.

Both types of diabetics must control their diets. The American Diabetic Association currently recommends a diet consisting of:

50–60 percent of Calories from complex carbohydrates

30–35 percent of Calories from fat

12–15 percent of Calories from protein

The carbohydrates should be of the complex type, such as fruits, vegetables, and whole grain products. An increased fiber content, found naturally in these products, may also be helpful because it may slow down the absorption of carbohydrates in the intestine. Simple sugars should be avoided. Although these general guidelines have been developed for the individual who has diabetes, they may also be very important in its prevention. Excessive intake of simple sugars stimulates the pancreas to release insulin in greater quantities. Prolonged consumption of simple sugars may possibly impair the ability of the pancreas to produce insulin. The diet should also be balanced in Calories in order to maintain the recommended body weight. One of the contributing factors to maturity-onset diabetes is excessive body fat. Excessive caloric intake decreases the number of active insulin receptors in body cells so insulin does not function properly. Decreasing caloric intake helps to reactivate these receptors.

Properly prescribed exercise may be an effective adjunct to insulin and diet for the diabetic patient. Exercise facilitates the utilization of glucose by the muscle cells, helping to lower blood glucose levels. For insulin-dependent diabetics, this may decrease the insulin requirement. Exercise also lowers blood lipid levels associated with diabetes, for muscle cells also use these lipids for energy. In addition, exercise increases energy expenditure, thus helping the individual to lose weight—of benefit to the maturity-onset diabetic. These beneficial effects of exercise for the diabetic may also help prevent the initial development of diabetes. Physically trained individuals normally have lower insulin secretions, which may help them to maintain normal pancreas functioning for a longer period of time. Moreover, some evidence is available to suggest that glucose tolerance, or the ability of the body to metabolize glucose, is improved in trained individuals, particularly if they are lean.

However, exercise may be harmful to the insulin-dependent diabetic if it is not carefully prescribed. The major problem in the exercising diabetic is **hypoglycemia,** or low blood sugar. Exercise stimulates blood flow and, thus, can increase the blood levels of insulin by mobilizing the insulin from its injection site. This increased insulin, and the effect of exercise itself, will increase the transport of glucose into the muscle rapidly, and possibly create hypoglycemia. The exercising diabetic should always carry something sweet to eat in case of a hypoglycemic episode. It is important that diabetics discuss a proper exercise program with their physicians.

Musculoskeletal Disorders

As the name suggests, musculoskeletal disorders afflict either the muscular system, the skeletal system, or both. Although there is a wide variety of these disorders—muscle strains, bone fractures, and muscular dystrophy to name a few—three types of musculoskeletal disorders that may be influenced by a Positive Health Life-style are of special interest. These disorders, or diseases, are low back pain, osteoporosis, and arthritis.

Low Back Pain

The skeletal spine is a remarkable structure, designed to support a good portion of the body's weight, to transmit this weight to the lower part of the body, to protect the delicate spinal cord of the nervous system, to serve as a shock absorber, and to provide for movement in all directions. Figure 2.10 is a lateral view of the spine, with a section showing the intervertebral discs. The discs of cartilage between each vertebra serve as shock absorbers and are also one of two types of joints in the spine where all movement can occur. The curves in the spine develop naturally, and are necessary for the spine to perform its major functions. Unfortunately, the lower part of the back, particularly the lumbar-sacral area, may be subjected to excessive stresses that may lead to a **low back pain syndrome,** which is characterized by dull aching pain in the lumbar region

Figure 2.10 Lateral View of the Spine. (*a*) Among the five segments of the spine, the cervical region curves forward in the neck area, the thoracic backward in the upper back, and the lumbar curve is forward in the low back region. (*b*) A disc of fibrocartilage, the intervertebral disc, is located between each of the vertebrae in the spinal column.
Source: From Hole, John W., Jr., *Human Anatomy and Physiology,* 3d. ed. © 1978, 1981, 1984. Wm. C. Brown Publishers, Dubuque, Iowa. All Rights Reserved. Reprinted by Permission.

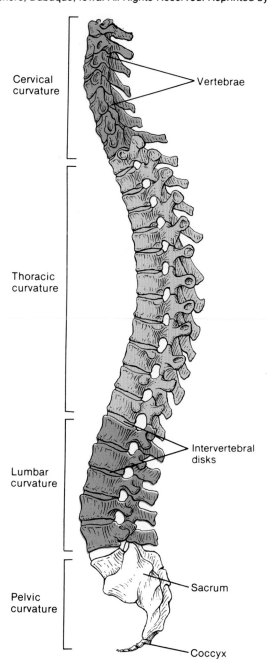

Cervical curvature

Vertebrae

Thoracic curvature

Intervertebral disks

Lumbar curvature

Pelvic curvature

Sacrum

Coccyx

and occasional bursts of sharp pain when certain movements of the low back area are performed. Low back pain may have several different general causes, including biomechanical imbalances, improper development, infection, or trauma. Medical advice should be obtained in cases of persistent pain.

The stability of the spine is due to the discs (between the vertebral bodies), the ligaments, and the extensive musculature. Excessive stresses may damage any of these tissues and cause pain. The usual cause of low back injury is mechanical trauma due to improper lifting techniques, lifting too heavy a load, or improper posture. The ligaments and muscles may be torn, and, in cases of very heavy loads or older discs, a herniation may occur. In this situation, the outer surface of the disc ruptures and exerts pressure on the nerves in the vicinity. In some cases, pain may radiate through the hip and back of the thigh. This situation is often termed *sciatica,* because the sciatic nerve is subjected to pressure.

Low back pain is a disease of civilization, and occurs in over 80 percent of the population at some time in their lives. In a recent year, it has been estimated that 14 billion dollars was spent on the treatment of industrial back injuries alone. There is a greater likelihood of experiencing low back pain as one gets older, for after the age of thirty the vertebral discs begin to lose some of their elasticity and become more prone to injury. However, low back pain also occurs in younger individuals, particularly those involved in vigorous sports in which harmful forces may be applied to the low back area.

Positive Health Life-style

Excessive pressure in the low back area must be avoided in order to prevent the development of a low back pain syndrome. One of the key behaviors is proper lifting techniques. Do not attempt to lift anything without bending your knees, nor lift an object that is too far in front of your body. Also, avoid positions that exaggerate the forward curve in the lumbar area, including exercises that may force your body into such a position. See figures 8.1 and 8.19 for examples.

A proper exercise program may help to prevent low back pain and may also be an effective treatment technique. The abdominal muscles must be strengthened and the flexibility of the muscles in the low back region must be increased. Another important consideration is the avoidance of exercises that may contribute to low back injury.

Osteoporosis

Osteoporosis is a disorder characterized by increased thinness and fragility of the bone structure, making them more susceptible to fractures. Osteoporosis results from a decreased bone density, mainly because calcium is lost from the bones faster than it is replaced. It usually occurs in older individuals, particularly women, and is associated with an increased susceptibility to hip fractures. Although osteoporosis may be caused by several things, two major contributing factors are a calcium-deficient diet and a sedentary life-style.

Positive Health Life-style

Although osteoporosis is primarily a disorder that manifests itself later in life, it may be prevented by a Positive Health Life-style in the early adult years. One of the major problems is a calcium-deficient diet, which is usually due to a decreased consumption of dairy products (particularly milk) as we get older. Dairy products represent the major source of calcium in the American diet, and adults should have at least two servings daily. Other foods that are high in calcium content are the dark-green, leafy vegetables.

Exercise, particularly weight-bearing exercise such as jogging or aerobic walking, may not only help to maintain normal bone structure, but may actually increase the bone-mineral content in body segments that are exercised.

It is important to realize that these two preventive measures—adequate calcium intake and physical activity—need to be continued throughout life. However, even if they are not implemented until later in life (even at age sixty to seventy), they may still help to maintain or increase bone density, thus preventing osteoporosis.

Arthritis

A *joint* is located wherever two bones come together in the body. There are a number of different types of joints, but most are of the diarthrodial (moving) type. A typical joint (fig. 2.11) is surrounded by a synovial membrane, which secretes a lubricant (synovial fluid) to help reduce friction in the joint. The ends of the bones are covered with cartilage, which serves to provide a smoother surface and, as a result, creates less friction.

Arthritis, translated literally, means inflammation of the joint, but the term is used to cover a number of different conditions (over 100) that cause pain in the joints. Over 30 million Americans experience some form of arthritis serious enough to necessitate medical care. An extensive discussion of the various forms of arthritis is beyond the scope of this book, but the two major types are highlighted in relation to the Positive Health Life-style.

Rheumatoid arthritis is the most serious form, and may cause crippling. It may occur at any age (even in children), and may affect almost all body tissues. It affects more women than men. The disease causes inflammation to the synovial lining surrounding the joint. The inflammation may eventually invade and destroy the cartilage, increasing friction within the joint and causing pain. The cause of rheumatoid arthritis is still a mystery, but infection and a malfunctioning immune system in the body are two current theories. There is no known cure, although certain medications may help to control the disease. Proper exercise is recommended therapy. Some recent research has revealed that exercise training decreases the progression of destructive changes within the joints of individuals with rheumatoid arthritis.

Osteoarthritis is the most common form of arthritis, and usually occurs later in life. There are basically two forms. *Primary osteoarthritis* occurs without any apparent cause, usually appears in women, and affects the smaller joints. *Secondary osteoarthritis* may result from excessive wear and tear, or mechanical stress, of a joint.

Figure 2.11 Structure of a Joint. (*a*) A simplified schematic of a typical diarthrodial (movable) joint. (*b*) The onset of arthritis, and the progressive destruction of the articular cartilage.

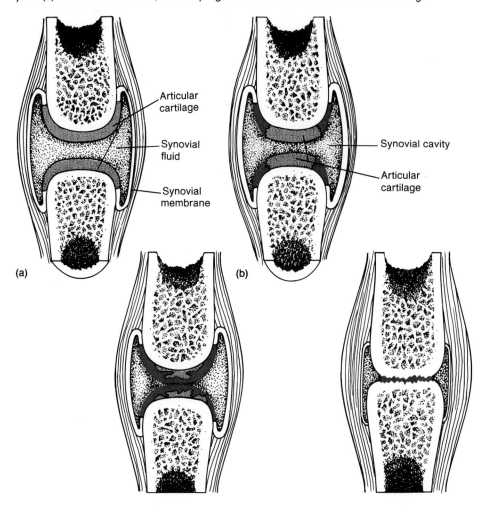

It usually affects the weight-bearing joints such as the knee and hip. The cartilage in the joint simply wears out, creating increased friction and pain. No cure for osteoarthritis exists and damage done cannot be undone, but the disease process may be controlled with medication and a rest-exercise rehabilitation program.

Positive Health Life-style

Exercise appears to be the one component of the Positive Health Life-style that may be helpful to the individual with arthritis. In most cases, exercises are prescribed by a physician and may be done either with the help of a physical therapist or by the individual alone. The major purpose of these exercises is to maintain or increase the current range-of-motion or flexibility of the joint. The exercises are specific to the joint that is affected. Moreover, recent research has revealed that rheumatoid arthritic patients may exercise aerobically on a stationary bicycle and increase their cardiovascular fitness, while decreasing their perceived pain level, with no increase in joint inflammation.

A question is often raised concerning the possibility that habitual exercise programs may contribute to the development of osteoarthritis, due to an increased rate of wear and tear. Athletes may develop arthritis specific to a joint that is particularly stressed in their sports. Baseball pitchers may have problems with their elbows; football players may have problems with their knees; and ballet dancers may have problems with their ankles. However, several recent studies have indicated that osteoarthritis is not an inevitable consequence of long-term training. A radiological (X ray) study of the upper and lower limbs of experienced weight lifters revealed significant degenerative changes in 20 percent of those investigated, but the percentage was no different from that found in the general population for that age group. This suggests that habitual weight training neither increases nor decreases the possibility of developing osteoarthritis. A study of Finnish runners also revealed that primary osteoarthritis of the hip joint was slightly less in the runners as compared to a control group. These investigators noted that the physical strain to which runners' hips are exposed does not contribute to the development of osteoarthritis. They suggested that rhythmical compression and release of the joint cavity by running motion stimulates the flow of synovial fluid and benefits the nutrition of the joint cartilage.

Based upon these studies, it would appear that normal, habitual exercise does not accelerate the development of osteoarthritis. However, joints that are excessively stressed and injured may be more prone to become arthritic. Whether the legion of individuals who are physically active now will be more likely to develop arthritis later in life remains to be seen, since we have very little data at this point. It seems, however, that the increased risk is minimal compared with the other benefits of habitual exercise.

Substance Abuse Problems

The evolutionary process has prepared the human body to assimilate most chemical components found in the natural environment. Our body is able to digest and metabolize the various nutrients found in the foods we eat—such as carbohydrate, fat, protein, vitamins, and minerals—that are all found in a complex chemical structure. The ability to extract and utilize nutrients from food is essential for human survival. Some chemical substances that may be toxic to humans, such as poisonous mushrooms, do occur in nature. However, the senses of taste and smell, along with acquired experience, have helped us to avoid them. Still other chemical substances that may create a specific physiological or psychological effect in humans, such as marijuana, coca leaves, and coffee beans, exist naturally.

As chemical technology developed over the past century, many of these naturally occurring chemical components could be processed or synthesized more rapidly, making them more readily available for public consumption. Combined with the changing social structure in an industrialized society, such as the United States, the availability of such drugs as amphetamines, cocaine, heroine, and other hard narcotics has lead to the serious health problem of **substance abuse.** The social and health problems associated with the use of illegal substances are beyond the scope of this text. However, two substances that are not illegal, but are abused by millions of Americans, are discussed briefly, as they may have a significant impact on health. These two substances are alcohol and cigarettes.

Alcohol-related Health Problems

The form of **alcohol** we consume is ethyl alcohol, also known as ethanol. Alcohol has existed from earliest times, and almost all societies include a traditional alcoholic beverage as part of their culture. In the United States, nearly 100 million people consume alcohol in one form or another, primarily for its mood-modifying effects. However, alcohol is a drug, a potent depressant that may exert harmful health effects on the human body if consumed in excessive amounts.

Alcohol, like other drugs, is metabolized by the liver. However, the rate at which the liver can process alcohol is limited—averaging about one drink per hour in the average-size individual. For the purpose of this discussion, one drink is equivalent to 12 ounces of beer, 4 ounces of wine, or 1½ ounces of regular bar whiskey. Alcohol consumed at a rate in excess of this amount accumulates in the blood and exerts depressant effects upon the brain. These effects vary depending upon a number of different factors, such as body size, amount of food in the stomach, and the individual's state of mind. In general, however, the following symptoms may be typical.

Number of Drinks Consumed in Two Hours	Typical Effects
2–3	Reduced tension; relief from daily stress
4–5	Coordination and fine motor ability impaired
6–8	Gross motor coordination impaired; staggering gait
9–12	Loss of control of voluntary motor ability; sleep
13 and above	Coma; depression of respiratory centers; death

Positive Health Life-style

Is alcohol consumption detrimental to your health? The answer appears to be dependent upon how much alcohol you consume. In moderation, alcohol consumption appears not to be detrimental to your health. Moderate drinking is interpreted as no more than two or three drinks per day. In some individuals, it may be beneficial, for a drink or two may serve as a relaxant and a stress reducer. Also, some studies have shown that moderate consumption of alcohol may raise HDL-cholesterol levels and, thus, provide a degree of protection against the development of atherosclerosis. On the other hand, even moderate drinking may be a health risk to some. According to a recent report from the National Academy of Sciences' Committee on Nutrition of the Mother and Preschool Child, even small amounts of alcohol intake by a pregnant woman, particularly in the first months of pregnancy, may be harmful to her unborn child. For those individuals who are dieting to lose weight, the additional Calories in alcohol make weight loss more difficult.

Major health problems are, however, associated with acute and chronic ingestion of excessive amounts of alcohol. As noted in the chart, the acute effects of excessive alcohol consumption include impairment of both motor coordination and judgment—two factors that are extremely important in the safe operation of an automobile. Drunk driving is the cause of nearly one-half of all automobile fatalities—more than 20,000 deaths per year in the United States alone. Alcohol is also a major cause of many household accidents, suicides, and homicides.

Over a period of years, chronic consumption of excessive amounts of alcohol may have detrimental effects on various body organs, particularly the liver. The liver begins to accumulate fatty deposits and, eventually, the liver cells degenerate and are replaced by nonfunctioning scar tissue, a condition known as *cirrhosis*. Alcoholism has also been associated with an increased incidence rate of heart disease, gastrointestinal disease, and cancer of the mouth and throat.

How does alcohol fit into a Positive Health Life-style? The following are some general recommendations:

Drink moderately or not at all.

Know your capacity and do not exceed it.

Eat some food, particularly some protein and fat, before or while you drink.

Drink slowly. Remember your body can metabolize only about one drink per hour.

Do not drink alcohol if you are taking other drugs that may also be depressants or cause drowsiness.

Do not drive after drinking and do not let your friends do so either.

Get professional help if you have a problem with alcohol.

Cigarette-related Health Problems

You see it almost every day—cigarette smoking can be dangerous to your health. Yet, millions of Americans smoke cigarettes, which is the most harmful of all habits that we voluntarily undertake. Literally thousands of studies have documented the fact that cigarette smoking is a leading cause of three major lung diseases. It can cause emphysema and chronic bronchitis (both of which may make breathing very difficult), and is the major cause of lung cancer, being responsible for nine out of every ten cases. As noted earlier in this chapter, it is also one of the three main risk factors for coronary heart disease. Due to these effects upon both the heart and lungs, the American Lung Association has noted that cigarette smoking is responsible for the premature deaths of 340,000 Americans each year. Women under age fifty have some degree of protection against CHD, but a recent report in the *Journal of the American Medical Association* indicates that women below the age of fifty who smoke thirty-five or more cigarettes a day have a ten times greater risk of having a heart attack than those who do not smoke. Moreover, a woman who smokes while pregnant may retard the growth of her unborn child, and make it more susceptible to respiratory diseases.

Smoking also impairs aerobic endurance capacity. Particles in the smoke constrict bronchial pathways to the lungs. This increases the air resistance and, thus, increases the muscular effort needed to ventilate the lungs. In addition, carbon monoxide from the smoke combines more readily with hemoglobin, and interferes with oxygen transport by the blood.

Positive Health Life-style

Needless to say, cigarette smoking is incompatible with a Positive Health Life-style. If you do not currently smoke, resolve never to start. If you are a smoker and want to improve your health, you must *want to quit* and you must *decide to quit*. There are a number of different techniques to use, but there is no one best way. You must determine what will work for you. The following are some suggestions:

Quit cold turkey. Use your willpower to avoid a substance harmful to your health.

Set a date to quit and gradually reduce the number of cigarettes you smoke per day.

Make a pact with a friend to quit together.

Join a quit-smoking program.

Use one of the commercial stop-smoking products on the market.

It may take several attempts to quit smoking, but do not quit trying. Your health depends on it.

Laboratory Inventory 2.1 will help you determine whether or not you really want to quit smoking.

Laboratory Inventory 2.1
Do You Really Want to Quit Smoking?

Answer each question, circling the number that most accurately indicates how you feel.

	Completely Agree	Somewhat Agree	Somewhat Disagree	Completely Disagree
A. Cigarette smoking might give me a serious illness.	4	3	2	1
B. My cigarette smoking sets a bad example for others.	4	3	2	1
C. I find cigarette smoking to be a messy kind of habit.	4	3	2	1
D. Controlling my cigarette smoking is a challenge to me.	4	3	2	1
E. Smoking causes shortness of breath.	4	3	2	1
F. If I quit smoking cigarettes, it might influence others to stop.	4	3	2	1
G. Cigarettes cause damage to clothing and other personal property.	4	3	2	1
H. Quitting smoking would show that I have willpower.	4	3	2	1
I. My cigarette smoking will have a harmful effect on my health.	4	3	2	1
J. My cigarette smoking influences others close to me to take up or continue smoking.	4	3	2	1
K. If I quit smoking, my sense of taste or smell would improve.	4	3	2	1
L. I do not like the idea of feeling dependent on smoking.	4	3	2	1

Source: U.S. Department of Health, Education and Welfare. *The Smoker's Self-Test.* Public Service Publication No. 2013. Washington, DC: U.S. Government Printing Office, 1969.

Enter the numbers you have circled to each test question in the appropriate space below, entering the number you circled to answer question A over line A, to question B over line B, and so on.

$$\frac{}{A} + \frac{}{E} + \frac{}{I} = \frac{}{\text{Health}}$$

$$\frac{}{B} + \frac{}{F} + \frac{}{J} = \frac{}{\text{Example}}$$

$$\frac{}{C} + \frac{}{G} + \frac{}{K} = \frac{}{\text{Esthetics}}$$

$$\frac{}{D} + \frac{}{H} + \frac{}{L} = \frac{}{\text{Mastery}}$$

Total the three scores across on each line to get your totals. For example, the sum of your scores over line A, E, and I gives your score on Health; lines B, F, and J give your score on Example, and so on.

Scores can vary from three to twelve. Any score nine and above is high; any score six and below is low. A *high* score on any of the following indicates that you are motivated by that factor to help you quit smoking.

Health—You believe smoking is potentially hazardous to your health.

Example—You believe you are an example to others and may influence their smoking behavior. By not smoking, your younger brother or sister may follow your example.

Esthetics—You believe that smoking is a bad habit that may be esthetically damaging. It smells and creates a mess.

Mastery—You want to be able to control your behavior and not be dependent upon smoking.

References

Aggrawal, N.; Kaur, R.; Kumar, S.; and Mathur, D. "A Study of Changes in the Spine in Weight Lifters and Other Athletes." *British Journal of Sports Medicine* 13:58–61 (1979).

Aloia, J. "Exercise and Skeletal Health." *Journal of the American Geriatric Society* 29:104–107 (1981).

American College of Sports Medicine. *Guidelines for Graded Exercise Testing and Exercise Prescription*. Philadelphia: Lea and Febiger, 1980.

American Heart Association. *About Your Heart and Bloodstream*. New York: AHA, 1962.

———. *Heart Disease in Children*. New York: AHA, 1961.

———. *Heart Facts—1983*. Dallas, TX: AHA, 1983.

———. *How to Stop Smoking*. Dallas, TX: AHA, 1982.

American Lung Association. *Cigarette Smoking*. ALA, 1982.

Arthritis Foundation. *Arthritis. The Basic Facts*. Atlanta: The Arthritis Foundation, 1981.

Berger, M., and Berchtold, P. "The Role of Physical Exercise and Training in the Management of Diabetes Mellitus." *Bibliotheca Nutritio et Dieta* 27:41–54 (1979).

Black, H. "Nonpharmacologic Therapy for Hypertension." *American Journal of Medicine* 66:837–42 (1979).

Blush, K. "From the Clinic: Back School." *American Corrective Therapy Journal* 33:23–25 (1979).

Bonnano, J. "Coronary Risk Factor Modification by Chronic Physical Exercise." In *Exercise in Cardiovascular Health and Disease,* edited by E. Amsterdam, et al. New York: Yorke Medical Books, 1977.

Bruce, R. "Primary Intervention against Coronary Atherosclerosis by Exercise Conditioning." *New England Journal of Medicine* 305:1525–26 (1981).

Camaione, D. N., and Sinatra, S. "Beneficial Effects of Exercise and Current Concepts in Adult Fitness." *Connecticut Medicine* 45:620–25 (1981).

Campaigne, B.; Gilliam, T.; Spencer, M.; and Lampman, M. "The Effects of a Physical Activity Program on Children with Insulin Dependent Diabetes." *Medicine and Science in Sports and Exercise* 15:149 (1983).

Clark, M., and Gosnell, M. "Battling Diabetes." *Newsweek* 94:117–24 (December 1979).

Clarke, H. H. "Health Practices, Physical Health Status, Diet and Exercise in Relation to Peripheral Vascular Disease." *Physical Fitness Research Digest* 6(2):11–17 (April 1976).

Coates, T.; Jeffery, R.; and Slinkard, L. "Heart Healthy Eating and Exercise: Introducing and Maintaining Changes in Health Behaviors." *American Journal of Public Health* 71:15–23 (1981).

Corrigan, B., and Kannangra, S. "Rheumatic Disease: Exercise or Immobilization." *Australian Family Physician* 7:1007–14 (1978).

Craig, J. "Clinical Implications of the New Diabetic Classification." *Postgraduate Medicine* 68:122–33 (October 1980).

Dressendorfer, R.; Amsterdam, E.; and Odland, T. "Adolescent Smoking and Its Effect on Aerobic Exercise Tolerance." *The Physician and Sportsmedicine* 11:109–19 (May 1983).

Dufaux, B.; Assmann, G.; and Hollmann, W. "Plasma Lipoproteins and Physical Activity: A Review." *International Journal of Sports Medicine* 3:123–36 (1982).

Felig, P. "Exercise." *Current Concepts in Nutrition* 10:165–72 (1981).

Fitzgerald, B., and McLatchie, G. "Degenerative Joint Disease in Weightlifters. Fact or Fiction." *British Journal of Sports Medicine* 14:97–101 (1980).

Fletcher, G. F. "Exercise and Coronary Risk Factor Modification in the Management of Atherosclerosis." *Heart and Lung* 10:811–13 (1981).

Froelicher, V. F. "Does Exercise Protect from Coronary Heart Disease?" *Advances in Cardiology* 27:237–42 (1980).

———. "Exercise and Health." *American Journal of Medicine* 70:987–88 (1981).

Goldberg, H.; Kohn, H.; Dehn, T.; and Seeds, R. "Diagnosis and Management of Low Back Pain." *Occupational and Health Safety* 49:14–31 (June 1980).

Grieve, D. "The Dynamics of Lifting." *Exercise and Sport Science Review* 5:157–79 (1977).

Guyton, A. *Textbook of Medical Physiology.* Philadelphia: W. B. Saunders, 1981.

Hartung, G. "Physical Activity and Coronary Heart Disease—A Review." *American Corrective Therapy Journal* 31:110–15 (1977).

Hartung, G.; Farge, E.; and Mitchell, R. "Effects of Marathon Running, Jogging, and Diet on Coronary Risk Factors in Middle Aged Men." *Preventive Medicine* 10:316–23 (1981).

Hartung, G.; Foreyt, J.; Mitchell, R.; et al. "Effect of Alcohol Intake on High-Density Lipoprotein Cholesterol Levels in Runners and Inactive Men." *Journal of the American Medical Association* 249:747–50 (1983).

Horton, E. "The Role of Exercise in the Treatment of Hypertension in Obesity." *International Journal of Obesity* 5 (Suppl. 1):165–71 (1981).

James, D. "What about Blood Pressure?" Burlington, N.C.: Carolina Biological Supply Co., 1981.

Kannel, W., and Sorlie, P. "Some Health Benefits of Physical Activity. The Framingham Study." *Archives of Internal Medicine* 139:857–61 (1979).

Kaplan, N. "Non-Drug Treatment of Hypertension." *Australian and New Zealand Journal of Medicine* 11 (Suppl): 73–75 (1981).

Kent, S. "Does Exercise Prevent Heart Attacks?" *Geriatrics* 33:95–104 (1978).

Korcok, M. "Add Exercise to Calcium in Osteoporosis Prevention." *Journal of American Medical Association* 247:1106 (1982).

———. "Pritikin vs AHA Diet: No Difference for Peripheral Vascular Disease." *Journal of the American Medical Association* 246:1871 (1981).

Kramsch, D.; Aspen, A.; Abramowitz, B.; Kreimendahl, T.; and Hood, W. "Reduction of Coronary Atherosclerosis by Moderate Conditioning in Monkeys on an Atherogenic Diet." *New England Journal of Medicine* 305:1483–89 (1981).

Kraus, H.; Melleby, A.; and Gaston, S. "Back Pain Correction and Prevention." *New York State Journal of Medicine* 77:1335–38 (1977).

Kroner, R. "Beware of Exercises That Do More Harm Than Good." *Occupational and Health Safety* 49:32–35 (June 1980).

Krzentowski, G.; Pirnay, F.; Pallikarakis, N.; Luyckx, A.; Lacroix, M.; and Lefebvre, P. "Glucose Utilization during Exercise in Normal and Diabetic Subjects. The Role of Insulin." *Diabetes* 30:983–89 (1981).

LeBlanc, J.; Nadeau, A.; Richard, D.; and Tremblay, A. "Studies on the Sparing Effect of Exercise on Insulin Requirements in Human Subjects." *Metabolism* 30:1119–24 (1981).

Lee, G.; Amsterdam, E.; DeMaria, A.; Davis, G.; Lafave, T.; and Mason, D. "Effect of Exercise on Hemostatic Mechanisms." In *Exercise in Cardiovascular Health and Disease,* edited by E. Amsterdam, J. Wilmore, A. DeMaria. New York: Yorke Medical Books, 1977.

Lohmann, D.; Liebold, F.; Heilmann, W.; Senger, H.; and Pohl, A. "Diminished Insulin Response in Highly Trained Athletes." *Metabolism* 27:521–24 (1978).

Milvy, P.; Forbes, W. F.; and Brown, K. "A Critical Review of Epidemiological Studies of Physical Activity." In *The Marathon: Physiological, Medical, Epidemiological and Psychological Studies,* edited by Paul Milvy. *Annals of the New York Academy of Sciences* 301:519–49 (1977).

Morris, J.; Pollard, R.; Everitt, M.; and Chave, S. "Vigorous Exercise in Leisure-time. Protection Against Coronary Heart Disease." *Lancet* 6:2(8206):1207–10 (1980).

Nordemar, R. "Physical Training in Rheumatoid Arthritis: A Controlled Long-Term Study." *Scandinavian Journal of Rheumatology* 10:25–30 (1981).

Nordemar, R.; Ekblom, B.; Zachrisson, L.; and Lundovist, K. "Physical Training in Rheumatoid Arthritis: A Controlled Long-Term Study." *Scandinavian Journal of Rheumatology* 10:17–23 (1981).

North, T.; Brammel, H.; Dickinson, A.; and Tran, Z. "Cardiorespiratory Exercise With Rheumatoid Arthritis Patients." *Medicine and Science in Sports and Exercise* 15:125 (1983).

Oscai, L. "Exercise and Lipid Metabolism." *Progress in Clinical and Biological Research* 67:383–90 (1981).

Parfrey, P.; Wright, P.; and Ledingham, J. "Prolonged Isometric Exercise. Part I: Effect on Circulation and on Renal Excretion of Sodium and Potassium in Mild Essential Hypertension." *Hypertension* 3:182–87 (1981).

Puranen, J.; Ala-Ketola, L.; Peltokallio, P.; and Saarela, J. "Running and Primary Osteoarthritis of the Hip." *British Medical Journal* 2(5968):424–25 (1975).

Richter, E.; Ruderman, N.; and Schneider, S. "Diabetes and Exercise." *American Journal of Medicine* 70:201–9 (1981).

Russell, C. "Doctors Warn of Pregnancy Hazards, From Foods to Nonfoods." *Washington Post* (4 November 1982).

Schwaid, M. "Advice to Arthritics; Keep Moving." *American Journal of Nursing* 78:1708–9 (1978).

Shephard, R., and Sidney, K. "Exercise and Aging." *Exercise and Sport Science Review* 6:1–57 (1978).

Sherwin, R., and Koivisto, V. "Keeping in Step: Does Exercise Benefit the Diabetic?" *Diabetologia* 20:84–86 (1981).

Siconolfi, S.; Carlton, R.; and Elder, J. "Acute Effects of Exercise and Relaxation on Blood Pressure." *Medicine and Science in Sports and Exercise* 14:181 (1982).

Skyler, J. "Diabetes and Exercise: Clinical Implications." *Diabetes Care* 2:307–11 (1979).

Smith, E.; Reddan, W.; and Smith, P. "Physical Activity and Calcium Modalities for Bone Mineral Increase in Aged Women." *Medicine and Science in Sports and Exercise* 13:60–64 (1981).

Stanitski, C. "Low Back Pain in Young Athletes." *The Physician and Sportsmedicine* 10:77–91 (October 1982).

Tran, Z., and Weltman, A. "Differential Effects of Exercise on Blood Lipids and Lipoproteins Seen with Changes in Body Weight. A Meta-Analysis." *Medicine and Science in Sports and Exercise* 15:90 (1983).

Tran, Z.; Weltman, A.; Glass, G.; and Mood, D. "The Effects of Exercise on Blood Lipids and Lipoproteins: A Meta-Analysis of Studies." *Medicine and Science in Sports and Exercise* 14:110 (1982).

U.S. Department of Health, Education and Welfare. Public Health Service. National Institute of Health. NIH publication No. 80–1822, 1980.

———. *The Smoker's Self Test.* Public Service Publication No. 2013. Washington, DC: U.S. Government Printing Office, 1969.

Vranic, M.; Horvath, S.; and Wahren, J., eds. "Proceedings of a Conference on Diabetes and Exercise." *Diabetes* 28 (Suppl 1):1–113 (1979).

Weltman, A., and Stamford, B. "Evaluating Your Risk for Heart Disease." *The Physician and Sportsmedicine* 10:202 (August 1982).

——— . "Exercise and the Cigarette Smoker." *The Physician and Sportsmedicine* 10:153 (December 1982).

——— . "Secondary Risk Factors for Heart Disease." *The Physician and Sportsmedicine* 10:191 (September 1982).

Williams, P.; Wood, P.; Haskell, W.; and Vranizan, K. "The Effects of Running Mileage and Duration on Plasma Lipoprotein Levels." *Journal of the American Medical Association* 247:2674–79 (1982).

Woo, S.; Kuei, S.; Amiel, D.; Gomez, M.; Hayes, W.; White, F.; and Akeson, W. "The Effect of Prolonged Physical Training on the Properties of Long Bone: A Study of Wolff's Law." *Journal of Bone and Joint Surgery* 63A:780–87 (1981).

Wood, P., and Haskell, W. "The Effect of Exercise on Plasma High Density Lipoproteins." *Lipids* 14:417–27 (1979).

Wood, P.; Haskell, W.; Stern, P.; et al. "Plasma Lipoprotein Distribution in Male and Female Runners." *Annals of the New York Academy of Sciences* 301:758 (1977).

Wood, P.; Haskell, W.; Terry, R.; Ho, P.; and Blair, S. "Effects of a Two-Year Running Program on Plasma Lipoproteins, Body Fat and Dietary Intake in Initially Sedentary Men." *Medicine and Science in Sports and Exercise* 14:104 (1982).

General Guidelines for Exercise Prescription

3

Key Terms

ATP-PC system
Calorie
energy
fatigue
lactic acid system

maximal oxygen uptake ($\dot{V}O_2$ max)
overload principle
oxygen system
principle of specificity

Key Concepts

With the proper knowledge of the principles underlying physical fitness, you should be able to design and implement your own personalized physical fitness program.

The most important physical fitness components related to personal health include cardiovascular-respiratory fitness, body composition, abdominal strength, and low back-hamstring musculoskeletal function.

The human body has three basic systems to produce energy for exercise: the ATP-PC system, the lactic acid system, and the oxygen system.

Two commonly used methods of expressing energy expenditure are by measuring Calories and oxygen consumption.

The two major principles of physical conditioning are the principles of specificity and overload.

The principle of specificity deals with the mode of exercise to be used. The body adapts to the energy system and neuromuscular patterns involved in a specific exercise mode.

The major components of the overload principle that are utilized in the design of any physical fitness program are intensity, duration, frequency, and progression of exercise.

In a Positive Health Life-style, exercise is a lifelong principle.

Introduction

The past ten years have witnessed a phenomenal physical fitness boom in the United States. Millions of Americans have taken to jogging, bicycling, swimming, and other forms of exercise in attempts to improve their appearance and physical condition. A number of factors have been involved in this increased emphasis on physical fitness, but probably one of the most influential was the 1968 publication of *Aerobics* by Dr. Kenneth Cooper. Based upon his research with thousands of subjects, Cooper developed a simple exercise test to evaluate an individual's level of cardiovascular physical fitness and described an aerobic exercise program to improve it where necessary. For a couple of dollars and a few hours of reading, the average person was presented with the necessary guidelines for developing a personalized exercise program for cardiovascular fitness.

At that time, aside from the YMCA and YWCA, there were only a few companies that operated fitness or health spas on a national level. Most were operated on a local or a regional level. However, since the fitness boom, hundreds of new companies have developed, both nationally and locally, in attempts to capitalize financially on America's increased interest in physical fitness. Today, we have centers specializing in aerobics to music, such as aerobic dancing or jazzercize, which advertise improved aerobic fitness through fun-type exercise; we have weight training programs with highly sophisticated and expensive equipment, which are advertised to develop strength and cardiovascular endurance; and we have numerous weight reduction spas, or salons, which advertise quick and easy weight loss.

From reputable firms of these types, the customer can expect to receive the advertised benefits. For example, one national company specializing in aerobic dancing has a certification program for its instructors, and several of the national weight loss centers monitor weight loss under medical supervision. Moreover, many individuals need the social atmosphere and/or facilities and equipment of an exercise spa or dance class to motivate them to exercise or lose weight. On the other hand, many of these operations are supervised by individuals who have very little background in proper exercise programs. At the present time there is no certification requirement for individuals employed in most commercial fitness organizations in the United States, although the Association of Fitness in Business (AFB) has developed certification requirements for its members, and the American College of Sports Medicine (ACSM) is working on a certification procedure for other commercial centers. At the present time, an unsuspecting customer at some of these establishments may receive improper advice relative to exercise and weight control. Additionally, this advice may be rather expensive, ranging to hundreds of dollars per year.

In general, you do not need to join a health spa or similar operation in order to initiate your own health-related physical fitness program. With appropriate knowledge, you can develop your own program.

Personal Fitness Goals

The design of any physical fitness program is based upon the ultimate purpose or goals that have been established by or for any given individual. In some cases, goals are established for individuals. A physician may design an exercise program for a post-cardiac patient who is entering a rehabilitation program, with the ultimate goal of regaining normal cardiovascular efficiency. Similarly, a coach may design a strenuous training program for a high school athlete with the potential to run a 4 minute mile. Although we may recognize the differences in the health status of the individuals in these two cases, similar principles are used in the design of the two vastly different training programs. Our concern in this book is not with rehabilitative exercise for patients, nor with training of athletes for high levels of competition, but rather for the normal, healthy individual who desires to improve his or her physical fitness levels.

Personal Fitness Needs

Before you are able to design a comprehensive personal physical fitness program for yourself, you should know what your current physical fitness status is. Physical fitness represents a complex assortment of components that may be grouped as either motor skill-related or health related. Motor skill-related components include such factors as strength, power, speed, agility, reaction time, and balance. Although important to physical performance, they are more related to athletics than they are to the health of the average individual. On the other hand, cardiovascular-respiratory function, body composition, and abdominal and low back-hamstring musculoskeletal function and flexibility are important health-related components. Since the thrust of this book is toward health-related physical fitness, personal fitness needs will only be addressed in relation to health-related physical fitness components. Thus, you will need to know your current status in the following areas:

1. Cardiovascular-respiratory function
2. Body composition
3. Abdominal and low back-hamstring musculoskeletal function: flexibility and abdominal strength

How do you determine what your physical fitness needs are in each of these areas? You will be presented with some guidelines and assessment experiments in chapter 4 for cardiovascular-respiratory function, in chapter 6 for body composition, and in chapter 8 for abdominal and low back-hamstring musculoskeletal function.

Personal Fitness Objectives

A popular advertising slogan urges you to "be all that you can be." Once you have determined your current physical fitness status, how do you know "all that you can be?" What are your physical limitations and how may these guide you in determining personal fitness objectives?

Figure 3.1 Health-related Fitness Components. The most important physical fitness components related to personal health include cardiovascular-respiratory fitness, body composition, and training of abdominal strength and low back-hamstring muscle flexibility to prevent low back problems.

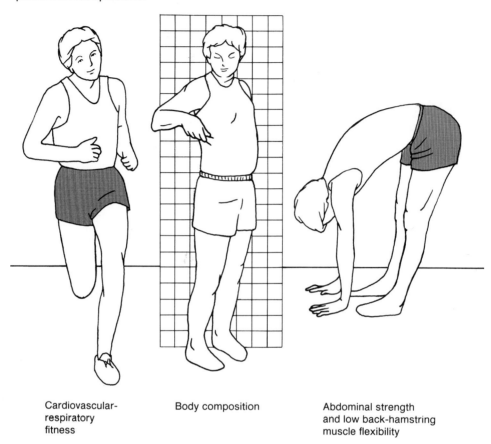

Cardiovascular-respiratory fitness

Body composition

Abdominal strength and low back-hamstring muscle flexibility

Genetics, the traits and characteristics we inherit from our parents, endow some of us with the physical ability to be very strong or very fast, while others may have inherited the capability for endurance activities. Somatotype, or body build, is also inherited. Some individuals are predisposed toward a muscular body, while others may have a tendency toward leanness or heaviness. The upper limits of such factors as maximal oxygen uptake and muscle fiber type, which are important determinants of endurance capacity, are estimated to be over 90 percent determined by your genetic endowment.

What do these genetic limitations mean to you? Let us explore the role of genetic endowment relative to maximal oxygen uptake, which, as mentioned above, is a very important determinant of endurance capacity. **Maximal oxygen uptake, or $\dot{V}O_2$ max,** represents the maximal ability of the body to use oxygen for the production of energy.

Individuals such as Steve Jones and Joan Benoit, male and female world record holders for the marathon, inherited a high maximal oxygen uptake capacity and, hence, the potential for world class performance. However, they would not have become world record holders if they had not undergone an intensive program of physical training to not only develop their maximal oxygen uptake to its greatest capacity, but also to exercise at a high percentage of their maximum without inducing early fatigue. The rest of us, even if we trained as intensively as Steve and Joan, would not be able to reach their performance levels because we do not have their genetic potential. However, with a proper training program, almost everybody could complete a 26.2 mile marathon. A proper training program increases your maximal oxygen uptake toward its genetic potential, and increases your ability to perform at a higher percentage of that maximum without fatigue. Thus, although genetics may set the upper limits, an optimal performance within your own genetic limitations can still be attained with proper training.

One of the distinguishing characteristics of the health-related physical fitness components is that they can be improved through a proper training program. Later on in this text you perform several tests that provide an evaluation of your fitness level in each of the health-related physical fitness components. For each of these areas, you are provided with norms and/or other data to determine your current fitness status. Based upon this information, you are able to establish specific objectives, if you so desire. You may establish short-term and long-term objectives, but it is important in the initial stages of a training program to establish personal fitness objectives that are attainable. For example, you may set a short-term goal to lose 5 pounds in a month, or run a mile nonstop, while long-term goals may be to lose 40 pounds and complete a 10 kilometer race. Guidelines are presented for each major health-related physical fitness component.

A properly designed aerobic exercise program may make a significant impact on your health: it may help reduce several risk factors associated with coronary heart disease (CHD) and other chronic diseases, it may be an effective means to control body weight, and it may also serve as a stress-reduction method. These are the major health-related reasons why millions of Americans have joined the fitness revolution and have initiated their own personal aerobic exercise programs. Although improvement of your personal health or appearance may be the primary motivation for initiating a fitness program, it appears that the motivational stimulus may change as the fitness revolution goes through several evolutionary stages. Hal Higdon, an accomplished runner and a popular writer on the running scene, described three levels of consciousness through which many runners progress after initiating their personal fitness program (see table 3.1). Although accomplishment and success may replace health and appearance as the primary motivational factors for exercising, the health-related benefits will be the same, and possibly of a greater magnitude.

The ultimate goal is to feel good about yourself, both physically and emotionally. Exercise can be an effective means to achieve this goal, but other factors such as sound nutrition and relaxation techniques also play important roles, and will be included as major components of a Positive Health Life-style.

Table 3.1
Motivation for Running at Different Levels of Consciousness

	Consciousness I	Consciousness II	Consciousness III
Activity	Jogging	Running	Racing
Weekly Mileage	5–15	30–50	50 and up
Type of Training	Jog/walk	Long slow distance	Hard day/easy day
Short-Term Goal	Aerobic points	Finish a marathon	Qualify for Boston Marathon
Long-Term Goal	Avoid heart disease	Improve best times	Age-group awards
Primary Motivation	Health and appearance	Accomplishment	Success

Source: From Hal Higdon, in *The Runner,* 4:52–53. Copyright by Hal Higdon. Reprinted by permission of the author.

Human Energy

Before discussing the principles of training, it is important to provide an overview of the human energy processes, for they serve as the basis for all training programs. A knowledge of energy storage and production in the human body is also an essential background for the chapters on weight control.

Energy Forms in the Body

Energy is the capacity to do work and, although energy may exist in six different forms, our concern is primarily with chemical energy, mechanical energy, and thermal energy. One of the major characteristics of energy is that one form may be transformed into another. For example, the chemical energy that is stored in a gallon of gas can be converted into thermal energy in an automobile engine, and then into mechanical energy to drive the pistons and move the car.

The sun is the ultimate source of energy. Solar energy is harnessed by plants, through photosynthesis, to produce either plant carbohydrates, fats, or proteins, which are all forms of stored chemical energy. When humans consume plant and animal products, the carbohydrates, fats, and proteins undergo a series of metabolic changes, and are utilized to develop body structure, regulate body processes, or provide a storage form of chemical energy. Chemical energy may be stored in a variety of forms in the human body. Carbohydrate may be found in the blood as glucose, a simple sugar. Carbohydrate may also be stored in the muscle or liver as glycogen, a combination of glucose molecules. Fat may be stored as triglycerides, primarily in the blood, muscle tissue, and adipose tissue. Although protein is not usually a major source of human energy, it may be under certain conditions such as starvation. Most of the soft tissue of the body, such as the muscles, consists of protein. Although chemical energy may be stored as carbohydrate, fat, or protein, the body cannot use them as an immediate source of energy for such functions as muscle contraction. They must be converted into **ATP** (adenosine triphosphate) another form of chemical energy in the human body. ATP is a high-energy compound, which is the immediate source of energy in humans.

Figure 3.2 The solar energy from the sun is utilized by plants through the process of photosynthesis, converting it to chemical energy in the form of carbohydrates, fats, or proteins. Animals eat plants, and convert the chemical energy into their own stores of chemical energy—primarily fat and protein. Humans ingest food from both plant and animal sources, and convert the chemical energy for their own stores and use.

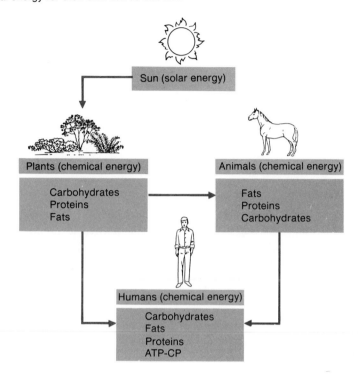

Another compound, PC (creatine phosphate), also formed in the body, serves to replace ATP very rapidly as it is used up.

In order to do mechanical work (exercise), ATP must be utilized. The faster you work, the more ATP is needed. However, since the ATP available in the muscle is only sufficient for about one second of maximal work, it must be restored rapidly if work is to continue. The faster or harder you work, the more rapidly the ATP must be replenished.

Exercise is classified as being aerobic or anaerobic. Aerobic refers to ATP production by utilizing oxygen in the body. Carbohydrates and fats combine with oxygen in a series of complex metabolic reactions to produce ATP. Anaerobic ATP production occurs in the absence of oxygen, by one of two processes. ATP, itself, may provide energy anaerobically, and be resynthesized by the utilization of PC. Or, ATP may be formed anaerobically when carbohydrate (muscle glycogen), in the absence of adequate oxygen, breaks down into lactic acid. Note that carbohydrate may be a source of ATP production under both aerobic and anaerobic conditions.

Table 3.2
Characteristics of Human Energy Systems

Characteristic	ATP-PC	Lactic Acid	Oxygen
Aerobic/anaerobic	Anaerobic	Anaerobic	Aerobic
Rate of ATP production	Fast	Fast	Slow
Time limits for maximal exercise	4–5 seconds	1–2 minutes	Hours
Capacity for ATP production	Low	Low	High
Lactic acid production	No	Yes	No
Fatigability	High	High	Low
Energy source	ATP-PC	Carbohydrate	Carbohydrate, fat
Track event	100 yards	½ mile	2 miles
Expected time for elite athlete	(0:09)	(1:45)	(8:25)

Human Energy Systems

Why does the human body store chemical energy in a variety of different forms? If we look at human energy needs that developed through the evolutionary process, the answer becomes rather obvious. Sometimes humans needed to produce energy at a rapid rate, such as when sprinting to safety in order to avoid dangerous animals. Thus, a fast rate of energy production was an important human energy feature that helped to insure survival. At other times, our ancient ancestors may have been deprived of adequate food for long periods of time, and, thus, needed a storage capacity for chemical energy that would sustain life throughout these periods of deprivation. Hence, the ability to store large amounts of energy was also important for survival. These two factors—rate of energy production and energy capacity—appear to be determining factors in the development of human energy systems.

There are three major classifications of energy systems in the human body. The major characteristics of these systems are presented in table 3.2. All three systems are designed to replenish ATP. Although all systems appear to operate under a wide variety of exercise intensities, one system usually predominates. In sprinting activities, lasting less than 10 seconds, the **ATP-PC system** predominates. In maximal exercise of about 1 to 2 minutes duration, such as running a fast ¼ mile or ½ mile, the **lactic acid system** predominates. In low levels of activity, such as at rest and during long slow-distance running, the **oxygen system** predominates. Thus, the ATP-PC and lactic acid system can produce ATP rapidly, while the oxygen system produces ATP at a slower rate but can sustain production for a longer time. It is important to keep in mind that, in most exercises, all the energy systems are used to one degree or another. The lactic acid system may predominate in a fast ¼ mile, but it is not the exclusive energy system, as the oxygen system also contributes some portion of the energy demand.

An important distinction between the oxygen (aerobic) energy system and the anaerobic energy systems is the rate of fatigue. **Fatigue** is a complex phenomenon that may have a variety of causes. For our purposes here, it is important to note that the

Figure 3.3 The Three Human Energy Systems. ATP is the immediate source of energy for most processes in the human body, and needs to be replenished.

The ATP-PC Energy System. ATP and PC are high-energy phosphates, stored in the muscle, that can provide energy very rapidly. ATP (adenosinetriphosphate) is stored in the muscle in limited amounts, and can be used for many body processes including muscular contraction. The ATP stores are used for fast, all-out bursts of power that last about one second. ATP must be replenished from other sources in order for muscle contraction to continue. PC (phosphocreatine) is stored in the muscle in limited amounts, and can be used to rapidly synthesize ATP. ATP and PC are called *phosphagens* and together represent the ATP-PC energy system. This system is utilized for quick, maximal exercises, such as sprinting, lasting about one to six seconds.

The Lactic Acid Energy System. Muscle glycogen can be broken down without the utilization of oxygen. This process is called *anaerobic glycolysis.* ATP is produced rapidly, but lactic acid is the end product. Lactic acid can be a major cause of fatigue in the muscle. The lactic acid system is utilized during exercise bouts of very high intensity, which are conducted at maximal rates for about one to two minutes.

The Oxygen System. The muscle stores of carbohydrates and fats, through complex changes, can enter the Krebs cycle. Glucose and free fatty acids may enter the cell from the bloodstream. When they eventually combine with oxygen, large amounts of ATP may be produced. The oxygen system is utilized during endurance exercises lasting longer than four or five minutes.

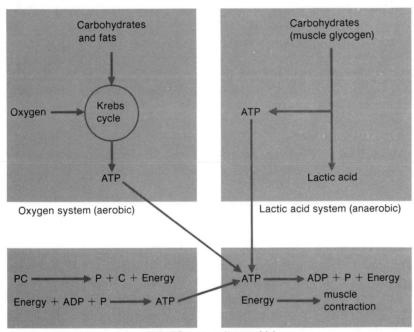

anaerobic processes involving the lactic acid system result in fatigue within a relatively short period of time, largely due to the accumulation of lactic acid in the muscle cell, which may disrupt normal functioning. On the other hand, aerobic exercise does not lead to lactic acid accumulation, and may be continued for longer periods of time, although fatigue may also occur due to other factors, such as fuel depletion or dehydration.

Energy Equivalents

The oxygen system is utilized as the main energy source during rest and at low levels of exercise. It may also be the major energy source for high levels of sustained activity. For the time being, however, we are concerned about the relationship of oxygen to energy expenditure.

Through a series of complex metabolic processes in the body, oxygen is eventually utilized in order to release the chemical energy in the body stores of carbohydrate and fat. During rest, most of this chemical energy is utilized to provide the energy for our basic metabolic functions. In the process heat is liberated (thermal energy), which helps to keep our body temperature at about 98.6°F. When we exercise, about 25 percent of the energy we produce by the oxidation of carbohydrate and fat is converted into mechanical energy (muscle contraction to actually move the body). However, about 75 percent of the energy produced during exercise is still released as heat, or thermal energy.

In the human body then, chemical energy can be converted to either thermal or mechanical energy. Since oxygen is the key to the energy release, the amount of oxygen used can be equated to measures of chemical, thermal, and mechanical energy. There are numerous units of measurement used to express energy in the different forms in which it exists. An international system of units has been developed in order to standardize measurements. However, in the United States, the Calorie still appears to be the most popular means of expressing energy, both for exercise and food. For practical purposes, we shall use it as the basic unit of measurement for human energy. The Calorie is especially relevant when exercise is used as a means to control body weight.

A calorie, or gram calorie, is the amount of heat necessary to raise the temperature of 1 gram of water one degree Celsius. A kilocalorie, or **Calorie,** is 1000 gram calories. We shall refer only to the Calorie in this text. Oxygen, in itself, does not contain any Calories, but carbohydrate and fat do. Oxygen releases the Calories from the carbohydrate and fat. For a given amount of oxygen, carbohydrate provides a slightly greater amount of Calories than fat. For example, 1 liter (1000 milliliters) of oxygen will release 5.05 Calories from carbohydrate and 4.70 from fat. However, for simplicity sake, without losing a great deal of accuracy, we can state that 1 liter of oxygen equals approximately 5.0 Calories. The average person consumes about .25 of a liter (250 milliliters) of oxygen per minute at rest, and about 3–3.5 liters per minute during maximal exercise. Highly trained athletes may consume as much as 6.0 liters per minute during exercise. Thus, the caloric expenditure may vary from 1.25 per minute during rest (.25l × 5 = 1.25 Calories) to 15–17.5 per minute during maximal exercise (3l × 5 = 15 Calories) in the average individual.

The **MET** is another related energy concept. One MET represents energy consumption during rest. By technical definition, 1 MET equals 3.5 milliliters (ml) of oxygen consumption per kilogram of body weight per minute (the resting metabolic rate).

Increasing oxygen consumption results in an increased caloric expenditure, which can have considerable value in a weight control program. In order for the oxygen to be utilized, it must be transported from the atmospheric air to the muscle tissues. This

Figure 3.4 Energy Equivalents in Oxygen Consumption and Calories. This figure depicts two means of expressing energy expenditure during four levels of activity. These values are for an average male of 154 pounds (70 kg). If you weigh more or less, the values increase or decrease accordingly.

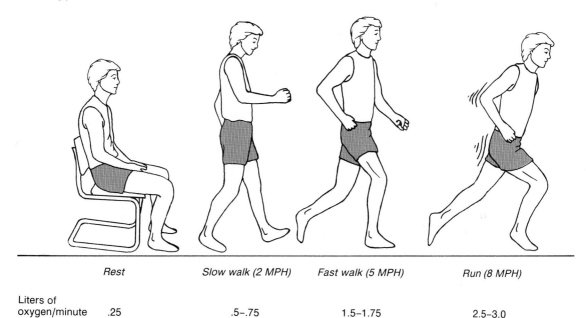

	Rest	Slow walk (2 MPH)	Fast walk (5 MPH)	Run (8 MPH)
Liters of oxygen/minute	.25	.5–.75	1.5–1.75	2.5–3.0
Calories/minute	1.25	2.5–3.75	7.5–8.75	12.5–15.0

1 liter oxygen/minute = 5 Calories/minute

is the major function of the cardiovascular-respiratory system—the heart, lungs, and blood. Exercise programs designed to stress the oxygen system concomitantly benefit the cardiovascular-respiratory system.

General Principles of Training

Individuals undertake physical training programs for a variety of reasons. Some want to increase strength, power, or speed; others are interested in losing excess body weight and improving appearance; others may want to improve endurance capacity. No matter what physical fitness component an individual desires to improve, there are two basic principles that underlie the design of any training program.

Principle of Specificity

Unlike machines, which tend to deteriorate with use, the human body possesses the ability to adapt to use and increase the capacity and efficiency of the system being utilized. Thus, in relation to the three energy systems discussed previously, the **principle of specificity** is critical; a specific energy system must be used if it is to improve. If you

Figure 3.5 Specificity of Training. There are two general aspects of training specificity. First, if you want to improve a particular energy system, you must exercise at an intensity level that stresses that particular system. Second, the training effect is better if you use the actual activity for which you are training. For example, if you want to improve in swimming, you should swim to train the specific neural patterns and muscle groups involved.

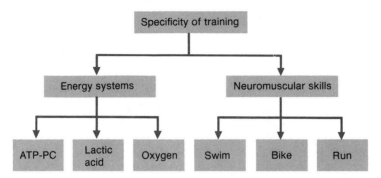

want to develop the oxygen system, you must design a training program that utilizes that particular energy system primarily. Physical activities that involve large muscle groups over sustained periods of time depend on the oxygen system and will eventually increase its efficiency and capacity. Conversely, if an energy system is not utilized, it deteriorates to a level congruent with the activity level of the individual. For example, bedridden individuals experience tremendous decreases in the oxygen energy system in relatively short periods of time, as do highly conditioned endurance athletes who go through a period of detraining. In order to achieve and maintain a desired level of fitness for a particular energy system, use of that energy system is paramount.

Another important aspect of the principle of specificity is the mode of exercise. Three common modes for conditioning the oxygen system are running, swimming, and cycling. Appropriate conditioning programs in each activity increase the capacity of the oxygen system in general, but the improvement in performance level is greatest for that activity in which the individual trains. One person training via a running program and another via a swimming program may make equal gains in utilization of oxygen. However, the swimmer will perform better in a swimming test, while the runner will do better in a running test. This indicates that specific neuromuscular involvement is extremely important if one is training for increased performance in a given activity. The particular muscles, including the neuromuscular pattern, involved in any given activity in which improvement is desired should be included in the conditioning program.

The Overload Principle

The **overload principle** is most important to all conditioning programs. It relates to the principle of use in that the energy system to be developed must be stressed beyond its normal limits of activity. The three major components of the overload principle are intensity, duration, and frequency of exercise. All three may be adjusted in order to impose an overload. Associated with the overload principle as applied to a conditioning program is the concept of progression, often referred to as progressive overload, or progressive resistance.

Figure 3.6 The Overload Principle in Action with Weight Training. In order to continue to improve strength, the weights must be increased.

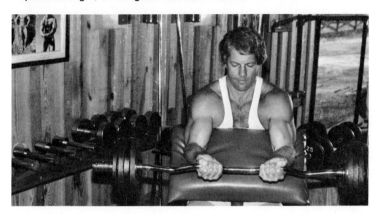

The intensity of the exercise is a very important component of the overload principle. Intensity is synonymous with rate of exercise, or tempo, in such activities as running and swimming. In weight lifting, intensity is related to the amount of resistance offered. There are a number of ways to express the intensity of an exercise task: amount of weight lifted, speed, Calories/minute, METS, percentage of maximal oxygen consumption, and heart rate. Heart rate is a commonly used method in many general conditioning programs for the oxygen system. Methods for determining proper intensity levels for specific exercise programs, including a newer technique involving psychological perception of exercise intensity (rating of perceived exertion), are presented in the next chapters.

A second component of the overload principle is duration. An overload may be imposed by simply increasing the length of time of the exercise period. The intensity of the exercise is generally inversely related to the duration—as intensity increases, duration decreases and vice versa. If duration of exercise is an important concern, the intensity level must be decreased correspondingly.

The frequency of training refers to the number of days per week that an individual exercises. For the average individual, 3–4 days per week is sufficient to elicit a training effect but increased frequency may be necessary for athletes training for competition.

Progression of overload is an important concept. The initial stages of the training program, especially for the habitually sedentary individual, should be mild to moderate. As the body begins to adapt to the exercise routine, the intensity, duration and/or frequency may be increased. However, it is important to progress slowly, as too rapid a progression may contribute to the development of overuse injuries.

Exercise Prescription

Your personal fitness goals and specific fitness objectives to meet these goals are the major determinants of your exercise prescription. As related to a Positive Health Lifestyle, exercise can be effective in the prevention or treatment of a variety of health disorders, including cardiovascular diseases, obesity, and low back problems. In this sense, exercise may be thought of as medication, and it can exert its effect upon the body in a number of ways. Exercise can increase the efficiency of the cardiovascular systems, oxidize body fats, expend energy, strengthen muscle tissues, and increase flexibility, to name but a few of its implications for health. However, just as a physician must prescribe an appropriate dose of a specific medication for a given disease, so too must a specific type of exercise and appropriate dosage be prescribed for different fitness goals. The principle of specificity deals with the type of exercise to be prescribed; the overload principle relates to the dosage.

In the succeeding chapters, you learn the details for prescribing your own exercise program. In chapter 4 you learn the specific types of exercises that may be used to train the cardiovascular system, and appropriate guidelines for the dosage of intensity, duration, and frequency. Other chapters cover exercise programs for losing body fat, increasing muscle mass, improving strength and flexibility, and even helping to reduce stress.

Some drugs are effective in a single dose; a shot of penicillin may help cure an infection somewhere in the body. Other drugs need to be taken repeatedly during the course of an illness; aspirin may be taken for a week or so to help reduce the symptoms of a cold. Still others must be taken for a lifetime; insulin must be administered daily to some diabetic patients. As a medication, exercise falls into this last category. A single dose elicits some physiological effects in the body, but does not produce any long-lasting changes in body structure or function. The body adapts to repeated doses of exercise, and, if the exercise is appropriate, many of these adaptations have beneficial health effects. However, these beneficial bodily adaptations revert back to normal if exercise is discontinued. Thus, for a Positive Health Life-style, exercise is a lifelong prescription.

References

American Alliance for Health, Physical Education, Recreation and Dance. *Lifetime Health Related Physical Fitness*. Reston, VA: AAHPERD, 1980.

American College of Sports Medicine. "Quantity and Quality of Exercise for Developing and Maintaining Fitness in Healthy Adults." *The Physician and Sportsmedicine* 6:35–41 (October 1978).

Bouchard, C.; Boulay, M.; Thibault, M.; Carrier, R.; and Dulac, S. "Training of Submaximal Working Capacity: Frequency, Intensity, Duration, and their Interactions." *Journal of Sports Medicine and Physical Fitness* 20:29–40 (1980).

di Prampero, R. "Energetics of Muscular Exercise." *Review of Physiology, Biochemistry and Pharmacology* 89:143–222 (1981).

Fox, E., and Matthews, D. *Physiological Basis of Physical Education and Athletics*. Philadelphia: Saunders College Publishing, 1981.

Morgan, W. "Psychophysiology of Self-Awareness during Vigorous Physical Activity." *Research Quarterly of Exercise and Sport* 52:385–427 (1981).

Weltman, A., and Stamford, B. "Designing a Safe, Sound Exercise Program." *The Physician and Sportsmedicine* 10:177 (July 1982).

Aerobic Exercise

4

Key Terms

aerobic dancing
aerobic fitness
aerobic walking
interval training
maximal heart rate reserve

mode of exercise
rating of perceived exertion (RPE)
steady-state threshold
target heart rate range (target HR)
threshold stimulus

Key Concepts

Aerobic fitness, (cardiovascular-respiratory efficiency) is the single most important health component of physical fitness.

Aerobic fitness involves the interaction of four physiological functions—respiration, central circulation, peripheral circulation, and muscle metabolism.

Maximal oxygen uptake ($\dot{V}O_2$ max), expressed in ml O_2/kg body weight/minute, is one important measure of aerobic fitness. Another is the ability to sustain exercise at a high percentage of $\dot{V}O_2$ max.

Indirect tests such as distance running, swimming, or bicycling are the most practical means available to evaluate aerobic fitness. Step tests are valuable in demonstrating the adaptation of the heart to aerobic training.

The four key components of an aerobic program are mode, intensity, duration, and frequency of exercise.

Exercise intensity is the most important component of an aerobic exercise prescription. Measurement of the threshold (target) heart rate is a valuable method for assessing exercise intensity.

Aerobic exercise programs must involve large muscle groups. Although a number of different modes of exercise may be used to achieve aerobic fitness, a walk-jog-run program is probably the most practical one available.

According to the American College of Sports Medicine (ACSM), the minimum amount of exercise for aerobic fitness is an intensity level of 60–90 percent of the heart rate reserve, for a duration of 15–60 minutes, at a frequency of 3–4 times per week.

It is important to take it easy when beginning an aerobic exercise program. Aerobic walking is a recommended approach, particularly for those who are habitually sedentary. The intensity of the exercise should gradually be increased, i.e., the principle of progression.

Although there are some risks associated with any aerobic exercise program, the benefits to your health appear to outweigh them, particularly if you are aware of potential problems, and take precautions to avoid them.

Heat is one serious problem that confronts the normal individual who exercises. You must be aware of means to avoid heat illnesses when exercising under hot and/or humid conditions.

Introduction

The purpose of this chapter is to discuss the principles for developing and implementing a personalized physical fitness program as they relate specifically to aerobic exercise programs. Although the major focus centers on the design of an aerobic exercise program for health purposes, some consideration is also given to aerobic training for competition and racing.

Aerobic Fitness

As you may recall from chapter 3, the body has three basic energy systems that may be used to provide biological energy (in the form of ATP) in order to do muscular work, or exercise. Two of the systems (the ATP-PC and lactic acid systems) are utilized to produce ATP very rapidly if the oxygen supply is inadequate, and are classified as anaerobic energy systems. Their capacity is limited, however, and fatigue will set in quickly (usually in minutes) at a very intense exercise level. The third energy system (the oxygen system) produces ATP only if oxygen is available, and is classified as the aerobic energy system. The oxygen system cannot produce ATP as rapidly as the anaerobic systems, but it has a greater capacity and can sustain exercise for hours. Although the basic principles for training the oxygen energy system have been established for a long time, it was not until 1968 that the term *aerobics* came into popular usage with the publication of a book of the same name by Dr. Kenneth Cooper. This classic fitness book served a major role in America's fitness revolution.

Aerobic fitness is probably the single most important health component of physical fitness. Aerobic fitness represents the ability of the cardiovascular and respiratory systems to accommodate the oxygen needs of the muscular system over a sustained period of time, as in such endurance events as distance running, swimming, and bicycling. A number of other terms are associated with aerobic fitness—cardiovascular endurance, cardiovascular fitness, cardiorespiratory fitness, aerobic endurance, and physical working capacity—and have the same essential meaning. Other associated terms are aerobic capacity and maximal oxygen uptake.

Aerobic fitness is a complex component of physical fitness. It involves the interaction of numerous physiological processes in the cardiovascular, respiratory, and muscular systems, including the capacity of the lungs to take up oxygen, the capacity of the blood in the lungs to pick up oxygen, the capacity of the heart to pump this oxygenated blood to the muscle tissues, and the capacity of the tissues to extract the oxygen from the blood and use it to generate energy in the form of ATP via the oxygen system. Thus, the combined cardiovascular and respiratory systems are the oxygen supply mechanism for the muscles. As the energy demands of the muscles increase, so do the demands on the cardiovascular and respiratory systems. Refer to figure 4.1 for an overall schematic of these systems as they relate to oxygen consumption.

A number of physiological processes are critical components of aerobic fitness. These physiological processes may be grouped under four general areas of physiological functioning during exercise: respiration, central circulation, peripheral circulation, and metabolism. The important aspects of each of these general areas to aerobic fitness

Figure 4.1 Physiological Processes Involved in Oxygen Uptake.

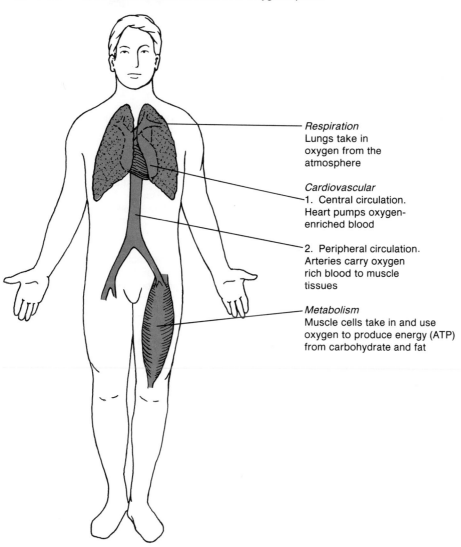

Respiration
Lungs take in
oxygen from the
atmosphere

Cardiovascular
1. Central circulation.
Heart pumps oxygen-
enriched blood

2. Peripheral circulation.
Arteries carry oxygen
rich blood to muscle
tissues

Metabolism
Muscle cells take in and use
oxygen to produce energy (ATP)
from carbohydrate and fat

are listed in table 4.1. Respiration is responsible for taking adequate amounts of oxygen into the lungs and blood; central circulation generates the force to pump the blood; peripheral circulation transports the oxygenated blood throughout the body; metabolism uses the oxygen in the muscle cells to produce ATP.

The interaction of these four physiological functions determines the level of aerobic fitness. The most common measure of aerobic fitness, which evaluates the effectiveness of these physiological functions, is maximal oxygen consumption, or $\dot{V}O_2$ max (pronounced as vee-oh-two-max), a term introduced in chapter 3. $\dot{V}O_2$ max is

Table 4.1
Human Physiological Functions Related to Aerobic Fitness

Respiration
1. Lung ventilation—Ability to take in sufficient air
2. Lung perfusion—Adequate blood distribution in lungs
3. Diffusion capacity—Ability of oxygen to go from lungs to blood rapidly

Central Circulation
1. Heart rate—Ability to sustain high heart rate
2. Stroke volume—Ability of heart to pump sufficient amounts of blood in each beat
3. Hemoglobin level—Sufficient to transport adequate amounts of oxygen
4. Blood volume—Optimal amount of blood in vascular system

Peripheral Circulation
1. Blood flow—Adequate blood to exercising muscles to deliver oxygen and nutrients
2. Capillary density—Adequate number of capillaries in muscle tissue
3. Diffusion capacity—Ability of oxygen to go from blood into muscle cells

Metabolism
1. Energy stores—Adequate energy present in muscle cells
2. Muscle fiber types—Proportion of aerobic muscle fibers to anaerobic fibers
3. Muscle myoglobin—Sufficient to transport oxygen within the muscle cell
4. Mitochondria and oxidative enzymes—Ability to use oxygen to produce ATP in muscle cell

the most accurate measure of aerobic fitness. It represents the interaction of the cardiovascular and respiratory systems to deliver oxygen to the muscles, and the ability of muscles to use the oxygen to generate energy. $\dot{V}O_2$ max is usually expressed in two ways: first, as liters of O_2 per minute (l O_2/min); and, second, as milliliters of O_2 per kilogram of body weight per minute (ml O_2/kg/min). $\dot{V}O_2$ max is partially dependent upon body weight. The larger the individual, the greater the potential $\dot{V}O_2$ max. All other things equal, a 200 pound man has twice the $\dot{V}O_2$ max of a 100 pound man (perhaps 4 liters versus 2 liters). For this reason, it is best to express $\dot{V}O_2$ max relative to body weight. Expressed in this way, a 132 pound person (Subject A) with a $\dot{V}O_2$ max of 3.0 liters is considered aerobically equivalent to a 176 pound person (Subject B) with a $\dot{V}O_2$ max of 4.0 liters. To illustrate:

Subject A

132 lbs ÷ 2.2 = 60 kg
3.0 liters = 3000 ml
3000 ml O_2 ÷ 60 kg = 50 ml O_2/kg/min

Subject B

176 lbs ÷ 2.2 = 80 kg
4.0 liters = 4000 ml
4000 ml O_2 ÷ 80 kg = 50 ml O_2/kg/min

Figure 4.2 Maximal Oxygen Uptake ($\dot{V}O_2$ max). The best way to express $\dot{V}O_2$ max is in milliliters of oxygen per kilograms (kg) of body weight per minute (ml O_2/kg/minute). As noted in the figure, the smaller individual has a lower $\dot{V}O_2$ max in liters, but a higher $\dot{V}O_2$ max when expressed relative to weight. In this case, the smaller individual has a higher degree of aerobic fitness.

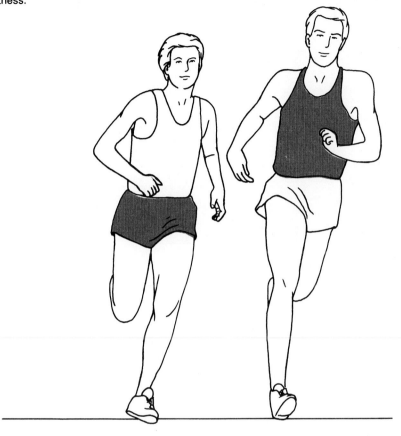

$\dot{V}O_2$ max: liters/minute	3.6 L (3600 ml)	4.0 L (5000 ml)
KG body weight	60	80
$\dot{V}O_2$ max: ml O_2/kg/minute	60	50

Both Subjects A and B have identical $\dot{V}O_2$ max, when expressed per unit of body weight.

Although $\dot{V}O_2$ max is a very important measure of aerobic fitness, it does not represent the total concept of aerobic fitness. Of equal or greater importance is the ability to exercise at a higher percentage of $\dot{V}O_2$ max. Figure 4.3 explains this concept. The figure represents the possible effects of an aerobic exercise training program over a 6 month period of time. Note that the $\dot{V}O_2$ max does increase somewhat—a 10–20 percent increase is all that can be expected in most normally active individuals. However, the ability to perform at a greater percentage of $\dot{V}O_2$ max increases much more

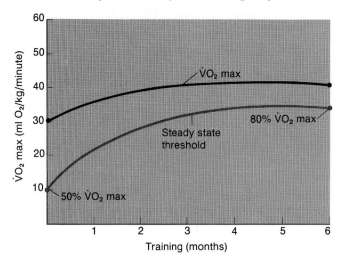

Figure 4.3 The Effect of Training upon $\dot{V}O_2$ Max and the Steady-state Threshold. Training increases both your $\dot{V}O_2$ max and your steady-state threshold, which is the ability to work at a greater percentage of your $\dot{V}O_2$ max without producing excessive lactic acid—a causative factor in fatigue. For example, before training, the $\dot{V}O_2$ max may be 40 ml, while the steady-state threshold is only 20 (50% of $\dot{V}O_2$ max). After training, $\dot{V}O_2$ max may rise to 50 ml, but the steady-state threshold may rise to 40 ml (80% of the $\dot{V}O_2$ max).

as the steady-state threshold is raised. If you are exercising in a steady state, then you have an adequate supply of oxygen to meet your energy needs. The **steady-state threshold** is that point in exercise intensity at which the contribution of energy from the lactic acid system increases very rapidly. As you may recall, this increased production of lactic acid speeds up the onset of fatigue. By raising your steady-state threshold through training, you may be able to perform at 80 percent of your $\dot{V}O_2$ max, as compared to only 50 percent before training. You will be able to perform at a greater percentage of your maximal ability without producing excessive amounts of lactic acid which could cause you to fatigue or slow down.

What are the implications of this concept? Figure 4.4 illustrates the effect of oxygen uptake on the ability to run long distances at a particular speed without the early onset of fatigue. At an oxygen delivery rate of 30 ml/kg, running speed is only about 5.6 miles per hour (MPH); at 60 ml/kg, speed doubles—to about 11.1 MPH. For an individual who could only do a 14 minute mile before training, this effect reduces the time to approximately 7 minutes.

In summary, we can see that aerobic fitness may be expressed in terms of $\dot{V}O_2$ max and the percentage of $\dot{V}O_2$ max at which an individual is able to sustain exercise. Both of these factors may be improved by a proper training program. More importantly, the major determinants of $\dot{V}O_2$ max are the physiological functions of the cardiovascular, respiratory, and muscular systems, which will also improve and bring significant benefits to the health of the individual.

Figure 4.4 Oxygen Uptake Necessary to Prevent Fatigue at Different Running Speeds. The greater your running speed, the more oxygen you need. In order to prevent fatigue, the amount of oxygen needed should be under your steady-state threshold.
Source: From Daniels, J., R. Fitts, and G. Sheehan. *Conditioning for Long Distance Running.* © 1978 by John Wiley and Sons, Inc. Reprinted by permission.

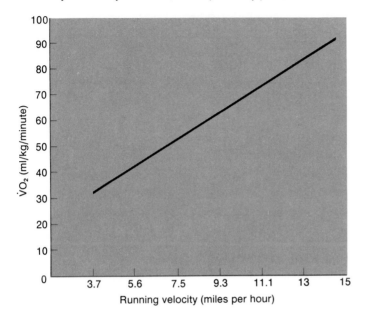

Measurement of Aerobic Fitness

Now that we know what aerobic fitness is, how do we measure it in a given individual? As mentioned previously, $\dot{V}O_2$ max is probably the best single indicator of aerobic fitness, and should be expressed in relation to the body weight of the individual (ml O_2/kg/min). The two general means to measure aerobic fitness include direct tests of $\dot{V}O_2$ max and indirect tests that are utilized to predict aerobic fitness or $\dot{V}O_2$ max.

There is a variety of test protocols that are used to measure $\dot{V}O_2$ max directly, but the general procedure is to monitor oxygen consumption while an individual exercises to exhaustion. This test is usually done on a motor-driven treadmill bicycle ergometer, although other exercise modes may also be used. The work load is gradually increased and, through the use of sophisticated monitoring devices and gas analyzers, the maximal level of oxygen uptake is recorded at or near exhaustion. This type of test requires considerable time and expense, making it impractical for use with large numbers of individuals. However, if the facilities are available this test does provide the most valid measure. With the increasing popularity and decreased cost of computers that are combined with electronic means to analyze respiratory gases, it is anticipated that direct tests will become increasingly more available for aerobic fitness assessment.

Figure 4.5 A Laboratory Stress Test. A laboratory stress test with a 12-lead EKG and measurement of maximal oxygen uptake (VO$_2$ max) can provide some highly technical data related to cardiovascular-respiratory function.
Source: From L. Zohman, MD, *Beyond Diet: Exercise Your Way to Fitness and Heart Health,* CPC International, Englewood Cliffs, NJ.

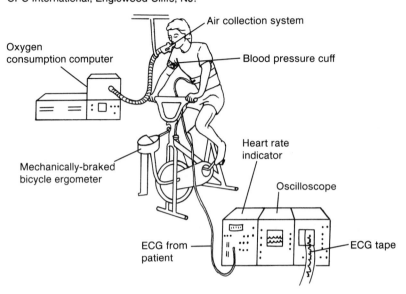

At the present time, however, a number of indirect tests are used to assess aerobic fitness. The two most common techniques in assessing aerobic fitness are distance runs and step tests.

Over the years, Dr. Kenneth Cooper has collected and analyzed data on thousands of individuals relative to $\dot{V}O_2$ max and performance in distance running, distance swimming, and distance cycling. Based upon his analysis, Cooper suggests that a given performance on his running, swimming, or bicycling test is indicative of a certain level of $\dot{V}O_2$ max. His research, and resultant fitness programs, are presented in a series of books. The most recent of these is *The Aerobics Program for Total Well-Being.*

Cooper's tests are designed for men and women between the ages of thirteen and sixty. An individual may take any of the following tests:

1. 3 mile walking test (no running)
2. 1½ mile running test
3. 12 minute walking/running test
4. 12 minute swimming test
5. 12 minute cycling test

For the 12 minute tests, the goal is to cover as great a distance as possible during the allotted time; finishing in the shortest time possible is the criterion in the 1½ and 3 mile tests. All that are needed to conduct these tests are accurately measured distances and a stopwatch. An indoor and outdoor track are excellent for the running, walking, and cycling tests; a 25 yard (or longer) pool is appropriate for swimming. Scoring tables for the 3 mile walking test and the 1½ mile running test are presented in appendix D.

Although there is general agreement that these types of indirect tests do measure the ability to produce aerobic energy over a prolonged period of time, they may not be highly accurate predictors of $\dot{V}O_2$ max. The factors that contribute to running, swimming, and bicycling performance are complex, and include not only $\dot{V}O_2$ max, but other factors such as the steady-state threshold, body fatness, and mechanical efficiency. Nevertheless, they appear to be some of the best practical means available to assess aerobic fitness. Moreover, since the steady-state threshold is a component of aerobic fitness, and body fat is a health-related component of fitness, these indirect tests do appear to be useful as fitness measuring techniques. Improved performance would most likely be due to increased fitness levels.

Laboratory Inventory 4.3 (at the end of this chapter) may be used to predict $\dot{V}O_2$ max and assess aerobic fitness. Be sure to read the instructions prior to taking any of the distance tests. Sedentary individuals should exercise regularly for several weeks before taking any of the tests. A recommended sequence is:

1. Train 2 weeks—take 3 mile walking test
2. Train 4 more weeks—take 3 mile walking test or 1½ mile running test
3. Train 6 more weeks—take 1½ mile running test
4. Repeat 1½ mile running test about once a month to check on progress

Another commonly used indirect technique to measure aerobic fitness involves the heart rate response during the recovery period after an exercise step test. Since the heart rate is the most readily obtainable measure of the cardiovascular response to exercise, it has commonly been used to predict $\dot{V}O_2$ max, or assesss aerobic fitness. Unfortunately, research has shown that the heart rate response to various step tests is not a good predictor of $\dot{V}O_2$ max or even of performance on the other indirect tests such as distance runs. However, they may be useful in evaluating the effect of a conditioning regimen on a given individual. One of the beneficial effects of training is a lower resting heart rate and a lower heart rate response to a submaximal exercise task. Hence, the results of a step test administered prior to the initiation of a conditioning program could be compared with the results of a test administered towards the conclusion of the program. A lowered heart rate response would be indicative that the heart has become more efficient. This should serve to motivate the individual to continue the training program. This may be the most valuable use of the step test. Laboratory Inventory 4.4 describes the protocol for a step test.

In order to achieve valid and reliable results for these tests, as well as for any fitness test, identical protocol must be used each time the test is taken. The same course should be used, if possible, and the step height and stepping cadence should remain the same. Extraneous factors such as the environmental temperature and wind conditions may influence test results. Try to minimize these extraneous influences whenever possible.

Exercise tests can be used to establish short-term and long-term goals. The results of these tests may provide excellent data for evaluating progress during an exercise program.

Prescription for Aerobic Exercise

When you are seriously ill you usually consult a physician, who may write you a prescription for a drug to help treat or cure your illness. However, many of us often treat minor health problems by prescribing our own medication, such as when we take aspirin for a headache or cold. A similar analogy may be used with exercise. A cardiac patient must have an exercise program specifically prescribed by a cardiologist, or other medical personnel, while the basically healthy individual without any major risk factors may prescribe his or her own exercise program.

A general outline for an exercise prescription for aerobic fitness should include goals, mode of exercise, warm-up, warm-down, and stimulus period. Before considering these points, however, let us first discuss whether or not you should seek medical clearance before you prescribe your own exercise program.

Medical Clearance

One concern is the type of medical clearance you should have before initiating an exercise program or taking an exercise test, particularly one that stresses the cardiovascular system. There appears to be some controversy over who needs to see a physician before initiating or increasing the intensity of an exercise program, particularly when the physical examination includes an exercise ECG stress test. The National Heart, Lung, and Blood Institute (NHLBI), American Heart Association (AHA), and American College of Sports Medicine (ACSM) have all developed guidelines relative to this issue, and some differences do exist in their recommendations. No thorough review of these guidelines is presented here, as they are rather extensive and beyond the scope of this text. However, some practical suggestions that represent a synthesis of these and other viewpoints are offered.

1. If you have any concern about any facet of your health, it would be a good idea to check with your physician before starting an exercise program.
2. No matter what your age, if you have any of the coronary heart disease risk factors noted in table 4.2 you should have a physical examination.
3. If you are young (twenties or early thirties) and healthy, and have no risk factors, it is probably safe to initiate an exercise program. As a matter of fact, it is probably more dangerous to your health in the long run not to exercise than it is to remain inactive simply because you have not had a physician's examination.
4. Above age thirty-five is where the controversy begins. If you are physically active and have no risk factors, you may continue with your customary program and even progressively increase the intensity on a gradual basis. If you possess any risk factors, see your physician. If you are sedentary without any risk factors, it would be a good idea to check with your physician, although you may be able to initiate a gradual, sensible exercise program with minimal risk. The older you are, the better the idea to get a medical examination.

Table 4.2
Risk Factors Associated with Coronary Heart Disease

Major Risk Factors
1. High blood pressure
2. Cigarette smoking
3. High blood lipid levels: cholesterol and triglycerides
4. ECG abnormalities

Predisposing Risk Factors
1. Family history of coronary heart disease before age sixty
2. Sedentary life-style
3. Stressful life-style and personality
4. Diabetes
5. Obesity

Source: American College of Sports Medicine. *Guidelines for Graded Exercise Testing and Exercise Prescription,* 2d. ed. Philadelphia: Lea and Febiger, 1980.

For individuals who do have a physical examination, the physician may recommend an exercise ECG stress test. An exercise ECG stress test may serve a very useful purpose, and is usually prescribed in suspected cases of coronary heart disease. It can be used to diagnose the presence and severity of coronary heart disease, to prescribe a safe exercise program, and to evaluate the rehabilitative effects of such a program. In essence, the patient exercises on a treadmill under the supervision of trained medical personnel. The ECG is monitored continuously, and the individual exercises to the point of exhaustion or to some other predetermined termination point. The tests are rather costly, ranging from $175–$500. You should take an ECG stress test only if it is prescribed by a physician and conducted under proper medical supervision. Some fitness organizations advertise a heart rate stress test without medical control for a lesser cost, but they are not to be regarded as a substitute for the ECG test.

Goals

The goals you set for yourself should be of two types—short-term and long-term. They should be personal goals and reflect the reasons why you are initiating an aerobic fitness program. For example, a short-term goal may be to lose 5 pounds of body fat in 1 month, while a long-term goal may be to lose 60 pounds in a year. Another example is a short-term goal of nonstop jogging for 1 mile, with a long-term goal to enter and complete a 10 kilometer road race. When you achieve your short-term goal, a new short-term goal should be established as you progress towards your long-term goal.

Mode of Exercise

The **mode of exercise** represents the choice of an activity of an aerobic nature that you participate in to achieve aerobic fitness. A wide variety of physical activities may be used for this purpose. A later section of this chapter is devoted to this topic.

Figure 4.6   Goal setting is an important factor in an exercise program.

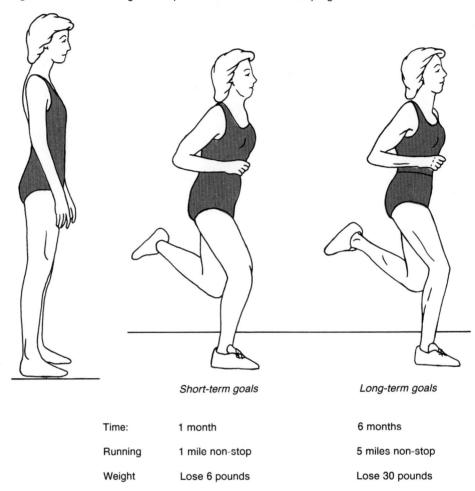

	Short-term goals	*Long-term goals*
Time:	1 month	6 months
Running	1 mile non-stop	5 miles non-stop
Weight	Lose 6 pounds	Lose 30 pounds

Warm-up

The **warm-up** precedes the stimulus period and may be done in a variety of ways. It usually is 5–10 minutes long. It may consist of general calisthenics, stretching exercises, or a lower intensity level of the actual mode of exercise. The goals of the warm-up phase are to gradually increase the stress on the cardiovascular system and loosen up the muscles as a possible preventive measure against injury. For example, a jogger may do several of the stretching exercises for the legs illustrated in chapter 8 and then jog at a slower-than-normal pace for several minutes.

Warm-down

The **warm-down** phase follows the stimulus period and is primarily designed to help restore the cardiovascular system to normal. If one stops exercising abruptly, blood may pool in the exercised body parts, thereby decreasing return of blood to the heart.

Figure 4.7 The Exercise Prescription. The exercise prescription is divided into three phases: warm-up, stimulus period, and warm-down. The stimulus period is the key.

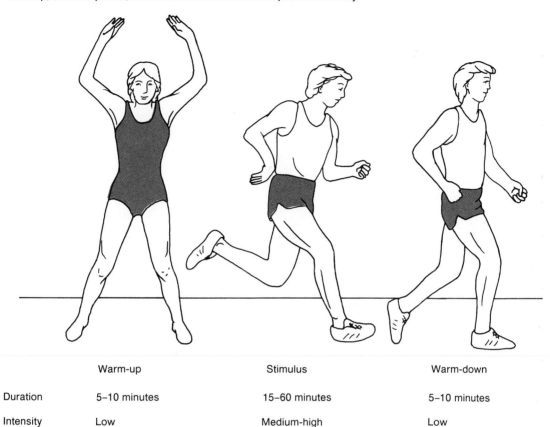

	Warm-up	Stimulus	Warm-down
Duration	5–10 minutes	15–60 minutes	5–10 minutes
Intensity	Low	Medium-high	Low

With less blood coming into the heart, less will be pumped to the brain, resulting in dizziness. By gradually warming down after strenuous exercise, such as walking or jogging after a strenuous run, the muscles help massage the blood through the veins back to the heart. Recent research has also noted that abrupt cessation of exercise may increase certain blood hormone levels, which may cause abnormal rhythm of the heart—emphasizing the importance of a gradual warm-down.

Stimulus Period

The **stimulus period** is based upon the overload principle and is the most important part of any exercise program. It is the heart of the exercise prescription for aerobic fitness. The two major components of the stimulus period are intensity and duration of exercise. Frequency (the number of exercise sessions per week) is also an important

Figure 4.8 The Relationship between Various Measures of Energy Expenditure. Caloric expenditure, oxygen consumption, RPE, and heart rate are, in general, directly related to the intensity of the exercise under steady-state conditions, i.e., when the oxygen supply is adequate for the energy cost of the exercise.

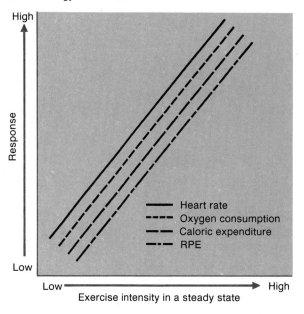

part of the exercise prescription. Following an exhaustive review of the pertinent research, the American College of Sports Medicine recommends the following guidelines to develop and maintain cardiovascular (aerobic) fitness in healthy adults.

1. Intensity of training: 60–90 percent of maximum heart rate reserve or 50–85 percent of maximum oxygen uptake ($\dot{V}O_2$ max)
2. Duration of training: 15–60 minutes of continuous aerobic activity
3. Frequency of training: 3–5 days per week

The Threshold Stimulus

The intensity of exercise is the most important component of the stimulus period, and, in order to receive the optimal benefits from the exercise program, you must attain a certain **threshold stimulus,** which is the minimal stimulus intensity that will produce a training effect. The intensity of exercise can be expressed in a number of different ways, such as percentage of $\dot{V}O_2$ max, calories/minute, or heart rate. In general, there is a high degree of relationship between these variables during exercise at a steady state. For example, the heart rate may reflect a certain level of oxygen consumption or caloric expenditure. Since the heart rate is easily obtained, it is usually used to determine the threshold level of exercise intensity. Another means to judge exercise intensity is the **RPE,** or **rating of perceived exertion,** your own perception of how strenuous the exercise is that you are doing.

The Target Heart Rate

How do you determine your threshold level? Let's look at two ways—the heart rate and RPE. To obtain the heart rate, press lightly with the index and middle fingers on the carotid artery, which is located just under the jawbone and beside the Adam's apple. Do not use your thumb as it also has a pulse, and do not press hard on the carotid artery for it may cause a reflex slowing of the beat. The radial artery pulse is obtained by placing all four fingers on the inside of the wrist on the thumb side. These are the two most common locations for monitoring pulse rate, but other locations (the temple, inside the upper arm, and directly over the heart) may be used.

To obtain the heart rate per minute, simply count the pulse rate for 10 seconds and multiply by six. Resting and recovery heart rates are easily obtainable since they may be taken while the individual is motionless, but it is difficult to manually monitor the heart rate while exercising. Research has shown that the exercise heart rate correlates very highly with the heart rate during the early stages of recovery. Hence, to monitor exercise heart rate, secure the pulse *immediately* upon cessation of exercise and count the beats for 10 seconds. This provides a reliable measure of exercise heart rate, although it may be slightly lower due to the beginning of the recovery effect. Laboratory Inventory 4.1 gives you some practical experience in palpating your heart rate.

There is rather widespread general agreement that, in order to obtain a conditioning effect, the heart rate response should be in the range of 60–90 percent of the **maximal heart rate reserve** (the difference between the resting heart rate and the maximal heart rate). Although there are individual variations, a general guide for the prediction of the HR max is 220 minus a person's age. Thus, a forty-year-old individual would have a predicted HR max of 180. Keep in mind, however, that there is considerable individual variation relative to predicted HR max: For example, a forty-year-old man may predict a HR max of 180, yet it may be 200, 160, or even much lower if he was a victim of coronary heart disease.

Continuing with our example of the forty-year-old man, we can calculate the heart rate range needed to elicit a training effect. This is called the **target heart rate range,** or **target HR.** In order to complete the calculations, we need to know the age-predicted HR max and the resting heart rate (RHR); the latter should be determined under relaxed circumstances. If we assume a RHR of 70 and a HR max of 180, the following formula would give us the target range:

Target HR = X% (HR max − RHR) + RHR

For the 60 percent threshold level, the target heart rate for our example would be calculated as follows:

.6 (180–70) + 70 = 136

For the 90 percent level, the target heart rate would be:

.9 (180–70) + 70 = 169

Thus, in order to achieve a training effect, our forty-year-old man needs to train within a target HR range of 136–169.

Figure 4.9 Palpation of the Heart Rate. The pulse rate may be taken at a variety of body locations (*a*), but the two most common locations are the neck (*b*) (carotid artery) and the wrist (*c*) (radial artery).

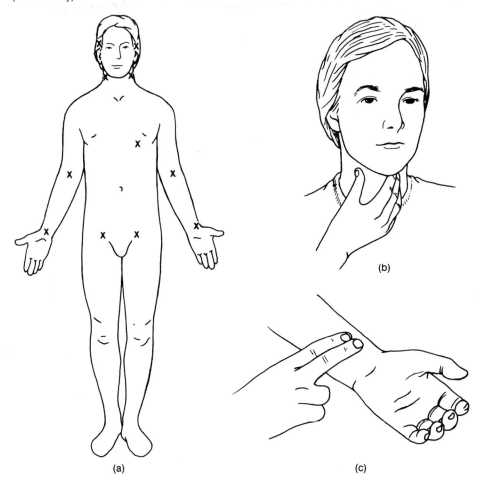

(a)

(b)

(c)

If you wish to bypass the calculations, table 4.3 presents the target HR ranges for various age groups with RHR between 50 and 90 beats/minute. Simply find your age group and RHR in the headings and locate your target HR range. The table is based on a predicted HR max of 220 − age.

In general, this table offers a useful guide to the threshold heart rate and target HR range. However, there is considerable variability in HR max among individuals, particularly in the older age groups. If your true HR max is below the predicted value (220 − age), the target HR range in the table would be higher than the recommended level. If your true HR max is higher than the predicted value, the target HR range in the table is lower than the recommended level. Although the target HR range might vary by a few beats, if your actual HR max is slightly higher or lower than the predicted value, you will still receive a good training effect—assuming you are in the middle of the range.

Table 4.3
Target Heart Rate Zones

Resting Heart Rate	Age											
	15–19	20–24	25–29	30–34	35–39	40–44	45–49	50–54	55–59	60–64	65–69	70–74
45–49	141–187	138–183	135–178	132–174	129–169	126–165	123–160	120–156	117–151	114–147	111–142	108–138
50–54	143–188	140–183	137–179	134–174	131–170	128–165	125–161	122–156	119–152	116–147	113–143	110–138
55–59	145–188	142–184	139–179	136–175	133–170	130–166	127–161	124–157	121–152	118–148	115–143	112–139
60–64	147–189	144–184	141–180	138–175	135–171	132–166	129–162	126–157	123–153	120–148	117–144	114–139
65–69	149–189	146–185	143–180	140–176	137–171	134–167	131–162	128–158	125–153	122–149	119–144	116–140
70–74	151–190	148–185	145–181	142–176	139–172	136–167	133–163	130–158	127–154	124–149	121–145	118–140
75–79	153–190	150–186	147–181	144–177	141–172	138–168	135–163	132–159	129–154	126–150	123–145	120–141
80–84	155–191	152–186	149–182	146–177	143–173	140–168	137–164	134–159	131–155	128–150	125–146	122–141
85–89	157–191	154–187	151–182	148–178	145–173	142–169	139–164	136–160	133–155	130–151	127–146	124–142

The target zone (60–90 percent threshold) is based upon the median figure for each age range and resting heart rate range.

Table 4.4
The RPE Scale

6	14
7 very, very light	15 hard
8	16
9 very light	17 very hard
10	18
11 fairly light	19 very, very hard
12	20
13 somewhat hard	

It is a good idea to determine your own HR max (Laboratory Inventory 4.2.) Recent research has revealed that HR max is lower bicycling and swimming, so the target HR may be slightly lower if one of these two modes of exercise is used.

The Target RPE

Although the target heart rate approach is a sound means for monitoring exercise intensity, you may also wish to use the RPE scale developed by Gunnar Borg. This scale was originally designed to reflect heart rate responses, by adding a zero to the rating. You simply rate the perceived difficulty or strenuousness of the exercise task according to the scale in table 4.4.

Figure 4.10 Aerobic mode exercises must involve large muscle groups, such as running, swimming, or bicycling.

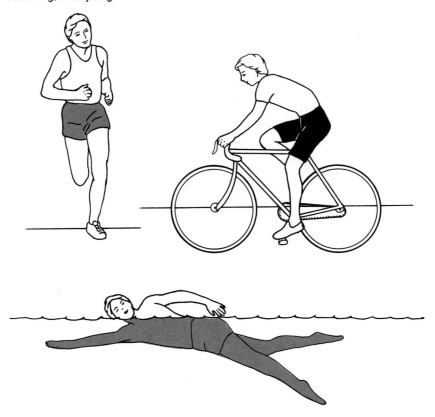

When you determine your exercise heart rate, it is a good idea to associate an appropriate RPE value with it. For example, at an exercise heart rate of 150 you might make a mental note of the exercise difficulty and assign a value of 15, or hard, to that level of exercise intensity. Research has shown that the RPE can be an effective means to measure exercise intensity in healthy individuals, particularly at heart rates above 150 beats/minute. A general rule of thumb is: If you cannot maintain a conversation with a friend while exercising, you are probably exercising too hard.

Modes of Aerobic Exercise

Aerobic exercises must involve large muscle groups in a rhythmical manner. The muscles of the legs and of the arms comprise a good portion of the total body mass. The major muscles in the chest and back are attached to the upper arm and are actively involved in almost all arm movements. Running and bicycling provide rhythmical exercise for the legs. Most types of swimming strokes do the same for the arms. There are many other good large muscle rhythmical activities.

Table 4.5
The Potential of Various Physical Activities for the Development of Aerobic Fitness

High Potential	Moderate Potential	Low Potential
Aerobic dancing	Basketball	Baseball
Aerobic walking	Calisthenics	Bowling
Bicycling	Downhill skiing	Football
Cross country skiing	Field hockey	Golf
Hiking uphill	Handball	Softball
Jogging	Racquetball	Volleyball
Rope jumping	Soccer	
Rowing	Squash	
Running	Tennis (singles)	
Running in place		
Skating		
Stationary bicycling		
Swimming		

Another important factor is your enjoyment of the exercise. To be effective in the long run, you should select an activity that you enjoy, that has a recommended intensity level, and that can be performed over a long period of time. If you do not enjoy jogging or running, other activities may be substituted. Fast walking (with vigorous arm action), swimming, bicycling, tennis, handball, racquetball, or a variety of other activities may produce a greater feeling of enjoyment, and elicit an aerobic fitness training effect. Enjoy your exercise. Try to make it a lifelong habit.

Practicality is also important. You may enjoy swimming, tennis, racquetball, and a variety of other sports, but lack of facilities, poor weather conditions, no partner, or high costs may limit your ability to participate. For the person who travels frequently, this may be a major concern. Practicality is the major reason that a walking-jogging-running program is stressed in this book. This mode of aerobic training is not superior to other modes of equal intensity, duration, and frequency, but it can be done almost anytime and anywhere—which is not the case for many other types of aerobic activities. All you need are a good pair of shoes and proper clothing to suit the weather. Nothing short of an injury should deter you from your daily exercise routine, be it fast walking, jogging, or running. You may not learn to enjoy jogging, but it can be a very practical substitute on those days when you cannot participate in your regular physical activity. Other practical modes of aerobic exercise include aerobic dancing and rope jumping.

Table 4.5 presents some physical activities that are grouped according to their potential for development of aerobic fitness. Again, keep in mind that in order for these activities to be effective, they must adhere to the overload principle. The exercise intensity must pass the threshold level, that level must be maintained for a set duration, and the exercise must be done frequently. Although many different types of activities develop the cardiovascular system, under the principle of specificity, the muscles that develop are specific to the type of exercises used.

Implementing an Aerobic Fitness Program

Now that you have all this information about aerobic exercise, how do you begin your own personal program? In this section, we discuss some general guidelines for selecting your aerobic exercise program, show you a technique to determine the exercise intensity necessary to elicit your target heart rate, discuss the concept of progression, and provide you with some sample exercise programs that satisfy the principles set forth in the preceding section.

At the end of this section, you should be able to complete Laboratory Inventory 4.5, which is an aerobic exercise prescription and contract.

General Guidelines

One of the most important factors to consider before beginning your aerobic fitness program is your current level of physical fitness. If you have been inactive for some time, you should begin with a less vigorous activity, such as aerobic walking. As you improve your physical fitness, the intensity of the exercise program may be increased. Review the practical suggestions in chapter 3 concerning health status and the initiation of an aerobic fitness program. In general, if you are young and healthy (twenties or early thirties) and have no coronary risk factors, it is probably safe to begin an aerobic exercise program without a medical examination.

The time of the day you exercise is immaterial, for the effects will be the same if you train in the morning, afternoon, or evening. The key point is to schedule your exercise as a part of your regular daily activities. Allot yourself that 40–60 minutes at least 3 days each week. If you regularly exercise in the evening, but have something else scheduled on the evening of your exercise day, then try to work the exercise into your schedule earlier in the day, maybe getting up an hour earlier than usual. Commitment is a key to developing a lifetime fitness program. Make exercise a part of your life-style.

Learn a variety of modes of aerobic exercise. You may prefer handball as your exercise mode, but lack of a partner or playing facilities may eliminate this means to exercise. Jogging is a good substitute. You may enjoy running outdoors because of the variety of scenery and the fresh air, but inclement weather may force you to exercise indoors. Aerobic dancing, rope jumping, and stationary running are good indoor substitutes.

Determination of Your Target Heart Rate

As you may recall from our previous discussion, exercise intensity is a key factor in developing aerobic fitness, along with duration and frequency. Duration and frequency are basically self-evident, that is, you exercise for 15–60 minutes on 3 or 4 days per week. However, you must determine the intensity of exercise necessary to elicit your target heart rate. Laboratory Inventory 4.1 introduces you to heart rate palpation techniques; Laboratory Inventory 4.2 enables you to determine the level of exercise intensity for your target zone.

Figure 4.11 Rope jumping may be an excellent indoor aerobic exercise.

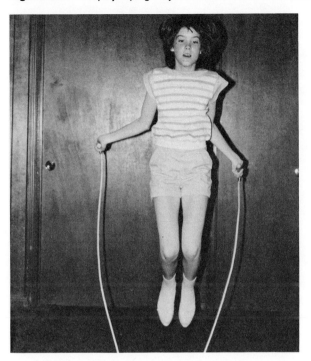

Since the concept of the target HR or RPE is so important, let us illustrate with an example of Laboratory Inventory 4.2 for someone who is twenty years old and has an RHR of 70. From table 4.3, the target range is 148 (60 percent) to 185 (90 percent).

This person takes the test outlined in Laboratory Inventory 4.2 with the following results:

Test	Time	RPE	HR	Minutes/Mile
1	7:30	12	125	15:00
2	6:00	15	150	12:00
3	4:00	17	174	8:00
4	3:15	19	193	6:30

Obviously, as the speed increases for each test, so do the heart rate and RPE. In this case, the RPE correlates fairly well with the heart rate, i.e., adding a zero to the RPE approximates the heart rate response. In this example, the first test at a pace of 7½ minutes for a ½ mile does not produce a training effect because the heart rate of 125 is below the 60 percent threshold of 148. Test two does reach the threshold value with a heart rate of 150, which is close to the minimal speed at which this person should walk or jog. Tests three and four lead to higher heart rates, with test four exceeding the 90 percent level of the target HR range. The data are plotted in figure 4.12. The RPE offers a means of judging the intensity of the exercise when you do not have a known distance or watch.

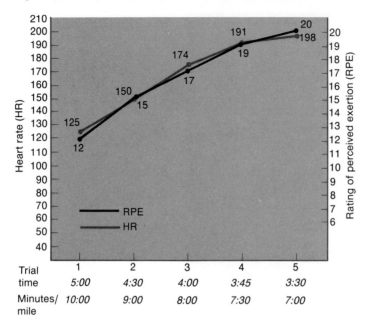

To determine speed for these tests, simply double the time for the ½ mile and you have the time per mile. In our example, the first test was a 15 minute mile, and subsequent tests were 12, 8, and 6½ minute miles.

The exercise intensity necessary to achieve the target heart rate should be developed specific to the type of exercise program you are going to do. For example, if you plan to swim for your aerobic exercise, then you should use the swim test protocol at different speeds to determine your heart rate response. It should be noted that the HR max is generally lower when swimming than running so that the target HR range for swimming might be 8–10 beats lower. This is due to the different body position for exercise in swimming. The heart can pump more blood per beat while the body is in a horizontal position than in a vertical position as in running. A lower HR max has also been noted during bicycling. Thus, it may be advisable to determine your HR max specific to your mode of exercise once you become conditioned. Using your RHR and your HR max for a specific type of exercise, you can calculate your target HR range from the table on page 87.

Progression

Progression of exercise intensity is an important concept. The intensity of exercise necessary to elicit the target heart rate at the higher levels of the target HR range may be too severe for some beginners, hence the initial stages of the training program, especially for the habitually sedentary individual, should be mild to moderate. For a forty-year-old individual with an RHR of 72, the target HR might be in the range of 136–167. Obviously, the intensity of exercise needed to produce an HR of 136 is much less than that needed for an HR of 167. During the early stages of training, the 136

Figure 4.13 As you become trained over several months, the heart rate response to a standard exercise, such as running a nine-minute mile, decreases significantly. Thus, to hit the target HR, your exercise intensity may have to be increased somewhat.

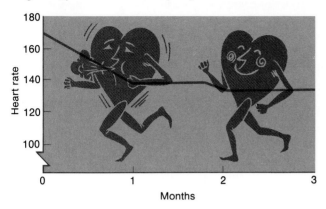

HR may be tolerated easily, while 167 may produce a rapid onset of fatigue or intolerance. Hence, the intensity of the exercise may be regulated towards the lower end of the target range during the early weeks of training, increasing gradually so that the HR begins to approach the upper limits of the target range.

It is important to reiterate that individuals who have been sedentary should begin their exercise programs no higher than the 60 percent level of the heart rate reserve. Many individuals start out at too high a work load and experience problems. It will take time to get back in shape and improve your fitness level. Start slowly, following the progressive programs offered later in this chapter.

A modified interval training program, such as the walk-jog-walk program described below, to produce a varying HR response during the exercise period may be advisable. For example, the individual may walk at a pace sufficient to achieve an HR of 136 for several minutes; increase the intensity by jogging to achieve an HR of 167 for several minutes; then walk again to reduce the heart rate to the lower levels of the target range. By alternating intensity levels, the HR can be made to vary from the lower to upper levels of the target HR range. Let your RPE also serve as a guide to exercise intensity.

As the body begins to adapt to the exercise routine over the weeks, the intensity, duration, and/or frequency may be increased. For example, one of the effects of training is a decrease in both the resting HR and the HR and RPE responses to a given work load. For example, you may be able to reach a target heart rate of 160, initially, by running a mile in 10 minutes. However, as you become conditioned, that same speed may elicit a heart rate of only 140. Hence, you must increase your intensity, or speed, in order to continue to elicit the target heart rate of 160. Eventually, you progress to a training level that helps maintain the desired target heart rate. The resting HR also decreases as you become better conditioned, and this decrease then modifies the heart rate reserve. Check your RHR periodically in order to calculate the changes in your threshold HR. Mathematically, the minimal threshold decreases, but, as that happens, you become able to work at higher threshold levels (70–80 percent), so that a good training effect still occurs.

Figure 4.14 Aerobic dancing can be an effective means to improve cardiovascular fitness for both males and females.

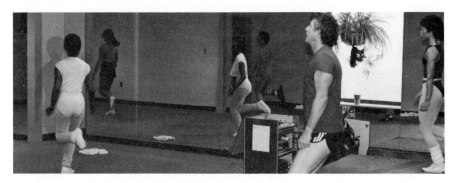

Aerobic Exercise Programs

Although diverse modes of aerobic exercise may be used to elicit a training effect for the cardiovascular system, only three of the more practical ones are described here. They are practical in the sense that they can be done alone and with a minimum of equipment.

Walk-Jog-Run Programs

There is a wide variety of methods to initiate an aerobic exercise program of walking, jogging, or running. The key is to begin slowly, gradually increasing the exercise intensity as you become better conditioned. Jogging and running are strenuous activities and usually will be effective means for reaching your target HR. Leisurely walking is not usually an adequate stimulus, so the walking pace must be brisk. Walking at a faster-than-normal pace is often called **aerobic walking.** In tables 4.6 and 4.7 you will find two sample programs. The first (table 4.6) is for those individuals who are at a low level of fitness, such that jogging may be too strenuous for them. The target heart rate method is used here, and is adjusted downward during the initial weeks. The second (table 4.7) is a rapid progression to jogging, using an interval training approach. **Interval training** was developed primarily for athletes, but its principles of alternating rest and exercise periods may also be applied to aerobic training for the nonathlete. Again, the heart rate should be palpated during this program to check whether you are within the target HR range.

Aerobic Dancing

By now, you should know the meaning of the word *aerobic* as it relates to exercise. And, for most of us, dancing is fun. Combining the two, we have a fun way to exercise. Exercise to music has been around for years, but it was not until the 1970s that aerobic dancing was developed. In essence, aerobic dancing is simply exercise to music. In a stricter sense, such as the method pioneered by Jackie Sorensen, aerobic dancing has been choreographed to contain certain percentages of (1) simple vigorous dance steps to improve aerobic capacity, (2) stretching movements to improve flexibility, and (3) muscle-toning movements.

Aerobic dancing has become increasingly popular in the past ten years, particularly among women. As a result, a number of organizations have been developed to

Table 4.6
Sample Aerobic Walking Program*

	Warm-up	Target Zone Exercising	Warm-down	Total Time
Week 1*	Walk slowly 5 minutes	Walk briskly 5 minutes	Walk slowly 5 minutes	15 minutes
Week 2	Walk slowly 5 minutes	Walk briskly 7 minutes	Walk slowly 5 minutes	17 minutes
Week 3	Walk slowly 5 minutes	Walk briskly 9 minutes	Walk slowly 5 minutes	19 minutes
Week 4	Walk slowly 5 minutes	Walk briskly 11 minutes	Walk slowly 5 minutes	21 minutes
Week 5	Walk slowly 5 minutes	Walk briskly 13 minutes	Walk slowly 5 minutes	23 minutes
Week 6	Walk slowly 5 minutes	Walk briskly 15 minutes	Walk slowly 5 minutes	25 minutes
Week 7	Walk slowly 5 minutes	Walk briskly 18 minutes	Walk slowly 5 minutes	28 minutes
Week 8	Walk slowly 5 minutes	Walk briskly 20 minutes	Walk slowly 5 minutes	30 minutes
Week 9	Walk slowly 5 minutes	Walk briskly 23 minutes	Walk slowly 5 minutes	33 minutes
Week 10	Walk slowly 5 minutes	Walk briskly 26 minutes	Walk slowly 5 minutes	36 minutes
Week 11	Walk slowly 5 minutes	Walk briskly 28 minutes	Walk slowly 5 minutes	38 minutes
Week 12	Walk slowly 5 minutes	Walk briskly 30 minutes	Walk slowly 5 minutes	40 minutes

From week 13 on, check your pulse periodically to see if you are exercising within your target heart rate range. As you become more fit, walk faster to increase your heart rate toward the upper levels of your target range. Follow the principle of progression.

Note: If you find a particular week's pattern tiring, repeat it before going on to the next pattern. You do not have to complete the walking program in 12 weeks. Remember that your goal is to continue getting the benefits you are seeking and enjoying your activity. Listen to your body and progress less rapidly, if necessary.

*Program should include at *least* three exercise sessions per week.

Source: U.S. Department of Health and Human Services.

capitalize on this trend—some reputable, others not. If you are interested in joining a commercial aerobic dance program, you should ask questions to see if it meets the guidelines set forth in this chapter and in chapter 3.

What are the qualifications of the instructor?

Do they screen for medical problems?

Do they use the ACSM exercise prescription guidelines in relation to intensity, duration, and frequency?

Is the program progressive in nature?

Does it allow for a warm-up and a warm-down period?

Table 4.7
Sample Aerobic Jogging Program (Interval Training)*

	Warm-up	Target Zone Exercising	Warm-down	Total Time
Week 1*	Stretch and limber up 5 minutes	Walk (nonstop) 10 minutes	Walk slowly 3 minutes; stretch 2 minutes	20 minutes
Week 2	Stretch and limber up 5 minutes	Walk 5 minutes; jog 1 minute; walk 5 minutes; jog 1 minute	Walk slowly 3 minutes; stretch 2 minutes	22 minutes
Week 3	Stretch and limber up 5 minutes	Walk 5 minutes; jog 3 minutes; walk 5 minutes; jog 3 minutes	Walk slowly 3 minutes; stretch 2 minutes	26 minutes
Week 4	Stretch and limber up 5 minutes	Walk 5 minutes; jog 4 minutes; walk 5 minutes; jog 4 minutes	Walk slowly 3 minutes; stretch 2 minutes	28 minutes
Week 5	Stretch and limber up 5 minutes	Walk 4 minutes; jog 5 minutes; walk 4 minutes; jog 5 minutes	Walk slowly 3 minutes; stretch 2 minutes	28 minutes
Week 6	Stretch and limber up 5 minutes	Walk 4 minutes; jog 6 minutes; walk 4 minutes; jog 6 minutes	Walk slowly 3 minutes; stretch 2 minutes	30 minutes
Week 7	Stretch and limber up 5 minutes	Walk 4 minutes; jog 7 minutes; walk 4 minutes; jog 7 minutes	Walk slowly 3 minutes; stretch 2 minutes	32 minutes
Week 8	Stretch and limber up 5 minutes	Walk 4 minutes; jog 8 minutes; walk 4 minutes; jog 8 minutes	Walk slowly 3 minutes; stretch 2 minutes	34 minutes
Week 9	Stretch and limber up 5 minutes	Walk 4 minutes; jog 9 minutes; walk 4 minutes; jog 9 minutes	Walk slowly 3 minutes; stretch 2 minutes	36 minutes
Week 10	Stretch and limber up 5 minutes	Walk 4 minutes; jog 13 minutes	Walk slowly 3 minutes; stretch 2 minutes	27 minutes
Week 11	Stretch and limber up 5 minutes	Walk 4 minutes; jog 15 minutes	Walk slowly 3 minutes; stretch 2 minutes	29 minutes
Week 12	Stretch and limber up 5 minutes	Walk 4 minutes; jog 17 minutes	Walk slowly 3 minutes; stretch 2 minutes	31 minutes

*Program should include *at least* three exercise sessions per week.
Source: U.S. Department of Health and Human Services.

Table 4.7
continued

	Warm-up	Target Zone Exercising	Warm-down	Total Time
Week 13	Stretch and limber up 5 minutes	Walk 2 minutes; jog slowly 2 minutes; jog 17 minutes	Walk slowly 3 minutes; stretch 2 minutes	31 minutes
Week 14	Stretch and limber up 5 minutes	Walk 1 minute; jog slowly 3 minutes; jog 17 minutes	Walk slowly 3 minutes; stretch 2 minutes	31 minutes
Week 15	Stretch and limber up 5 minutes	Jog slowly 3 minutes; jog 17 minutes	Walk slowly 3 minutes; stretch 2 minutes	30 minutes

From week 16 on, check your pulse periodically to see if you are exercising within your target zone. As you become more fit, try exercising within the upper range of your target zone.

Note: If you find a particular week's pattern tiring, repeat it before going on to the next pattern. You do not have to complete the jogging program in 15 weeks. Remember that your goal is to continue getting the benefits you are seeking and enjoying your activity.

Research has shown that aerobic dancing is an effective means to reach the target HR range, but the movements must usually be very vigorous.

It may be quite expensive to enroll in a commercial aerobic dance class. One option is to design your own aerobic exercise program to music. Simply follow these steps:

1. Select a record with a strong 4 beat count.
2. Count the total number of 4 beat counts in the record. This total will give you the total number of exercises you will do.
3. Select a series of 4 count exercises; arrange them in a logical sequence.
4. Divide the number of exercises in Step three into the total number of 4 beat counts in Step two. This gives you the number of repetitions for each exercise. For example, if you have 400 total 4 count beats in your record, and you have 10 different exercises, you will have 40 repetitions of each exercise. You might organize your exercise sequence into 10 repetitions of each exercise in sequence, and repeat each sequence 4 times to get the total 40 repetitions.
5. Design a 5–10 minute aerobic dance exercise routine.
6. Check your heart rate responses before and after your dance or exercise routine. (Determine your target HR range from table 4.3.)

Rope Jumping

A number of recent research studies have shown that rope jumping may be a very effective means to achieve the target HR range and thus is an effective mode for an aerobic fitness program. In fact, it may be too strenuous for the sedentary individual who is just beginning an exercise program. For such a person, a walking-jogging program might precede a rope jumping program. In the studies, the turn rates for the rope varied from 66–160 per minute (RPM). In order to individualize a rope jumping program in relation to your target HR range, simply follow the protocol of Laboratory Inventory 4.2 and vary the RPM of the rope for each test.

Other Aerobic Activities

Although the emphasis here has been on a walk-jog-run mode of training, the fact is that a wide variety of activities may be utilized to elicit an aerobic training effect. The interested student should consult Dr. Kenneth Cooper's *The Aerobics Way* for aerobic data on such activities as basketball, bicycling, swimming, stationary running, and many others. In essence, the application of the overload principle, using the target HR as the method to determine exercise intensity, may be used with any mode of exercise to develop your personal exercise program. Exercise in your target zone for 15–60 minutes for 3–4 days per week.

An alternative method is to select exercises presented in chapter 6 as means to control body weight. These exercises are based upon approximate caloric expenditure per minute. Appendix F has been developed to facilitate the implementation of this approach.

Benefit-Risk Ratio

Medicines are developed because they provide some benefits to us. For example, penicillin and other antibiotics help to cure infections. However, medicines may also be associated with a certain degree of risk to the patient. Some individuals are allergic to penicillin. For them the allergic reaction may be more serious than the infection it was designed to cure. As we note in the first two chapters, exercise brings significant benefits to our health, but it may also pose some risks to certain individuals.

Benefits

You may wish to review chapters 1 and 2 for a more detailed discussion relative to the potential benefits of aerobic exercise.

Potential Benefits of Aerobic Exercise
1. Reduces risk of heart attack by
   a. increasing HDL cholesterol levels
   b. reducing high blood pressure
   c. reducing the desire to smoke
   d. improving the efficiency of the heart
2. Reduces risk of developing diabetes
3. Reduces excess body weight and helps to maintain optimal weight
4. Increases resistance to stress, anxiety, and fatigue
5. Increases stamina, strength, and working ability
6. Improves self-concept

A proper aerobic exercise program, in conjunction with a proper diet and other Positive Health Life-style practices, can produce lifelong health benefits.

Risks

The risks of exercise can be categorized under five general headings: hidden heart problems; muscular soreness and injuries; heat illnesses; cold weather running risks; and safety concerns.

Hidden Heart Problems

One of the most popular forms of exercise to sweep the United States in the past decade is an aerobic program of jogging and running. Periodically, however, the communications media questions the safety of such an exercise program by publishing such articles as, "Running is dangerous to your health," or "Jogging can kill you." Occasionally, you will also read in the newspaper that a jogger died while exercising. Such incidents are likely to raise a question in your mind as to the actual safety of an exercise program. The most startling incident was the cardiac death of Jim Fixx, author of a best-seller on running, while running on a country road.

This issue has been studied by several groups of researchers, and they suggest that a small (though not negligible) risk exists of acute cardiovascular problems (such as heart attack) for adults participating in a vigorous exercise program. The prevalence of such problems is most common in individuals who are susceptible to cardiovascular problems. In most cases, deaths while jogging are observed in middle-aged men with preexisting coronary heart disease. These deaths occur in susceptible individuals who may be participating in competitive events that overexcite the heart, who are heavy smokers, or who do not exercise on a regular basis. The death rate during jogging is about seven times greater than the estimated death rate during more sedentary activities, but only in susceptible individuals. There have been no deaths reported for those whose hearts were tested and found to be healthy. Most reported deaths during jogging are in middle-aged individuals who already had a diseased heart, such as Jim Fixx.

However, one often reads of sudden deaths in young, highly trained athletes, who do not appear to have diseased hearts. In a recent review of such deaths, atherosclerotic heart disease was not a very common occurrence, although it was noted in several cases. The most common cause was a structural cardiovascular abnormality that appeared to interfere with normal heart function. Again, although different in nature, a cardiovascular problem exists in these victims prior to exercise.

Exercise may aggravate existing hidden heart problems. Individuals who may be prone to coronary heart disease should consult a physician before initiating an exercise program. This topic was previously covered rather thoroughly so you may want to consult pages 80 to 81 for a review, particularly if you are over thirty-five years of age.

Whether or not you have had a medical examination, you should be aware of symptoms occurring during or after exercise that may be indicative of cardiovascular problems. Stop exercising and consult a physician if you experience any of the following:

1. Pain in the chest under the breastbone or in the arm
2. Irregular pulse rate (flutters, or changes rate very rapidly—either too fast or too slow)
3. Palpitations in the chest or throat
4. Dizziness, light-headedness, confusion, or fainting

Figure 4.15 Body Signals to Stop Exercising. If you experience any of these symptoms during exercise, stop immediately and rest. Consult a physician if they persist.

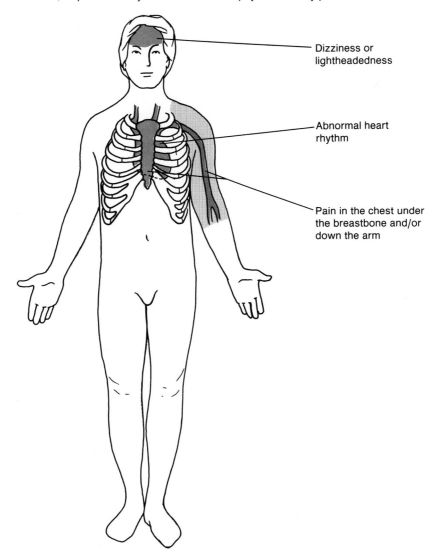

Dizziness or lightheadedness

Abnormal heart rhythm

Pain in the chest under the breastbone and/or down the arm

Muscular Soreness and Injuries

If you develop and implement an exercise program properly, you should experience little, if any, problems as you continue to train. The key to avoiding problems is to start easily and progress slowly. However, most individuals overdo it at one time or another, and eventually end up with either sore muscles or an injury.

Basically there are two types of muscle soreness. *Acute soreness* occurs during exercise and appears to be due to inadequate circulation to the exercising muscle. The lack of blood flow leads to an accumulation of metabolic by-products of exercise in the muscle. These by-products can stimulate pain receptors, and cause pain or soreness, which usually disappears when you stop exercising. A second type is called *delayed soreness*. This usually occurs 24–48 hours after an exercise period, and may persist for several days. This type of muscle soreness is usually caused by exercise bouts that involve repetitive, strenuous muscle contractions. For example, as you run downhill you put a tremendous stress on the leg muscles as they try to control your body from moving too fast (due to gravity's pull). This stress appears to tear the connective tissue and/or muscle fibers, causing inflammation that, according to the most current theory, may be the cause of the delayed soreness. A stretching program may be helpful for relief, but generally rest and/or reduced activity levels for several days are necessary to let the soreness run its course and gradually fade away.

Muscle soreness will usually limit exercise for a few days at the most. However, an injury may incapacitate you for months—depending upon its type and severity. All individuals who become physically active can, at one time or another, expect to be injured. Certain types of activities predispose to a specific injury (bruised palms in handball; heel bruises in running). In many cases, injuries can be prevented by the use of proper equipment, technique, and conditioning, but even these factors are not able to prevent some acute injuries that happen very suddenly (a sprained ankle due to uneven terrain; a sprained wrist incurred during a fall).

A common cause of several types of injuries is overuse, particularly during the early stages of an exercise program. As you begin an exercise program, you make rapid gains in fitness, which often encourages you to overexert yourself. For example, your normal progression on a jogging program may call for a 2 mile jog, but you may feel good and decide to do 5 miles that day. The next day, you feel some tenderness in your shin bone, Achilles tendon, or knee. It may not be sore enough to prevent you from running, so you continue to overdo it. Eventually, the pain gets so severe that you must stop training due to a case of shin splints, Achilles tendinitis, or chondromalacia of the knee. You are a victim of the overuse syndrome. Hence, one of the keys to injury prevention is to follow a proper progression in your training program and avoid sudden increases in the intensity and duration of exercise.

Space does not permit a full coverage of all the means to prevent injuries in all types of activities, but the following may be helpful.

1. Warm up thoroughly before your activity. Stretching exercises for the Achilles tendon and groin area are helpful before jogging or running. See chapter 8 for appropriate stretching exercises.
2. Do not progress too rapidly in the early stages of training. Take it easy and follow a gradual progression.
3. Listen to your body. Minor aches and pains are early warning signals. If they persist when you are resting, lay off for a day or so to help avoid developing a more serious condition. Minor aches and pains may be relieved by rest, aspirin, and ice applied directly to the injured area.

Figure 4.16 Exercise in the heat may lead to weakness or severe heat injury if proper precautions are not taken.

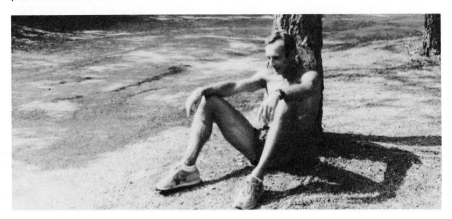

4. Try to avoid situations that may change your running biomechanics and lead to ankle, knee, or hip problems. Avoid running too much in one direction on a slanted road. Keep the soles of your shoes in good repair so that one side is not worn down excessively. Avoid a lot of downhill running. Check your shoes for proper fit so your foot does not roll in toward the inside excessively.

5. Avoid hard surfaces (concrete surfaces for jogging and hard floors for aerobic dancing and rope jumping) as persistent impact may contribute to shin splints.

Heat Illnesses

Be aware of the signs of heat illnesses when exercising in the hot weather. Excessive fatigue, weakness, nausea, and cramps may be indicative of heat exhaustion. Headache, disorientation, and a high body temperature may signal the onset of heat stroke. If you experience these symptoms, stop exercising, seek a cool place to rest, and drink cool fluids.

The following suggestions may be helpful in the prevention of heat illnesses.

1. Check the temperature and humidity conditions before exercising. Adjust your intensity as needed. Hot humid conditions cause fatigue sooner, so slow your pace or decrease the duration of your activity.

2. Exercise in the cool of the morning or evening in order to avoid the heat of the day.

3. Exercise in the shade, if possible, in order to avoid radiation from the sun.

4. Wear as little clothing as possible. That which is worn should be loose to allow air circulation, white to reflect radiant heat, and porous to permit evaporation to occur. In particular, avoid the use of plastic or rubberized sweatsuits.

5. Drink fluids periodically. If on a long training run, have your route planned so you know where some watering holes may be (gas stations or other public sources of water). Take frequent water breaks, consuming about 6–8 ounces of water every 15 minutes or so. During exercise, thirst is not an adequate stimulus to replace water losses, so you should drink before you get thirsty. To help cool down, pour water over your head and chest also.

6. Replenish your water daily. Keep a record of your body weight. For each pound you lose, drink 1 pint of fluid. Your body weight should be back to normal before your next exercise workout.

7. Hyperhydrate if you plan to perform prolonged strenuous exercise in the heat. This means drinking about 16–32 ounces of fluid 30–60 minutes prior to exercising.

8. Replenish lost electrolytes (salt) if you have sweated excessively.
Put a little extra salt on your meals, and eat foods high in potassium, such as bananas and citrus fruits. Additional information on nutrition is presented in chapter 5.

9. If you are sedentary, overweight, or older, you are less likely to tolerate exercise in the heat and should, therefore, use extra caution.

10. If you are going to compete in a sport that is held under hot environmental conditions, you must become acclimatized to exercise in the heat. You can do this by exercising in the heat for 7–9 days before the event, but at a much reduced intensity. Your body will gradually adjust to exercise in the heat, but you still will not be able to perform as well as you will in cooler weather.

If you are monitoring your heart rate as a guide to your training intensity, you will probably note that you have a higher exercise heart rate at a lower exercise intensity while performing in the heat. The need to channel extra blood to both your muscles and skin (for cooling purposes) imposes an additional work load on the heart. Consequently, exercise intensity must be reduced somewhat in order not to exceed the recommended target HR range.

Cold Weather Running

Cold weather does not usually pose a problem if you dress properly for it. Some general suggestions are:

1. Cover your head, hands, and wrists. Your head and neck can lose up to 40 percent of your body heat, and you feel warmer if your hands and wrists are warm.

2. Wear several layers of light clothing with a windbreaker on the outside. Some of the newer cold weather running gear is designed to be lightweight, yet very warm, and allows for sweat to dissipate without getting your clothing too wet.

Properly dressed, you can exercise outside in almost any weather. However, if you would prefer to stay inside and avoid the cold, home aerobic exercise programs such as stationary bicycling, treadmill running, jogging in place, stair climbing, rope skipping, and aerobic dancing can be beneficial alternatives.

Safety Concerns

As with injuries, space will not permit a full coverage of the safety concerns associated with all aerobic activities, but the following suggestions may be helpful.

1. Use proper equipment, such as eye goggles for handball and raquetball sports.
2. Joggers and runners should be on the lookout for cars. Be cautious at all intersections. If you must run on the road, run facing traffic. Wear light-colored clothing or reflective material at night. Do not assume that drivers see you. You should also avoid heavy traffic areas for another reason. Research has shown that running in polluted air exposes you to potentially harmful effects of carbon monoxide. If you must run in such areas, try to run on the side of the road where the wind is blowing the automobile pollutants away from you.
3. Bicyclists should use all safety devices available, including reflectors, flags, and a safety helmet. Ride in the direction of traffic. Seek out bike trails, not busy roads.
4. Never swim alone.

Practice taking the heart rate (HR) via the technique described on page 85. Practice finding the pulse as rapidly as possible so that it may be found readily when needed. Practice taking the HR in pairs, you (the subject) taking your own radial pulse while your partner takes your carotid pulse.

Take the HR under the following situations:

1. Lying down after 3 minutes
2. Sitting after 3 minutes
3. Standing after 3 minutes
4. After doing vigorous jumping jacks for 1 minute (same number each time), record the heart rate during:
   a. a 10 second period from 5–15 seconds after the cessation of exercise
   b. a 30 second period after 1 minute of recovery (1–1½ minutes after exercise)
   c. a 30 second period after 2 minutes of recovery (2–2½ minutes after exercise)

Record your heart rate results below:

	Date____	Date____	Date____	Date____	Date____
Lying down	____	____	____	____	____
Sitting	____	____	____	____	____
Standing	____	____	____	____	____
5–15 seconds after exercise	____	____	____	____	____
1–1½ minutes after exercise	____	____	____	____	____
2–2½ minutes after exercise	____	____	____	____	____

The following procedure is based upon a walk-jog-run mode of exercise, but it may be adapted to other modes such as bicycling, swimming, rope jumping, aerobic dancing, and others. Simply increase the intensity of the exercise and observe the effect on the heart rate.

1. Determine your resting heart rate (RHR) in a relaxed state, preferably just before getting up in the morning. The RHR should also be taken several times a day, after you have been resting for the previous hour or so.

2. Based upon your RHR and your age, consult table 4.3 to determine your target HR range.

3. Mark a ½ mile course. Two laps on a ¼ mile course is ideal. If you do not have an accurately measured track area available, you may have to design one yourself. There are measuring wheels available, but a simple technique is the following:
   a. Find a measured distance, such as a 100 yard football field.
   b. Walk the distance at your normal pace and count the number of steps you take. Do it several times to insure accuracy.
   c. Calculate the average number of yards you cover per step. For example, if you take 120 steps to walk 100 yards, your average distance per step is .833 yards (100 yards/120 steps).
   d. Using sidewalks, fields, or other areas by your home, mark off a circular or elliptical course, which measures ½ mile (880 yards). You may wish to place markers at 220 yard (⅛ mile) intervals to facilitate recording your pace. A steady pace is reflected by nearly equal times for each of the four 220 yard segments in the ½ mile.

4. Measure your RHR again before you begin to exercise.

5. Walk until you have settled into an even pace, and then time yourself for the ½ mile. Immediately measure your heart rate for 10 seconds at the conclusion of the exercise. It is important to measure your recovery heart rate immediately so that it very closely represents your exercise heart rate. Also, during your walk or run, mentally record your RPE as explained on page 87.

6. Record your heart rate and RPE in the chart and plot them on the graph. Try to relate the RPE to your heart rate.

7. If you do not reach your target heart rate, rest until your RHR returns to nearly normal (within 5–10 beats) and then repeat the ½ mile test at a faster pace. Again record your heart rate and RPE.

8. Repeat this procedure until you have plotted a pattern of your heart rate and RPE. You should be exercising at least to the 60 percent level. You may also use this technique to get to the 90 percent level.

9. You may use this technique to determine your true HR max. Keep increasing your speed for the ½ mile until you can go no faster. This procedure should be done only when you are fairly well-conditioned.

Record your results below:

	Date___	Date___	Date___	Date___	Date___
Target HR for training effect*					
Resting HR	___	___	___	___	___
Predicted HR max (220 − age)	___	___	___	___	___
60% of HR reserve	___	___	___	___	___
90% of HR reserve	___	___	___	___	___
½ mile test					
Trial 1					
Time	___	___	___	___	___
Minutes/mile	___	___	___	___	___
HR	___	___	___	___	___
RPE	___	___	___	___	___
Trial 2					
Time	___	___	___	___	___
Minutes/mile	___	___	___	___	___
HR	___	___	___	___	___
RPE	___	___	___	___	___
Trial 3					
Time	___	___	___	___	___
Minutes/mile	___	___	___	___	___
HR	___	___	___	___	___
RPE	___	___	___	___	___
Trial 4					
Time	___	___	___	___	___
Minutes/mile	___	___	___	___	___
HR	___	___	___	___	___
RPE	___	___	___	___	___

To calculate minutes/mile, simply double your ½ mile time. For example, ½ mile time of 5:40 is an 11:20 mile.

*Example: Individual 20 years old. RHR = 70. THR = X% (HR max − RHR) + RHR

60% Target HR = .60 (200 − 70) + 70 = 148
90% Target HR = .90 (200 − 70) + 70 = 187

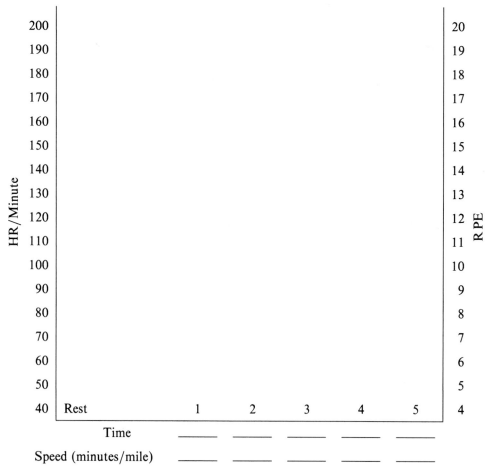

Record resting HR and RPE at rest, then plot HR and RPE at different speeds. See figure 4.12 for an example.

Administer one of the following tests:

a. 3 mile walking test (no running)

b. 1½ mile running test

The person taking the test should have medical clearance and should have been exercising for 6–8 weeks prior to the test. Some other guidelines for taking these tests are presented on pages 78–79. It is helpful if the person is instructed to keep an even pace throughout the test, rather than going out too fast or too slow in the early stages, since the test requires a nearly exhaustive effort.

Other helpful suggestions include:

1. Rest both the day before and the day of the test.
2. Practice at the actual distance or time several times before the test day.
3. Refrain from eating and smoking for at least 2–3 hours prior to the test.
4. Warm up adequately.
5. Have someone keep you aware of your pace time.
6. Warm down after the test by walking or reducing the intensity of the activity.

Tables in appendix D represent the fitness categories for two of the tests developed by Cooper. On the appropriate table for your test, find your age category across the top row, locate your sex in the second column, then find the entry that corresponds to your time or distance. For example, an eighteen-year-old female who walked 3 miles in 34 minutes is in the *excellent* fitness category. If a nineteen-year-old male ran the 1½ mile test in 11:22, in what fitness category would he be? The answer is *fair*.

Once you have determined the fitness category, consult Table D.3 to predict the $\dot{V}O_2$ max in ml O_2/kg/minute. For the eighteen-year-old female, you would predict 39.0–41.9 ml O_2/kg/minute. The nineteen-year-old male should be 38.4–45.1 ml O_2/kg/minute.

Test Taken:

_____ 3 mile walk (no running)

_____ 1½ mile running

	Date____	Date____	Date____	Date____	Date____
Time or distance	____	____	____	____	____
Fitness level	____	____	____	____	____
Predicted $\dot{V}O_2$ max (ml O_2/kg/min)	____	____	____	____	____

Step tests have been developed for two purposes—to predict aerobic fitness, and to help evaluate the effects of training. Keep in mind the limitations of step tests as a means to predict aerobic fitness, as discussed in this chapter. The 3 minute step test does have a fitness prediction scale, but is best utilized to evaluate a training effect. You may wish to design your own test for this purpose by using available equipment such as bleacher steps, chairs, locker room benches, etc. Simply establish a rate of stepping such as 18, 24, 30, or 36 4-count steps per minute, and an appropriate test length (3–5 minutes).

When administering any step test it is important that the individual maintain the cadence of the stepping. This is critical as it determines the work rate. A metronome or tape recording may be used to expedite maintenance of cadence. One step involves 4 beats on the metronome: left up, right up, left down, right down. The individual should completely straighten the knees when coming to the standing position on the bench. It may be advisable to alternate stepping legs so that one leg does not do all the work and develop soreness.

Three Minute Step Test
The 3 minute step test has been developed by Mead and Hartwig for men and women ages 18–26.

Bench height:	12 inches
Stepping cadence:	24 steps/minute
Duration:	3 minutes
Heart rate:	Sit down immediately and record heart rate for exactly 1 minute

Fitness Index	Males	Females
Superior	68	73
Excellent	69–75	74–82
Good	76–83	83–90
Average	84–92	91–100
Fair	93–99	101–107
Poor	100–106	108–114
Very poor	>107	>115

Figures represent heart rate response as measured for 1 minute immediately after the step test.

Source: From "A Comparison of the Exercise Tolerance of Post-Rheumatic and Normal Boys," by Frederick Kasch, in *Journal of the Association of Physical and Mental Rehabilitation* 15:35, 1961. © 1961 American Corrective Therapy Association. Reprinted by permission.

Record your step test results:

	Date____	Date____	Date____	Date____	Date____
Resting HR*	____	____	____	____	____
Recovery HR (1 minute)	____	____	____	____	____
Fitness index	____	____	____	____	____

*Resting heart rate is not necessary, but may be of interest to the student from test to test.

For your own individual step test, use the following form to tabulate your data.

	Date____	Date____	Date____	Date____	Date____
Individual step test					
Step height	____	____	____	____	____
Cadence	____	____	____	____	____
Duration	____	____	____	____	____
Resting HR	____	____	____	____	____
Recovery HR (1 minute)	____	____	____	____	____

Laboratory Inventory 4.5
Exercise Prescription and Contract

Name _____ Age _____

Inclusive dates _____ to _____

Training Heart Rate

Resting HR (RHR) _____

HR max
  Predicted _____
  Actual _____

Target HR Levels

Target HR = X%(HR max − RHR) + RHR

60% _____
70% _____
80% _____
90% _____

Fitness goals:
  Short-term _____
  _____
  Long-term _____
  _____

Exercise prescription:
  Mode _____
  Warm-up _____
  Warm-down _____

Stimulus period	Date____	Date____	Date____	Date____	Date____
Intensity	____	____	____	____	____
Duration	____	____	____	____	____
Frequency	____	____	____	____	____

By my signature below, I do hereby commit myself to this exercise prescription and will do everything in my power to complete this prescription and attain my short-term and/or long-term fitness goals. I know that the successful completion of this exercise prescription will help me to become a regular exerciser and may lead to a lifetime commitment to health through improved physical fitness.

_____   _____

Name (signed)   Date

_____

Witness

References

Abraham, W. "Exercise-Induced Muscle Soreness." *The Physician and Sportsmedicine* 7:57–60 (October 1979).

American College of Sports Medicine. "Quantity and Quality of Exercise for Developing and Maintaining Fitness in Healthy Adults." *The Physician and Sportsmedicine* 6:39–41 (October 1978).

American Medical Association Council on Scientific Affairs. "Indications and Contraindications for Exercise Testing." *Journal of the American Medical Association* 246:1015–18 (1981).

Astrand, P. O., and Rodahl, K. *Textbook of Work Physiology.* New York: McGraw-Hill, 1977.

Barnard, R. J. "The Heart Needs Warm-Up Time." *The Physician and Sportsmedicine* 4:40 (January 1976).

Baumgartner, T., and Jackson, A. *Measurement for Evaluation in Physical Education.* Dubuque, IA: Wm. C. Brown Publishers, 1982.

Borg, G. "Perceived Exertion: A Note on 'History' and Methods." *Medicine and Science in Sports* 5:90–93 (1973).

Brown, R. "Jogging: Its Uses and Abuses." *Virginia Medicine* 106:522–23 (1979).

CIBA Foundation. *Human Muscle Fatigue: Physiological Mechanisms.* London: Pitman Medical, 1981.

Clarke, H. "Jogging." *Physical Fitness Research Digest* 7:1–23 (January 1977).

——— . "Rope Skipping—Dancing—Walking and Golf-Pack Carrying." *Physical Fitness Research Digest* 7:1–21 (October 1977).

——— . "Swimming and Bicycling." *Physical Fitness Research Digest* 7:1–22 (July 1977).

Cooper, K. *The Aerobics Program for Total Well Being.* New York: M. Evans, 1982.

——— . *The Aerobics Way.* New York: M. Evans, 1977.

Cureton, K. "Distance Running Performance Tests in Children." *Journal of Health, Physical Education, Recreation and Dance* 53:64–66 (October 1982).

Daniels, J.; Fitts, R.; and Sheehan, G. *Conditioning for Distance Running.* New York: John Wiley & Sons, 1978.

Dimsdale, J.; Hartley, L. H.; Guiney, T; et al. "Postexercise Peril: Plasma Catecholamines and Exercise." *Journal of the American Medical Association* 251: 630–32 (1984).

Fisher, A. G. "How Can I Use Heart Rate to Prescribe an Exercise Program?" In *Conditioning and Physical Fitness,* edited by P. Allsen. Dubuque, IA: Wm. C. Brown Publishers, 1978.

Fox, E., and Mathews, D. *Interval Training.* Philadelphia: W. B. Saunders, 1974.

——— . *The Physiological Basis of Physical Education and Athletics.* Philadelphia: Saunders College Publishing, 1981.

Froelicher, V., and Grouse, D. "The Pluses and Minuses of Exercise Testing." *Geriatrics* 35:120–26 (1980).

Gardner, J., and Purdy, J. *Computerized Running Training Programs.* Los Altos, CA: TAFNEWS Press, 1970.

Gibbons, L.; Cooper, K.; Meyer, B.; and Ellison, C. "The Acute Cardiac Risk of Strenuous Exercise." *Journal of the American Medical Association* 244:1799–1801 (1980).

Greer, N., and Katch, F. "Validity of Palpation Recovery Pulse Rate to Estimate Exercise Heart Rate Following Four Intensities of Bench Step Exercise." *Research Quarterly for Exercise and Sport* 53:340–43 (1982).

Hage, P. "Air Pollution: Adverse Effects on Athletic Performance." *The Physician and Sportsmedicine* 10:126 (1982).

———. "Exercise Guidelines: Which to Believe?" *The Physician and Sportsmedicine* 10:23 (June 1982).

———. "Prescribing Exercise: More than Just a Running Program." *The Physician and Sportsmedicine* 11:123–31 (May 1983).

Hagerman, F.; Hikida, R.; Staron, R.; et al. "Muscle Fiber Necrosis in Marathon Runners." *Medicine and Science in Exercise and Sports* 15:164 (1983).

Henritze, J.; Weltman, A.; Schurrer, R.; and Barlow, K. "Effects of Training above and below the Onset of Blood Lactate Accumulation (OBLA) on Cardiovascular and Body Composition Parameters in Women." *Medicine and Science in Sports and Exercise* 14:114 (1982).

Higdon, H. "Training." *The Runner* 4:52–53 (August 1982).

Hubbard, R. "Effects of Exercise in the Heat on Predisposition to Heat Stroke." *Medicine and Science in Sports* 11:66–71 (1979).

Illinois Governor's Council on Health and Fitness. "Walking as an Exercise." Springfield, IL: IGCPF.

Johnson, J., and Siegel, D. "The Use of Selected Submaximal Step Tests in Predicting Change in the Maximal Oxygen Intake of College Women." *Journal of Sports Medicine and Physical Fitness* 21:259–64 (1981).

Karpovich, P. V., and Sinning, W. *Physiology of Muscular Activity.* Philadelphia: W. B. Saunders, 1971.

Kinderman, W.; Simon, G.; and Keul, J. "The Significance of the Aerobic-Anaerobic Transition for the Determination of Work Load Intensities during Endurance Training." *European Journal of Applied Physiology* 42:25–34 (September 1979).

Legwold, G. "Does Aerobic Dance Offer More Fun than Fitness?" *The Physician and Sportsmedicine* 10:147 (September 1982).

Londeree, B., and Moeschberger, M. "Effect of Age and Other Factors on Maximal Heart Rate." *Research Quarterly for Exercise and Sport* 53:297–304 (1982).

MacDougall, D., and Sale, D. "Continuous vs. Interval Training: A Review for the Athlete and Coach." *Canadian Journal of Applied Sport Sciences* 6:93–97 (1981).

Maron, B.; Roberts, W.; McAllister, M.; Epstein, S.; and Rosing, D. "Sudden Death in Young Athletes." *Circulation* 62:218–29 (1980).

Mead, W., and Hartwig, R. "Fitness Evaluation and Exercise Prescription." *Journal of Family Practice* 13:1039–50 (1981).

Morgan, W. P. "Psychophysiology of Self-Awareness during Vigorous Physical Activity." *Research Quarterly of Exercise and Sport* 52:385–427 (1981).

Myles, W.; Dick, M.; and Jantti, R. "Heart Rate and Rope Skipping Intensity." *Research Quarterly for Exercise and Sport* 52:76–79 (1981).

National Heart, Lung and Blood Institute. *Exercise and Your Heart.* Washington, DC: U.S. Government Printing Office, 1981.

Nicholson, J., and Case, D. "Carboxyhemoglobin Levels in New York City Runners." *The Physician and Sportsmedicine* 11:135–38 (March 1983).

Pearl, A. "Heat and Physical Activity." *Journal of the Florida Medical Association* 67:396–98 (1980).

Pollock, M.; Broida, J.; and Kendrick, Z. "Validity of the Palpation Technique of Heart Rate Determination and Its Estimation of Training Heart Rate." *Research Quarterly* 43:77–81 (1972).

President's Council on Physical Fitness and Sports. *Adult Fitness Manual.* Washington, DC: U.S. Government Printing Office.

——— . *Aerobic Dancing.* Washington, DC: PCPFS.

——— . *Jogging Guidelines.* Washington, DC: PCPFS.

Quirk, J., and Sinning, W. "Anaerobic and Aerobic Responses of Males and Females to Rope Skipping." *Medicine and Science in Sports and Exercise* 14:26–29 (1982).

Saltin, B., and Rowell, L. "Functional Adaptations of Physical Activity and Inactivity." *Federation Proceedings* 39:1506–13 (1980).

Shoenfeld, Y.; Keren, G.; Shimoni, T.; Birnfeld, C.; and Sohar, E. "Walking: A Method for Rapid Improvement of Physical Fitness." *Journal of the American Medical Association* 243:2062–63 (1980).

Smith, J.; Dressendorfer, R.; Borysyk, L.; Gordon, S.; and Timmis, G. "Failure of the Karvonen Formula to Accurately Estimate Training Heart Rate in Coronary Artery Disease Patients." *Medicine and Science in Sports and Exercise* 14:149 (1982).

Smutok, M.; Skrinar, G.; and Pandolf, K. "Exercise Intensity: Subjective Regulation by Perceived Exertion." *Archives of Physical and Medical Rehabilitation* 61:569–74 (1980).

Thompson, P.; Funk, E.; Carleton, R.; and Sturner, W. "Sudden Death during Jogging: A Study of the Rhode Island Population from 1975 through 1980." *Medicine and Science of Sports and Exercise* 14:115 (1982).

Weltman, A., and Stamford, B. "Home Aerobic Exercise Programs." *The Physician and Sportsmedicine* 11:210 (February 1983).

Williams, M. H. *Nutritional Aspects of Human Physical and Athletic Performance.* Springfield, IL: C. C. Thomas, 1976.

Wilmore, J. H. "Acute and Chronic Physiological Responses to Exercise." In *Exercise in Cardiovascular Health and Disease,* edited by E. Amsterdam, J. Wilmore, and A. DeMaria. New York: Yorke Medical Books, 1977.

——— . "Individual Exercise Prescription." In *Exercise in Cardiovascular Health and Disease,* edited by E. Amsterdam, J. Wilmore, and A. DeMaria. New York: Yorke Medical Books, 1977.

Zeppilli, P., and Venerando, A. "Sudden Death and Physical Exertion." *Journal of Sports Medicine and Physical Fitness* 21:299–300 (1981).

Zohman, L. *Run for Life.* Hartford: Connecticut Mutual Life Insurance Company, 1978.

5 Basic Nutrition for Healthful Eating

Key Terms

amino acids
Basic Four Food Groups
carbohydrates
cholesterol
complex carbohydrates
essential amino acids
fats
fatty acids
fiber
Food Exchange Lists
glucose
glycogen

hydrogenated fats
key nutrient concept
lipids
mineral
nutrient density
nutritional labeling
ovolactovegetarian
phytates
polyunsaturated fatty
  acids
protein
protein complementarity

Recommended Dietary
  Allowances (RDA)
*Recommended Dietary
  Goals*
saturated fatty acid
simple carbohydrates
triglycerides
United States
  Recommended Daily
  Allowances (U.S. RDA)
vegetarian
vitamins
water

Key Concepts

The human body has a need for over forty different nutrients that are found in six general classes—carbohydrates, fats, protein, vitamins, minerals, and water.

Carbohydrates, fats, and protein are the energy nutrients, while protein, vitamins, minerals, and water help to build body tissues and regulate metabolic processes.

The protein in foods from animal sources contains the eight essential amino acids we need to include in our diet, but proper combinations of different plant foods also provide these essential amino acids.

Vitamin and mineral supplements are not necessary for an individual on a well-balanced diet.

Water has a number of important roles in the body. For the physically active person, water is essential as a means to prevent excessive body temperature while exercising in the heat.

If your diet is adequate in the eight key nutrients—protein, vitamin A, vitamin C, thiamin, riboflavin, niacin, iron, and calcium—you should be receiving an ample supply of all the nutrients essential to humans.

Nutritional labeling can be a valuable asset in helping you select foods that have high nutrient density (significant amounts of the key nutrients in low-Calorie foods).

The Basic Four Food Groups and the Exchange Lists are two practical means to enable you to obtain a well-balanced diet.

Eight general recommendations for healthier nutrition include: (1) maintaining an ideal body weight, (2) consuming a wide variety of natural foods, (3) eating adequate amounts of protein, (4) decreasing the intake of total fat, saturated fat, and cholesterol, (5) reducing consumption of refined sugar, (6) increasing the dietary proportion of complex carbohydrates and natural sugars, (7) decreasing salt intake, and (8) moderating alcohol consumption.

Although a vegetarian diet may be a healthful way to obtain the nutrients you need, so too is a well-balanced diet containing wisely selected animal products.

Introduction

Within the past decade there has been a phenomenal increase in knowledge about all facets of life, including the science of nutrition. Thousands of studies have been and are being conducted in order to discover the intricacies of how the various nutrients function in the body, and their role in the overall health of the individual. All of the answers are not in, but sufficient evidence is available to provide us with some useful guidelines for healthful eating practices.

This chapter provides you with sufficient knowledge of the nutritional needs of healthy individuals so that you can plan and eat a healthier diet. The three major sections in this chapter deal with the major nutrients, the basis of dietary planning, and general guides to healthier eating.

The Major Nutrients

There are six general classes of nutrients that are considered necessary in human nutrition. They are carbohydrates, fats, protein, vitamins, minerals, and water. Within several of these general classes (notably protein, vitamins, and minerals), there are a number of specific nutrients necessary for life. For example, over a dozen vitamins are needed for optimal physiological functioning. Table 5.1 represents the specific nutrients that are essential to humans.

There are three major functions of food; the six nutrients are necessary to fulfill these functions. First, foods provide energy for human metabolism; carbohydrates and fats are the prime sources of energy. Although protein may also provide energy, that is not its major function. Vitamins, minerals, and water are not energy sources. Second, foods are used to build and repair body tissues; protein is the major building material for muscles and other soft tissues, while certain minerals such as calcium and phosphorus make up the skeletal framework. Third, foods are used to help regulate body processes; vitamins, minerals, and proteins work closely together in order to maintain the diverse physiological processes of human metabolism. Let us look briefly at each of the six nutrients and their roles in human nutrition.

Carbohydrate

Carbohydrates are the basic foodstuffs that are formed when the energy from the sun is harnessed in plants. They are organic compounds that contain carbon, hydrogen, and oxygen in various combinations. Their major function in human nutrition is to provide a source of energy.

Carbohydrates are one of the least expensive forms of Calories to produce, and, hence, represent one of the major food supplies for the vast majority of the world's population. In general terms, carbohydrates may be categorized as either simple or complex. **Simple carbohydrates** are usually known as sugars. Although there are many different types of sugars, the most common one is sucrose, or table sugar.

The **complex carbohydrates** are commonly known as starches. The vast majority of carbohydrates that exist in the plant world are in this form. Of prime interest to us

Table 5.1
Essential Nutrients

1. Protein (essential amino acids)

Isoleucine	Threonine
Leucine	Tryptophan
Lysine	Valine
Methionine	Histidine (for children, but not adults)
Phenylalanine	

2. Fats (essential fatty acids)

Linoleic

3. Carbohydrates

Fiber

4. Vitamins

Water-soluble	**Fat-soluble**
B Complex	A (Retinol)
B_1 (Thiamin)	D
B_2 (Riboflavin)	E (Tocopherol)
Niacin	K
B_6 (Pyridoxine)	
Pantothenic acid	
Folacin	
B_{12} (Cyanocobalamin)	
Biotin	
C (Ascorbic acid)	

5. Minerals

Calcium	Iron	Selenium
Chloride	Magnesium	Silicon
Chromium	Manganese	Sodium
Cobalt	Molybdenum	Sulfur
Copper	Nickel	Tin
Fluoride	Phosphorus	Vanadium
Iodine	Potassium	Zinc

6. Water

Essential nutrients are necessary for human life. An inadequate intake may result in disturbed body metabolism, certain disease states, or death.

Some of the nutrients listed have been shown to be essential for various animals, and are probably essential for humans. Essential nutrients, or nutrients from which they may be formed, must be obtained from the foods we eat.

are the plant starches, through which we obtain a good proportion of our daily Calories, along with a wide variety of nutrients. An important component of the complex carbohydrates is fiber. **Fiber** is found in all plants. In general, fiber is an inert substance that does not break down in the presence of human digestive enzymes. Hence, dietary fiber adds bulk to our diet, which is important for the health of the intestines.

Table 5.2
Foods High in Carbohydrate

Bread List	Fruit List	Vegetable List
Beans	Apples	Beets
Biscuits	Apricots	Carrots
Bread	Bananas	Cauliflower
Cereal	Cantaloupe	Eggplant
Corn	Cherries	Squash
Crackers	Dried fruits	String beans
Grits	Figs	Tomatoes
Macaroni	Oranges	Zucchini
Muffins	Peaches	
Noodles	Pineapple	
Peas		
Potatoes		
Rice		
Spaghetti		
Waffles		
Yams		

Some foods that are high in carbohydrate content are found in table 5.2. For the most part, all dietary carbohydrate is digested and eventually converted to **glucose,** a very simple carbohydrate. Blood glucose may have several metabolic fates. It may be utilized directly by some tissues for energy, or it may be stored as **glycogen** (a complex carbohydrate) in the liver and muscles. Excess blood glucose may be excreted in the urine, or converted into fat and stored in the body's adipose tissue. Figure 5.1 illustrates the general fates of blood glucose.

Fat

Although fat is one of the most criticized nutrients, it does play a rather significant role in human nutrition and in human physiological functioning. Dietary fat is a source of energy, and helps to provide the essential fatty acids and fat-soluble vitamins (A, D, E, and K) for the regulation of human metabolism.

The fat content in foods can vary from 100 percent, as found in most cooking oils, to less than 1 percent, as found in most fruits and vegetables. The fat content of some foods, such as butter, oils, shortening, mayonnaise, and margarine is obvious. In other foods, the fat content may be high but not as obvious, as in meat, milk, cheese, nuts, desserts, and some vegetables and cereals. The percentage of Calories in the fat contained in some common foods is presented in table 5.3.

Fats, also known as **lipids,** represent a general term for a number of different compounds found in the body in the forms of both solid fat and liquid oils. The three major classes are triglycerides, sterols (such as cholesterol), and phospholipids. The fats of major interest to us are the triglycerides, or neutral fats, for this is the primary form in which fats are eaten and stored in the human body. **Triglycerides** are composed of two different compounds—fatty acids and glycerol.

Figure 5.1 Fates of Blood Glucose. After assimilation into the blood, glucose may be stored in the liver or muscles as glycogen or be utilized as a source of energy by these and other tissues, particularly the nervous system. Excess glucose may be partially excreted by the kidneys, but major excesses are converted to fat and stored in the adipose tissues.
Source: From Williams, Melvin H. *Nutrition for Fitness and Sport.* © 1983, Wm. C. Brown Publishers, Dubuque, Iowa. All Rights Reserved. Reprinted by Permission.

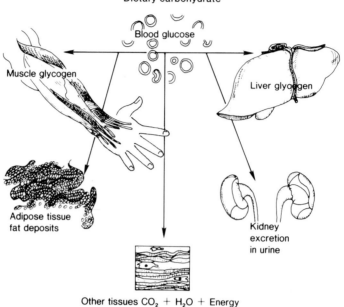

Dietary carbohydrate

Blood glucose

Muscle glycogen

Liver glycogen

Adipose tissue
fat deposits

Kidney
excretion
in urine

Other tissues CO_2 + H_2O + Energy

Fatty acids, one of the components of fat, are chains of carbon and hydrogen atoms that vary in the degree of hydrogen saturation. A **saturated fatty acid** contains a full quota of hydrogen; unsaturated fatty acids may absorb more hydrogen. These latter fatty acids may be classified as monounsaturated (capable of absorbing two more hydrogen ions), and **polyunsaturated fatty acids** (capable of absorbing four or more hydrogen ions). Saturated fats are usually solid; unsaturated fats are usually liquid. **Hydrogenated fats** or oils have been treated by a process that adds hydrogen to some of the unfilled bonds, thus hardening the fat or oil. In essence, the fat becomes more saturated. The health implications of these different types of fats are discussed later in this chapter.

Cholesterol is not a fat; it is a fatlike pearly substance found in animal tissues. Cholesterol is found only in animal products, and is not found in fruits, vegetables, nuts, grains, or other plant sources. Cholesterol is vital to human physiology, but since it may be manufactured in the body from either fats, carbohydrate, or protein, there is apparently little need for us to obtain it in the foods we eat. As you may recall from chapter 2, a positive relationship has been established between blood cholesterol levels and coronary heart disease, so reduction of dietary cholesterol has been advocated by a number of health-related associations. Refer back to chapter 2 for a discussion of

Table 5.3
Fat and Saturated Fat Content in Some Common Foods

Food Exchange	Total Fat (% Calories)	Saturated Fat (% Calories)
Meat List		
Bacon	80	30
Beef, lean only	32	13
Ham	70	23
Hamburger, regular	62	29
Chicken, breast	23	8
Sausage, pork	79	29
Haddock	32	6
Eggs, whole	67	22
Beans, dry navy	4	—
Peanut butter	76	19
Milk List		
Milk, whole	45	28
Milk, skim	trace	trace
Cheese, cheddar	62	39
Vegetable List		
Beans, green	trace	trace
Carrots	trace	trace
Potatoes	trace	trace
Fruit List		
Bananas	trace	trace
Oranges	trace	trace
Bread List		
Bread	12	—
Cake, plain sheet	31	8
Crackers	18	—
Doughnuts	43	7
Macaroni	5	—
Macaroni and cheese	46	20
Oatmeal	13	—
Pancakes, wheat	30	—
Rolls, dinner	22	7
Fat List		
Butter	99	54
Margarine	99	19
Oil, corn	100	10
Salad dressing, French	68	14

Dashes indicate no value was found, although it is believed some is present.

Source: U.S. Department of Agriculture.

the different ways cholesterol is transported in the body. The cholesterol content in some common foods is noted in table 5.4.

Dietary fat is digested into its constituents (fatty acids, glycerol, cholesterol, and phospholipids), which are eventually used for energy, incorporated in the formation of certain cell structures, or stored as fat. A diagram of the metabolic fates of dietary fat is presented in figure 5.2.

Table 5.4
Cholesterol Content in Some Common Foods

Food	Amount	Cholesterol (milligrams)
Meat List		
Beef	1 oz	25
Pork, ham	1 oz	25
Poultry	1 oz	23
Fish	1 oz	21
Shrimp	1 oz	45
Lobster	1 oz	25
Sausage	2 links	45
Tuna, salmon	1 oz	0
Frankfurter	1	50
Bacon	1 strip	5
Eggs	1	253
Liver	1 oz	120
Milk List		
Milk, whole	1 c	27
Milk, 2%	1 c	15
Milk, skim	1 c	7
Butter	1 tsp	12
Margarine	1 tsp	0
Cream cheese	1 tbsp	18
Ice milk	1 c	10
Ice cream	1 c	85
Bread List		

Whole grains and nuts contain no cholesterol, but cholesterol may be added in the preparation of some foods (such as eggs in French toast or other baked foods).

Bread	1 slice	0
Biscuit	1	17
Pancake	1	40
Sweet roll	1	25
French toast	1	130
Doughnut	1	28
Cereal, cooked	1 c	0
Fruit List		

Fruits contain no cholesterol.

Vegetable List
Vegetables contain no cholesterol.

Source: U.S. Department of Agriculture.

Protein

Protein is a complex chemical structure containing carbon, hydrogen, and oxygen—just as carbohydrates and fat do. However, protein has one other essential element, nitrogen. These four elements are combined into a number of different structures called **amino acids.** There are twenty amino acids, all of which can be combined together in a variety of ways to form the different proteins necessary for the structure and functions of the human body. Protein is one of our most essential nutrients, for it is the

Figure 5.2 Simplified Diagram of Fat Metabolism. After digestion, fats are carried in the blood as chylomicrons. Through the metabolic processes in the body, fat may be utilized as a major source of energy, used to help develop cell structure, or stored as a future energy source. **Source:** From Williams, Melvin H. *Nutrition for Fitness and Sport.* © 1983, Wm. C. Brown Publishers, Dubuque, Iowa. All Rights Reserved. Reprinted by Permission.

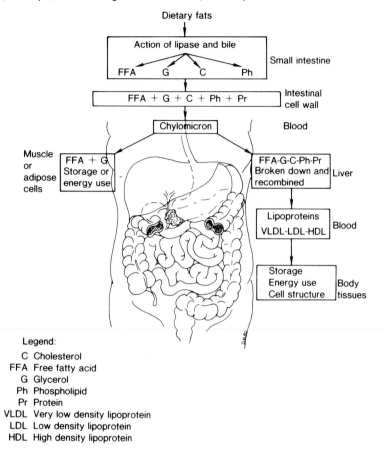

Legend:

C	Cholesterol
FFA	Free fatty acid
G	Glycerol
Ph	Phospholipid
Pr	Protein
VLDL	Very low density lipoprotein
LDL	Low density lipoprotein
HDL	High density lipoprotein

main structural component of all tissues in the body. Since all enzymes are derived from protein, all physiological processes are dependent upon this nutrient.

Protein is contained in foods from both animal and plant sources. Hence, humans obtain their supply of amino acids from these two general sources. However, the human body can synthesize some of the amino acids, but not others. The amino acids that cannot be manufactured in the body are called **essential amino acids,** and must be supplied in the diet. It should be noted that all twenty amino acids are necessary, and must be present simultaneously for optimal maintenance of body growth and function. Thus, the utilization of the term *essential* in relation to amino acids is to distinguish those that must be obtained in the diet. The nonessential amino acids are formed in the body.

Table 5.5
Protein Content in Some Common Foods

Food	Amount	Protein (grams)
Milk List		
Milk, whole	1 c	9
Milk, skim	1 c	9
Cheese, cheddar	1 oz	7
Yogurt	1 c	8
Meat List		
Beef, lean	1 oz	8
Chicken, breast	1 oz	8
Luncheon meat	1 oz	5
Fish	1 oz	7
Eggs	1	6
Navy beans, cooked	1/2 c	7
Peanuts, roasted	1/2 c	18
Peanut butter	1 tbsp	4
Vegetable List		
Broccoli	1/2 c	2
Carrots	1	1
Peas, green	1/2 c	4
Potato, baked	1	3
Fruit List		
Banana	1	1
Orange	1	1
Pear	1	1
Bread List		
Bread, wheat	1 slice	2
Bran flakes	1 c	4
Doughnuts	1	1
Spaghetti	1 c	5

In general, the proteins we ingest from animal products are superior to those found in plants. This is not to say that an amino acid found in a plant is inferior to the same amino acid found in an animal. They are the same. However, let's look at the distribution of all the amino acids in the two food sources, to see why animal protein is called a high-quality protein whereas plant protein is considered to be of low quality.

The reasons for the superiority of animal protein are twofold. First, it is a complete protein, since it contains all the essential amino acids. Second, it also contains the essential amino acids in the proper proportion. As noted previously, all amino acids must be present simultaneously in order for the body to synthesize them into necessary body proteins. If one essential amino acid is in short supply, protein construction may be blocked. Hence, having the proper amount of animal protein in the diet is a good way to ensure receiving a balanced supply of amino acids. Excellent sources include milk, cheese, meat, and eggs. However, since many animal products that are high in protein may also be high in cholesterol and fat, it may be desirable to restrict their intake.

Proteins usually exist in smaller concentrations in plants and may be lower in several of the essential amino acids. Hence, individually, most plant foods are unable to

Figure 5.3 Simplified Diagram of Protein Metabolism. After digestion, amino acids are metabolized in the liver, forming amino acids needed for new protein synthesis, being converted to glucose or fatty acids, or being converted to urea. These by-products are then transported by the blood for body use or, in the case of urea, excretion.
Source: From Williams, Melvin H. *Nutrition for Fitness and Sport.* © 1983, Wm. C. Brown Publishers, Dubuque, Iowa. All Rights Reserved. Reprinted by Permission.

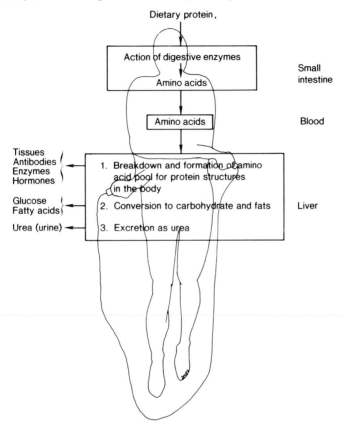

meet our total nutritional needs. However, if plant foods are eaten in proper combinations, they will provide a balanced supply of amino acids. An example of a good combination of plant foods that represents a complete protein is that of grain products and beans, such as rice and navy beans. This balanced intake is of extreme importance to strict vegetarians. Table 5.5 presents some common foods and their protein content. The average male needs about 56 grams of protein per day, while the average female needs about 44 grams.

After protein is digested, the amino acids are generally utilized to form body tissues and other protein substances, such as enzymes and hormones. Excess protein may be converted to glucose or fatty acids and protein waste products may be excreted as urea. Figure 5.3 represents a simplified description of protein metabolism in the human body.

Table 5.6
Essential Vitamins

Vitamin	Synonymous Terms	Body Functions
Fat-soluble Vitamins		
Vitamin A	Retinol; carotenoids	Growth and maintenance of body tissue; proper vision
Vitamin D	Calciferols	Calcium and phosphorus metabolism for strong bones and teeth
Vitamin E	Tocopherols	Prevention of oxidation of body cell membranes
Vitamin K	Phylloquinone	Proper blood clotting
Water-soluble Vitamins		
Vitamin B_1	Thiamin	Release of energy from carbohydrates; proper functioning of central nervous system
Vitamin B_2	Riboflavin	Metabolism of carbohydrate, fat, and protein; healthy skin
Niacin	Nicotinamide; nicotinic acid	Cellular metabolism for energy
Vitamin B_6	Pyridoxine	Metabolism of proteins
Pantothenic acid	—	Conversion of fat and carbohydrate to energy
Folacin	Folic acid	Production of genetic material
Vitamin B_{12}	Cyanocobalamin; corrinoids	Maintenance of healthy nervous system; RBC formation
Biotin	—	Metabolism of carbohydrates, fat, and protein
Vitamin C	Ascorbic acid	Maintenance of connective tissue

Vitamins

Vitamins continue to be one of the most used and abused nutrients in the United States today. Vitamin pill manufacturers and advertisers have perpetuated the myth that the average American diet contains insufficient amounts of vitamins, a potential cause of many diseases. We now have vitamin supplements on the market that have been designed, or so the manufacturers say, to help us combat the stress of everyday life, to help prevent the common cold, and to provide optimal energy for athletic performance. To be sure, vitamins are necessary nutrients. However, exaggerated claims by those with economic interests in vitamin supplements are not supported by factual data.

Vitamins represent a number of extremely complex organic compounds that are found in small amounts in most foods. They are essential for the optimal functioning of a great number of diverse physiological processes in the human body. Space limitations preclude a detailed discussion of each individual vitamin, but table 5.6 highlights the major vitamins, their synonyms, and their major functions in the human body. Later in this chapter the key nutrient concept is introduced. Five of these vitamins (A, B_1, B_2, niacin, and C) are key nutrients. If foods that contain these five vitamins and the other key nutrients are consumed in sufficient quantity, all the other vitamins will be obtained in the diet.

There are many questions you may ask about vitamins, but probably one of the most important is whether or not you should take a vitamin supplement. The vitamin industry, through its advertising media, has attempted to convince the American public that we are not receiving an ample supply of vitamins in the foods we normally eat and, thus, may experience certain diseases due to vitamin deficiency. In general, however, there is no solid evidence to indicate that the average healthy American on a balanced diet is suffering from vitamin deficiency and related diseases. A well-balanced diet contains all the necessary vitamins for the average individual. However, there may be certain situations where vitamin supplements are recommended.

Some recent national surveys note slight deficiencies in several nutrients, particularly the water-soluble vitamins, in the diets of some Americans. However, these surveys only indicate a deficiency in the diet and do not report any disease symptoms. If an individual feels he is not receiving a balanced diet for some reason, a simple balanced vitamin supplement will not do any harm. There are a number of preparations on the market that contain the daily RDA of most vitamins. The only damage sustained by consuming such products is to the pocketbook.

Minerals

You may recall the periodic table hanging on the wall in your high school or college chemistry class containing all the known elements on earth. At latest count, there are 103 known elements, 90 of them occurring naturally and the remainder man-made. A number of the natural elements were incorporated in humans through the process of evolution and became essential to body structure and function.

A **mineral** is an inorganic element found in nature. The term is usually reserved for solid elements. In nutrition, the term *mineral* is used to list those elements that are essential to life processes. Twenty-five minerals are currently known to be essential in human nutrition, and they perform a wide variety of functions in the body. Seven minerals (carbon, oxygen, hydrogen, nitrogen, sulfur, calcium, and phosphorus) are used as the building blocks for such body tissues as bones, teeth, muscles, and other organic structures. Minerals are also important in a number of regulatory functions in the body. Some of the physiological processes that are regulated or maintained by minerals include muscle contraction, nerve impulse conduction, acid-base balance of the blood, body water supplies, blood clotting, and normal heart rhythm. Table 5.7 lists the minerals essential to human nutrition and a brief coverage of their major physiological functions.

Generally, most minerals are widely distributed in many foods, so dietary deficiencies are rare. However, calcium and iron are key nutrients, and special attention should be given to including in the diet foods that are high in these two minerals. Consuming a diet that has adequate amounts of the key nutrients, including calcium and iron, will insure an adequate intake of the other essential minerals. On the other hand, one mineral, sodium, may need to be restricted in the diet. More information on these three minerals is given later in this chapter.

Table 5.7
Essential Minerals in Human Nutrition

Mineral (symbol)	Major Body Function
Calcium (Ca)	Muscle contraction; nerve impulse transmission; blood clotting; fat digestion
Chloride (Cl)	Water and electrolyte balance; formation of stomach acids
Chromium (Cr)	Glucose metabolism in cells; related to insulin action
Cobalt (Co)	Component of vitamin B_{12}; development of red blood cells
Copper (Cu)	Formation (with iron) of hemoglobin and iron enzymes
Fluoride (F)	Formation of bones and teeth
Iodine (I)	Formation of thyroxine (a thyroid hormone)
Iron (Fe)	Formation of compounds (such as hemoglobin) for the transportation of oxygen
Magnesium (Mg)	Activates a number of enzymes that are involved in the regulation of protein synthesis and muscle contraction
Manganese (Mn)	Many enzyme functions; bone formation; fat synthesis
Molybdenum (Mo)	Required in several enzymes
Phosphorus (P)	Acts with calcium to form bone tissue; part of high-energy compounds in body cells
Potassium (K)	Maintains acid-base balance; nerve impulse conduction; muscle contraction; many other functions in the body cells
Selenium (Se)	Functions with vitamin E; liver function
Silicon (Si)	Formation of connective tissue
Sodium (Na)	Maintenance of normal body fluid volume; nerve impulse transmission and muscle contraction; acid-base balance
Sulfur (S)	Formation of body tissues and enzymes
Zinc (Zn)	Component of many enzymes

Water

Water is a clear, tasteless, odorless fluid. It is a rather simple compound composed of two parts hydrogen and one part oxygen (H_2O). Yet, even with its simple chemical composition it is a very stable compound. Of all the compounds that are essential in the chemistry and functioning of living forms, water is the most important. Most of the other nutrients essential to life can be utilized by the human body only in their combination with water. It provides the medium within which the other nutrients may function.

In essence, water provides the essential building material for cell protoplasm; it is essential in the maintenance of a proper balance with the electrolytes; it is the main transportation mechanism in the body, conveying oxygen, nutrients, hormones, and other compounds to the cells for their use; it helps to regulate the acid-base balance in the body; and it plays a major role in the regulation of body temperature, particularly when exercising in the heat.

The requirement for body water depends upon the body weight of the individual. Under normal environmental temperatures and activity levels, the average adult needs about 2000 milliliters, or 2 liters (slightly more than 2 quarts), of water per day. This amount is sufficient to maintain adequate water balance in the body.

Table 5.8
Daily Water Loss and Intake for Water Balance

Water Loss

Source	Quantity
Urine output	1100 ml
Water in feces	100 ml
Lungs—exhaled air	200 ml
Skin—insensible perspiration	600 ml
Total	2000 ml

Water Intake

Source	Quantity
Fluids	1000 ml
Water in food	700 ml
Metabolic water	300 ml
Total	2000 ml

Body water balance is maintained when the intake of water matches the output of body fluids. Urinary output is the main avenue for water loss; a small amount is lost in the feces and through exhaled air in breathing. Insensible perspiration, which is not visible, is almost pure water and makes a significant contribution to body water losses. Sweat losses increase considerably during exercise and/or hot environmental conditions. Fluid intake of beverages is the main source of water to replenish losses. Solid foods also contribute water in two different ways. First, food contains water in varying amounts; certain foods, such as lettuce, celery, melons, and most fruits, contain about 90 percent water. Many others contain more than 60 percent—even bread, an outwardly dry-appearing food, contains 36 percent water. Second, the metabolism of foods for energy produces water; fat, carbohydrate, and protein all produce water when broken down into energy. This water is often called metabolic water. Table 5.8 summarizes daily water loss and intake for the maintenance of water balance.

The Basis of Diet Planning

Eating a well-balanced diet is the key to good nutrition. We have all heard this statement at one time or another, but what exactly is a well-balanced diet? In essence, a diet needs to be balanced in two aspects. First, it must contain an adequate amount of the forty or more essential nutrients to sustain growth and/or repair body tissues for a given individual during the various stages of life. Second, it must be balanced in caloric intake for control of body weight (weight maintenance, gain, or loss, depending upon the individual).

Although everyone needs the essential nutrients and a balanced caloric intake in their diet, the proportions differ at varying stages of the life cycle—the infant has different needs than his grandfather, and the pregnant or lactating woman has different needs than her adolescent daughter. Needs also differ between the sexes, particularly the iron content of the diet. Moreover, individual variations in life-style impose different nutrient requirements. A long-distance runner in training for a marathon has some distinct nutritional needs compared to a sedentary colleague. The individual trying to lose weight needs to balance Calorie losses with nutrient adequacy. The diabetic needs strict nutritional counseling for a balanced diet. Thus, there are a number of different conditions that influence nutrient needs and the concept of a balanced diet.

The Recommended Dietary Allowances (RDA)

As is noted in table 5.1, humans need to regularly consume over forty essential nutrients, but what is an adequate amount of each?

In the United States, the amounts of certain of these nutrients have been established by the Food and Nutrition Board, National Academy of Sciences—National Research Council. The **Recommended Dietary Allowances (RDA)** represent the levels of intake of essential nutrients considered (in the judgment of the Food and Nutrition Board on the basis of an extensive review of the available scientific knowledge) to be adequate to meet the known nutritional needs of practically all healthy persons in the United States. The current RDA are found in appendix A.

The RDA should not be construed as the recommended ideal diet. They are not guaranteed to represent total nutritional needs, for there is insufficient evidence relative to some essential trace elements. Moreover, they are designed for healthy persons, not those needing dietary modifications due to illness.

An individual's diet is not necessarily deficient if it does not include the full RDA daily. The daily RDA should average over a 5 to 8 day period, so that one may be deficient in iron consumption in one day's diet, but compensate for this during the remainder of the week. A general recommendation to help meet the daily RDA requirements is to select as wide a variety of foods as possible when planning the diet.

Although the RDA have not been designed to be used as individual requirements, they can be an effective guide for this purpose. The U.S. RDA, discussed in a subsequent section, are an extension of the RDA, and may be useful in determining nutrient intake.

Key Nutrient Concept

There are eight of the essential nutrients that, when found naturally in plant and animal sources, are usually accompanied by the other essential nutrients. These eight nutrients are:

protein	vitamin B_2 (riboflavin)
vitamin A	niacin
vitamin C	iron
vitamin B_1 (thiamin)	calcium

Thus, if your diet is adequate in these eight key nutrients, you probably receive an ample supply of all nutrients essential to humans. That is the **key nutrient concept.** An important point here is that the foods that contain these key nutrients should be obtained, as much as possible, from naturally occurring plant and animal food sources.

Table 5.9 presents the eight key nutrients along with the significant plant and animal sources of each.

Table 5.9
Eight Key Nutrients and Significant Food Sources
from Plants and Animals

Nutrient	Plant Source	Animal Source
Protein	Dried beans and peas, nuts	Meat, poultry, fish, cheese, milk
Vitamin A	Dark green leafy vegetables, yellow vegetables, margarine	Butter, fortified milk, liver
Vitamin C	Citrus fruits, broccoli, potatoes, strawberries, tomatoes, cabbage, dark green leafy vegetables	Liver
Vitamin B_1 (thiamin)	Breads, cereals, nuts	Pork, ham
Vitamin B_2 (riboflavin)	Breads, cereals	Milk, cheese, liver
Niacin	Breads, cereals, nuts	Meat, fish, poultry
Iron	Dried peas and beans, spinach, asparagus, prune juice	Meat, liver
Calcium	Turnip greens, okra, broccoli, spinach	Milk, cheese, mackerel, salmon

U.S. RDA and Nutritional Labeling

Although the two are related, the RDA should not be confused with the **United States Recommended Daily Allowances (U.S. RDA).** The U.S. RDA are a simplified RDA. They appear on the labels of food products and simply represent the percentage of the RDA provided by one serving of the food product. They serve as a useful guide in planning meals that contain the daily RDA.

With the tremendous increase in manufactured food products over the past twenty to thirty years, it has become increasingly difficult to determine the nutritional quality of the food we eat. Moreover, food manufacturers have often distorted nutritional facts, and have made rather extravagant claims for their particular products. The average consumer knows little about the nutrient value of even most natural foods, and these recent developments have compounded the problem of selecting foods that have high nutrient content. A law was passed in 1973 that established a set of standards so that Americans could choose what to eat based on sound nutritional information.

This set of standards resulted in **nutritional labeling,** whereby the major nutrients found in a food product are listed on its label. Although it is not the total solution to the problem of poor food selection by many Americans, combined with an educational program to increase nutritional awareness it may effectively improve the nutritional health of our nation.

Under nutritional labeling, the eight key nutrients must be listed on food labels. Carbohydrate and fat content are also usually listed, since the type of carbohydrate and fat may be important to your health. The content of simple refined sugar, fiber, saturated and polyunsaturated fats, and cholesterol should be included on the label. The sodium content is another important concern. Additional information on the label includes Calories, serving size, servings per container, and Calories per serving—valuable information in weight control programs. Other vitamins and minerals may also be listed.

Table 5.10
Nutritional Labeling for a Quart of Skim Milk

Nutrition Information per Serving

Serving size	8 oz
Servings per container	4
Calories	90
Protein	9 grams
Carbohydrate	12 grams
Fat	0 grams

Percentage of U.S. Recommended Daily Allowances (U.S. RDA)

Protein	20	Vitamin D	25
Vitamin A	10	Vitamin B_6	4
Vitamin C	4	Vitamin B_{12}	15
Thiamin	8	Phosphorus	25
Riboflavin	30	Magnesium	10
Niacin	*	Zinc	6
Calcium	30	Pantothenic acid	6
Iron	*		

*Contains less than 2% of the U.S. RDA of these nutrients.

In order to be of practical value to you, the nutrient content of the food is listed as a percentage of the U.S. RDA. However, you must interpret the U.S. RDA with care. In nutritional labeling, the U.S. RDA is based upon the nutrient requirements of the average adult male for seven of the key nutrients. The requirement for iron is based upon the female because her requirement is greater. This means that if you are a female, or a male who weighs less than the average male (70 kg or 154 pounds), a certain food will actually provide a greater percentage of the U.S. RDA for you than what is listed. If a glass of milk provides 20 percent of the protein requirement for an average size male, it may actually provide 25 percent for an average size female. On the other hand, if you weigh more than the average size male, then you will receive a slightly lower percentage of your protein requirement from that food.

Protein is listed twice on the label—as the amount in grams, and as a percentage of the U.S. RDA. The percentage amount reflects the fact that not all protein is of the same quality. For example, 9 grams of protein from milk (a complete protein) is listed as 20 percent of the U.S. RDA; however, a similar amount of protein in spaghetti (an incomplete protein) represents only 10 percent of the U.S. RDA.

Also recall that food manufacturers must list ingredients in order of their percent of the total volume of the product. A label that lists gravy, turkey, salt, and so forth, indicates there is more gravy than turkey in the product. Sometimes what may appear to be a good nutritional buy really is not what you may be led to believe.

A nutrition label for a quart of skim milk is presented in table 5.10. Skim milk is an excellent source of protein, vitamin A, riboflavin, calcium, vitamin D, vitamin B_{12}, phosphorus, and magnesium; it is a poor source of vitamin C, niacin, iron, and vitamin B_6.

Figure 5.4 The Concept of Nutrient Density. The key principle is to select foods that are high in nutrients and low in Calories. Compare the nutrient value of the three beverages in this figure. As you can see, orange juice and milk are significant sources of several key nutrients, while cola simply contains Calories in the form of simple carbohydrates.

Amount	8 ounces	8 ounces	8 ounces
Calories	120	145	100
Protein (grams)	2.5	10.3*	0
Fat (grams)	0.2	4.9	0
Carbohydrates (grams)	28.1	14.8	25
Calcium (milligrams)	27	352*	0
Iron (milligrams)	0.5	0.1	0
Vitamin A (IU)	500*	500*	0
Thiamin (milligrams)	0.2*	0.1	0
Riboflavin (milligrams)	0.07	0.5*	0
Niacin (milligrams)	1.0	0.2	0
Vitamin C (milligrams)	152*	2	0
	Orange juice	Milk, 2%	Cola

*Significant source of this key nutrient, over 10% of the RDA.

Nutrient Density

When buying food, you should attempt to select foods with significant amounts of the key nutrients, but with a low to moderate amount of Calories. This, in general, is the meaning of **nutrient density.** A food with high nutrient density provides a significant amount of a specific nutrient or nutrients per serving, or for a certain amount of Calories. An example of nutrient density is presented in figure 5.4.

The Basic Four Groups and the Food Exchange Lists

The RDA, key nutrients, and nutrient density are important concepts to apply when selecting foods for a balanced diet, but they are not practical approaches in educating the American public about sound nutrition. Hence, some time ago the *food group* approach was developed as a simple guide to eating that can be easily understood by the average American. The basis of the food group approach is that certain groups of foods contain significant amounts of several of the key nutrients in common. There were originally seven food groups, but they have been condensed to the **Basic Four Food Groups.** Foods of similar nutrient value are placed in either the Meat Group, the Milk Group, the Bread-Cereal Group, or the Fruit-Vegetable Group. Some publications list

Table 5.11
Key Nutrients Found in the Basic Four Food Groups

Meat Group	Milk Group	Bread-Cereal Group	Fruit-Vegetable Group
Protein	Calcium	Thiamin	Vitamin A
Thiamin	Protein	Niacin	Vitamin C
Niacin	Riboflavin	Riboflavin	
Iron	Vitamin A	Iron	
		Protein	

Table 5.12
Carbohydrate, Fat, Protein, and Calories in the Six Food Exchanges

Food Exchange	Carbohydrate	Fat	Protein	Calories
Vegetables	5	0	2	25
Fruits	10	0	0	40
Fat	0	5	0	45
Meat	0	3	7	55
Bread	15	0	2	70
Milk	12	0	8	80

Carbohydrate, fat, and protein in grams

1 g carbohydrate	= 4 Calories
1 g fat	= 9 Calories
1 g protein	= 4 Calories

a fifth group, the Fats, Sweets, and Alcohol Group. The Meat Group may also be described as the Meat, Poultry, Fish, and Bean Group, while the Milk Group is also known as the Milk and Cheese Group.

The value of the Basic Four Food Group approach is in its simplicity. Different patterns of nutrients are found in the four food groups and, since the American population has a tremendous variety of foods from which to select, it is not difficult to get the necessary amount of nutrients if we select our foods from across the four groups. Table 5.11 represents the key nutrients that are found in each of the four food groups. This listing represents the major nutrient content of each food group, but there is some variation in the proportion of the nutrients found between food groups as well as between different foods within each group. For example, the Bread-Cereal Group is a good source of protein, but not as good as the Meat or Milk Groups. Within the Fruit-Vegetable Group, oranges are an excellent source of vitamin C, but peaches are not.

An extension of the Basic Four Food Group plan is the Food Exchange Lists, which were developed by several national health organizations, including the American Dietetic Association. The **Food Exchange Lists** represent groups of foods, in specific measured amounts, that contain approximately the same amount of energy, carbohydrate, fat, and protein. It is similar in concept to the Basic Four Food Groups, but there are six Food Exchange Lists. The basic content of each food exchange is presented in table 5.12. Listings of specific foods and amounts are found in appendix B.

Table 5.13
Current Dietary Intake and Proposed Dietary Goals for Americans Expressed in Percent of Dietary Intake

	Current Dietary Intake		Proposed Dietary Goals	
Fat	42%		30%	
Saturated		16%		10%
Monounsaturated		13%		10%
Polyunsaturated		13%		10%
Carbohydrate	46%		58%	
Simple		24%		10%
Complex		22%		48%
Protein	12%		12%	
Cholesterol	500–1000 mg		< 300 mg*	
Salt	6–18 g		< 3 g*	

*Daily cholesterol and salt intake should be restricted to 300 mg and 3 g or less, respectively.

Although the use of the Food Exchange Lists is a valuable means to achieve a balanced diet, there may be some problems if the underlying concepts are not understood. It is easily possible to consistently choose the least nutritious foods from among the lists. This could lead to a nutrient deficiency. The key point to keep in mind is to eat a wide variety of natural foods within each of the groups or lists.

Since the Food Exchange Lists have been developed and utilized extensively as a means to balanced nutrition and weight control, it is the method utilized in the next chapter as a dietary means to control body weight. More details are presented about the Exchange Lists in chapter 6, but if you are interested in perusing the types of foods found in each of the six Food Exchange Lists, you may consult appendix B.

Healthier Eating

During the past fifty years or so there has been a gradual, but rather significant shift in the dietary habits of most Americans. Changing social customs, improvement in food processing technology, and the advent of the fast-food industry have been instrumental factors in producing changes in the types of food we eat. At the same time there has been a rather parallel increase in degenerative types of diseases, such as atherosclerosis, leading to coronary heart disease. Some epidemiologists who observed these parallel trends suggest that the dietary changes may be a contributing factor to the development of coronary heart disease and other health problems. For this reason, a study of the relationship of nutrition to health was initiated by the United States Senate in the 1970s. The result of this extensive study was the publication of *Recommended Dietary Goals* for Americans. Table 5.13 represents our current dietary intake and proposed dietary goals as percentages of Calories in the diet from carbohydrate, fat, and protein, as well as suggested limitations on several other dietary constituents. Although these dietary recommendations have been criticized by some, most nutritionists believe they are sensible changes toward a healthier diet.

Figure 5.5 The key to sound nutrition is a balanced diet that is high in nutrients and low in Calories. Select a wide variety of foods from among and within the Exchange Lists (appendix B) for balance.
(All photos, Bob Coyle)

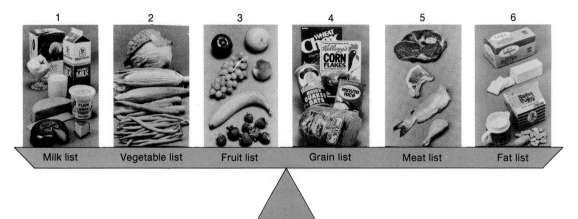

1	2	3	4	5	6
Milk list	Vegetable list	Fruit list	Grain list	Meat list	Fat list

Eight Guidelines for Healthier Eating

To make these recommendations more practical for the average American, the following guidelines have been developed to provide a sound means to achieve them.

1. Maintain a normal body weight.

   In order to avoid becoming overweight, you should consume only as many Calories as you expend daily. Methods of maintaining or losing weight are presented in chapter 6. Programs to gain weight are presented in chapter 7.

2. Eat a wide variety of natural foods from among the Exchange List food groups.

   This point is made repeatedly in this chapter as it is the best means to obtain an adequate supply of all the essential nutrients. Of special importance, especially for females and growing children, are foods high in calcium and iron. Milk and other dairy products are excellent sources of calcium, while iron is found in good supply in the Meat and Bread Groups.

3. Eat a sufficient amount of protein.

   The recommended dietary goal for protein is about 12 percent of the daily Calories. This averages out to about 50 to 60 grams of protein per day; the current American intake is about 100 grams, so we appear to be meeting this dietary goal. However, most of the protein we eat is of animal origin. Although animal products are an excellent source of complete protein, they may also contain substantial quantities of saturated fat and cholesterol.

4. Decrease your consumption of foods that are high in total fat, saturated fats, and cholesterol.

   There is no specific requirement for fat in the diet. However, a need exists for an essential fatty acid and vitamins that are components of fat. Since almost all foods contain some fat, sufficient amounts of the essential fatty acid and vitamins are found in the average diet. Even on a vegetarian diet of fruits,

Figure 5.6 Avoid excessive consumption of foods that are high in fats, cholesterol, saturated fats, simple sugars, and salt.

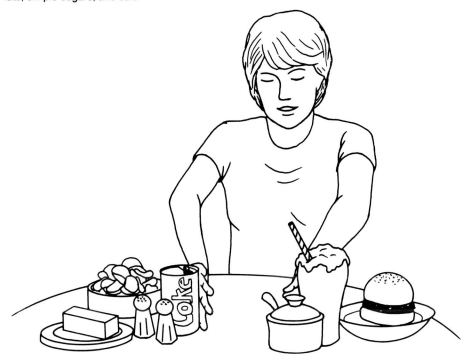

vegetables, and grain products, about 5–10 percent of your Calories are derived from fat, thus supplying enough of these essential nutrients. Fat, however, currently comprises over 40 percent of our Calories; the recommended dietary goal is less than 30 percent. In addition, the amount of saturated fat in the diet should be 10 percent or less, and cholesterol intake should be limited to 300 milligrams or less per day.

The basis for the reduction in dietary saturated fats and cholesterol is the assumption that they are associated with high blood levels of triglycerides and cholesterol, which is a risk factor associated with atherosclerosis and CHD. There appears to be enough medical evidence to justify a modification of the diet to lower high blood levels of triglycerides and cholesterol, or to prevent their rise in individuals with low to normal levels. The following practical suggestions will help you meet the recommended dietary goal.

a. Eat less meat that has a high fat content. Avoid hot dogs, luncheon meats, sausage, and bacon. Trim off excess fat before cooking. Eat only lean red meat and more white meat, such as turkey, chicken, and fish, which have less fat.

b. Eat only two to three eggs per week. One egg yolk contains about 250 milligrams of cholesterol, which is close to the limit of 300 milligrams per day. Egg whites have no cholesterol and are an excellent source of high-quality protein. You may also use commercially prepared egg substitutes.

c. Eat fewer dairy products that are high in fat. Switch from whole milk and hard cheeses to skim milk and soft cheeses. Eat other dairy products, such as yogurt and cottage cheese, made from low fat milk.

d. Eat less butter by substituting margarine made from liquid oils that are polyunsaturated. Try to avoid margarine made from hydrogenated oils.

e. Eat less commercially prepared baked goods that have been made with eggs and saturated fats. Check the labels for main ingredients.

f. Broil and bake your foods, rather than fry them. If you must fry your foods, use polyunsaturated liquid oils, rather than hard fats.

g. Consume less refined sugar and alcohol to help reduce blood triglycerides.

These suggestions should be modified somewhat for young children who may need the excellent nutritional protein of eggs and the Calories of whole milk to help support growth.

5. Reduce your consumption of refined sugar.

The recommended dietary goal is to reduce consumption of refined sugar from the current level of 24 percent of the daily Calories to 10 percent or less. Excessive consumption of refined sugar has been associated with high blood triglyceride levels. Sticky sugars are a major contributing factor to dental cavities. Sugars also significantly increase the caloric content of foods without an increase in nutritional value, so they may contribute to body weight problems.

In order to meet this goal you should reduce your intake of common table sugar and products that are high in refined sugar. Sugar is one of the major additives to processed foods so check the labels. If sugar is listed first then it is the main ingredient. Look also for terms such as corn syrup, dextrose, fructose, and malt sugar, which are also primarily refined sugars.

6. Increase your consumption of the complex carbohydrates and natural sugars found in vegetables, fruits, and whole grain products.

The dietary goals recommend that approximately 60 percent of your dietary Calories be derived from carbohydrate, with about 50 percent from the complex carbohydrates. The complex carbohydrates in vegetables and whole grain products are accompanied by significant quantities of vitamins and minerals, with small amounts of protein and little fat. Fruits are a good source of natural sugars, vitamins, and minerals. Increased intake of complex carbohydrates also naturally increases the amount of fiber (regarded as important for a healthy intestinal tract) in the diet.

7. Consume less sodium and high salt foods.

The recommended dietary goal is to reduce the current sodium intake to less than three grams, which is 3000 mg. This lower amount will provide sufficient sodium for normal physiological functioning. Increased sodium intake has been associated with high blood pressure (hypertension), but the National Research Council has indicated there is little or no direct evidence to suggest that high blood pressure can be produced in an individual with normal blood pressure and normal dietary intake of salt. On the other hand, hypertensive individuals may be able to reduce their blood pressure by decreasing the amount of salt in the diet.

Figure 5.7 Include in your diet foods that are high in plant starch and fiber. Eat more fruits, vegetables, and whole grain products. (Bob Coyle)

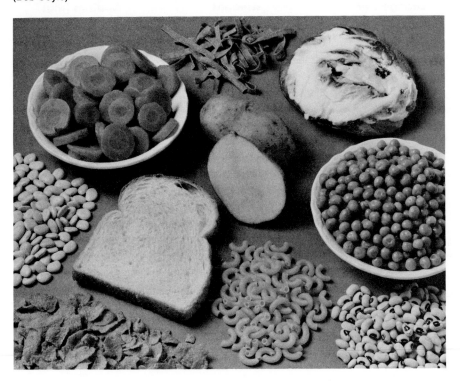

Sodium is found naturally in a wide variety of foods that we eat so it is not difficult to get an adequate supply. Several key suggestions may help you reduce the sodium content in your diet.

  a. Use your salt shaker less often. One teaspoon of salt is 2000 mg of sodium; the average well-salted meal contains about 3000–4000 mg. Put less salt on your food both in your cooking pot and on your table.
  b. Reduce the consumption of obviously high-salt foods, such as pretzels, potato chips, pickles, and other such snacks.
  c. Check food labels for sodium content. If salt is one of the ingredients listed first, you have a high-sodium food. Salt is a major additive in many processed foods.
  d. Eat more fresh fruits and vegetables, which are very low in sodium. Fruits, both fresh and canned, have less than 8 mg sodium per serving. Fresh vegetables may have 35 mg or less, but if canned may contain up to 460 mg. Table 5.14 lists the sodium content in some common foods.

8. Use moderation in the consumption of alcohol.

Table 5.14
Sodium Content of Common Foods

Food Exchange Item	Amount	Sodium (mg)
Milk		
Low fat milk	1 c	120
Cottage cheese		
Creamed	½ c	320
Unsalted	½ c	30
Cheese, American	1 oz	445
Vegetables		
Beans, cooked fresh	1 oz	5
Beans, canned	1 oz	150
Pickles, dill	1 medium	900
Potato, baked	1 medium	6
Fruits		
Banana	1 medium	1
Orange	1 medium	1
Bread-Cereal		
Bread, whole wheat	1 slice	130
Bran flakes	¾ c	340
Oatmeal, cooked	1 c	175
Pretzels	1 oz	890
Meat		
Luncheon meats	1 oz	450
Frankfurter	1 medium	495
Chicken	3 oz	40
Beef, steak	3 oz	70
Pork sausage	1 medium link	170
Tuna, in oil	3 oz	800
Fish (cod, flounder)	1 oz	35
Deviled crab-frozen	1 c	2085
Fats		
Butter, salted	1 tsp	50
Margarine, salted	1 tsp	50
Canned Foods and Prepared Entrees		
Chop suey, canned	1 c	1050
Spaghetti, canned	1 c	1220
Turkey dinner, frozen	1	1735
Chicken noodle soup	5 oz	655
Condiments		
Mustard	1 tbsp	195
Tomato catsup	1 tbsp	155
Soy sauce	1 tbsp	1320

As you can see in this table, the sodium content of foods can vary greatly. In general, canned and processed foods have much greater sodium content than fresh foods. Eat fresh meats, fruits, vegetables, and bread products whenever possible, and prepare them with little or no salt. Avoid highly salted foods like pickles, pretzels, soy sauce, and others. Look for low-sodium labels when you shop for canned foods.

Source: U.S. Department of Agriculture.

Although this was not a specific recommendation of the Senate report, it is important to include at this point because there are some health implications of alcohol consumption.

Alcohol is a transparent, colorless liquid derived from the fermentation of sugars in fruits, vegetables, and grains. The alcohol that is designed for human consumption is ethyl alcohol, also known as ethanol. Ethanol, although classified legally as a drug, is a component of many beverages served throughout the world. In the United States, alcohol is consumed mainly as a natural ingredient of beer, wine, and liquor. Though alcohol content may vary in different types, in general, beer is about 4–5 percent alcohol, wine is 12–14 percent, and liquor is 40–45 percent. The following amounts of these three beverages contain approximately equal amounts of alcohol (about 13 grams).

12 ounces (one bottle) of beer
4 ounces (one wine glass) of wine
1½ ounces (one jigger or shot glass) of liquor

The purposes of food are to supply energy, to build and repair body tissues, and to regulate body processes. In this sense, alcohol could be construed to possess food value as it is a concentrated source of energy. Alcohol contains about 7 Calories per gram, which is almost twice the value of an equal amount of carbohydrate or protein. Beer and wine also contain some carbohydrate, which is a source of additional Calories. In general, a bottle of regular beer has about 150 Calories, while a 4 ounce glass of wine or a shot glass of liquor have 100 Calories.

In general, the Calories found in beer, wine, and liquor are empty Calories. They do not provide substantial amounts of any nutrient. A 12 ounce bottle of beer does contain about one gram of protein, about one-tenth the RDA of niacin, smaller amounts of vitamins B_1 and B_2, and some calcium and potassium. Wine contains trace amounts of protein, niacin, vitamins B_1 and B_2, calcium, and iron. Liquor is void of any other nutrients. The nutrient content of beer and wine is considered to be low and does not make any significant contribution to the diet since the vitamins and minerals found in these beverages are distributed widely in other foods. Although alcohol may have a certain value to us as a social beverage, its value as a food and source of nutrients is extremely limited.

There is some controversy as to whether or not light to moderate alcohol drinking poses a significant health hazard. As a matter of fact, some epidemiological research has shown that moderate consumption of alcohol (about three beers or three glasses of wine per day) is associated with a lesser chance of developing coronary heart disease (CHD). Alcohol is known to relieve emotional tension and has also been associated with increased levels of high density lipoprotein cholesterol (HDL), both of which may help to prevent CHD. On the other hand, other research has shown that three or more drinks per day increase the risk of developing high blood pressure, another cardiovascular disorder. In addition, alcohol consumption is known to raise the lipid or fat levels in the blood, a risk factor for CHD. However, the current available evidence does not suggest that light to moderate consumption of alcohol (three bottles of beer, three glasses of wine, or two highballs per day) needs to be given up in order to prevent heart disease.

Consumed in moderation, along with a balanced diet, alcohol should not pose any health problems to the average individual. However, since alcohol is a significant source of Calories, it should be restricted in weight loss diets.

Heavy alcohol consumption is a different matter. It can produce significant health problems. One of the major body organs affected by alcohol is the liver. Even with a balanced diet high in protein, six drinks a day for less than a month has been shown to cause significant accumulation of fat in the liver. If continued, this could lead to irreversible liver disease, hepatitis and cirrhosis (the formation of scar tissue). As liver function deteriorates, fat, carbohydrate, and protein metabolism are not regulated properly with possible pathological consequences for other body organs such as the kidney and heart. The health hazards of prolonged excessive alcohol consumption have been well documented, and anyone with such a problem should seek professional help.

In this necessarily brief discussion, only some of the physiological effects of alcohol have been mentioned. As you know, alcohol affects the brain, which can have profound effects on thinking processes, motor performance, and emotional behavior. All three of these functions are important for the safe operation of motor vehicles. Excessive alcohol consumption disturbs all three functions and, unfortunately, is associated with nearly half the automobile accidents in our country. This is the major health hazard resulting from the behavioral effects of alcohol.

The Vegetarian Diet

The recommendation to eat less meat and more fruits, vegetables, and whole grain products is suggestive of a vegetarian diet. Vegetarianism is a complex topic and cannot be covered in any depth in this text, but the following information may be helpful to those who are thinking in that direction.

Vegetable, in a broader sense, is a term used for foods that have a plant origin. If we look at our Four Basic Food Groups, this excludes most foods normally found in the Milk and Meat Groups (which are primarily animal products), but includes those in the Bread and Cereal Group, as well as the Fruit and Vegetable Group.

There are a variety of types of **vegetarians.** A strict vegetarian, known also as a *vegan,* eats no animal products at all. Most nutrients are obtained from fruits, vegetables, breads, cereals, legumes, nuts, and seeds. *Ovovegetarians* include eggs in their diet, while *lactovegetarians* include foods in the Milk Group, such as cheese and other dairy products. An **ovolactovegetarian** eats both eggs and milk products. These latter classifications are not strict vegetarians, since eggs and milk products are derived from animals. Others may consider themselves vegetarians because they do not eat red meat, such as beef and pork products, although they may eat fish and other sea products. Others even add poultry to their diets. In practice, then, a vegetarian may range on a continuum from one who eats nothing but plant foods to someone who eats a typical American diet with the exception of red meat. The concern for obtaining a balanced intake of nutrients depends on where a vegetarian is on that continuum.

Although the individual who eats a typical American diet needs to be aware of sound nutritional principles, this knowledge is even more important for the vegetarian, particularly the vegan who eats no animal products whatsoever. If foods are not selected carefully, the vegetarian may suffer nutritional deficiencies of Calories, vitamins, minerals, and protein.

Caloric deficiency is one of the lesser concerns of a vegetarian diet. However, since plant products are generally low in caloric content, a vegetarian may be on a diet with insufficient Calories for proper body maintenance. This may be particularly true for the active individual who may be expending over 1000 Calories per day through exercise. The solution is to eat greater quantities of the foods that constitute the diet, and include more higher Calorie foods, like nuts, beans, corn, green peas, potatoes, sweet potatoes, avocadoes, orange juice, raisins, dates, figs, whole wheat bread, and pasta products. These foods may be used both in main meals and as snacks. On the other hand, the low caloric content of vegetarian diets may be a desirable attribute in weight reduction programs or in maintenance of proper body weight.

Strict vegetarians may incur a vitamin B_{12} deficiency, since it is not found in plant foods, and develop a severe form of anemia. B_{12} is found in many animal products, such as meat, eggs, fish, and dairy products, so the addition of these foods to the diet helps prevent a deficiency state. An ovolactovegetarian should have no problem getting required amounts. A B_{12} supplement is needed for the strict vegan.

Riboflavin (vitamin B_2) is low in many fruits, vegetables, breads, and cereals. Green leafy vegetables, such as beet greens, broccoli, collards, and turnip greens, are relatively good sources of riboflavin for the vegan. Dairy products, such as milk and cheese, add substantial amounts of riboflavin to the diet.

Mineral deficiencies of iron, calcium, and zinc may occur, particularly if the vegetarian diet contains large amounts of grains and legumes. During the digestion process, these foods form compounds called **phytates** that can bind these minerals so that they cannot be absorbed into the body. Avoidance of unleavened bread helps reduce this effect, as does thorough cooking of legumes such as beans. Foods rich in these minerals should also be included in the vegetarian diet. Iron-rich plant foods include nuts, beans, peanuts, split peas, green leafy vegetables (like spinach), dates, prune juice, raisins, and many iron-enriched grain products. Calcium-rich plant foods include many green vegetables like broccoli, cabbage, mustard greens, and spinach. Dairy products added to the diet supply very significant amounts of calcium. Zinc-rich plant foods include whole wheat bread, peas, corn, and carrots. Egg yolk and seafood also add substantial zinc to the diet.

The major concern of the vegetarian is to obtain adequate amounts of the right type of protein. If you recall our earlier discussion, proteins are classified as either complete or incomplete. A protein is complete if it contains all of the essential amino acids that the human body cannot manufacture. Animal products generally contain complete proteins, while plant proteins are incomplete. However, certain vegetable products may also provide good sources of protein. Grain products such as wheat, rice, and corn, as well as soybeans, peas, beans, and nuts have a substantial protein content. However, most vegetable products lack one or more essential amino acids in sufficient quantity. They are incomplete proteins and, eaten individually, are not generally adequate for maintaining proper human nutrition. But, if certain plant foods are eaten together, they may supply all the essential amino acids necessary for human nutrition, and be as good as meat protein.

Figure 5.8 It is important for the vegetarian to eat protein foods that complement each other (e.g., nuts and bread, rice and beans) so that all the essential amino acids are obtained in the diet. © David A. Corona

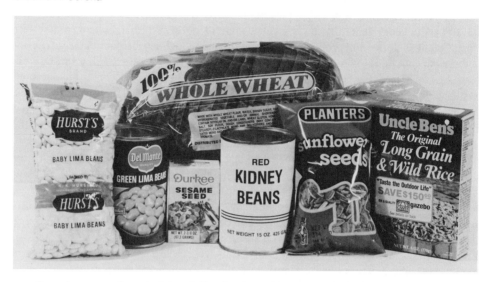

In order to receive a balanced distribution of essential amino acids, the vegan must eat vegetable foods that possess what is known as **protein complementarity,** in which a vegetable product that is low in a particular amino acid is eaten together with a food that is high in that same amino acid. Grains and cereals that are low in lysine need to be complemented by legumes, such as beans, that have adequate amounts of lysine. The low level of methionine in the legumes is offset by its high concentration in the grain products. These types of food combinations are practiced throughout the world. Mexicans eat pinto beans and corn; Chinese eat soybeans and rice. Through the proper selection of complementary foods, the vegan can get an adequate intake of the essential amino acids. It is important that the complementary foods be eaten together, or within a very short period of time. Eating them at one meal helps guarantee that they are properly utilized by the body.

Although the vegetarian diet has not been proven to be healthier than a diet that includes foods in the Meat and Milk Groups, it is based on certain nutritional concepts that may help in the prevention of some degenerative diseases common to industrialized society. First, the saturated fat content in a vegetarian diet is usually low, since fats found in plant foods are generally polyunsaturated. Second, plants do not contain cholesterol, since this compound is found only in animal products. These two factors account for the fact that vegetarians generally have lower blood triglycerides and cholesterol than meat eaters, which may be an important mechanism in the prevention of coronary heart disease. Third, plant foods possess a high fiber content that has been associated with reduced levels of serum cholesterol and the prevention of certain disorders in the intestinal tract. Fourth, if the proper foods are selected, the vegetarian diet supplies more than an adequate amount of nutrients and yet is rather low in caloric content. Plant foods can be high nutrient density foods, providing bulk in the diet without the added Calories of fat. Hence, the vegetarian diet can be an effective dietary regimen for losing excess body weight.

It should be emphasized, however, that the non-vegetarian who carefully selects foods from the Meat and Milk Group, including lean red meat, may attain the same health benefits as the vegetarian. The major difference between a vegetarian and a non-vegetarian diet appears to be the higher content of saturated fats and cholesterol in the latter. Selection of animal products with low-fat and low-cholesterol content helps to avoid this problem, and also assures consumption of a very high-quality protein.

Choosing a vegetarian diet is up to the individual, and represents a significant change in dietary habits. Anyone desiring to make an abrupt change to a vegetarian diet should do some serious reading on the matter beforehand. Once you have done some reading on vegetarianism, there may be several ways to gradually phase yourself into a vegetarian diet. You may become a partial vegetarian by simply decreasing the amount of red meat in your diet. You may have several meatless days per week, or one or two meatless meals each day (breakfast and lunch). For example, you may skip the ham or sausage at breakfast, and have a big salad for lunch. You may wish to substitute white meat, with its generally lower fat content, for red meat. Eat more fish, chicken, and turkey. You may wish to become an ovolactovegetarian, eating eggs and dairy products. These excellent sources of complete protein can be blended with many vegetable products or eaten separately. You may use the above methods as forerunners to a strict vegetarian diet, gradually phasing out animal products altogether as you learn to select and prepare vegetable foods with protein complementarity.

Remember, there is nothing magic about a vegetarian diet. It can be a healthful way to obtain the nutrients your physically active body needs, but so, too, is a well-balanced diet containing animal products that are selected wisely.

In summary, the dietary recommendations presented in this chapter, in combination with a properly designed exercise program, represent the two essential keys to a Positive Health Life-style. They complement each other nicely relative to the reduction of risk factors associated with the development of such diseases as diabetes, high blood pressure, and coronary heart disease. Moreover, as is noted in the next chapter, a combined exercise-diet program is the most effective type of program for losing or maintaining body weight. As noted in chapter 7, a modified exercise-diet program may also be utilized for gaining desirable body weight, particularly muscle mass.

As with a sound aerobic exercise program, sound nutritional habits need to be lifelong. The earlier in life you adopt such a sound exercise-nutrition life-style, the greater the possibility of preventing the onset of many of the chronic diseases discussed in chapter 2.

Keep a record of everything you eat and drink for one day, including the specific amounts. Be sure to note the ingredients of combination foods, such as casseroles, pizza, and sandwiches. Use the form below to record the type of food, the Exchange List it is on, and the amount. If you are uncertain as to which exchange it is in, consult appendix B.

Appendix B should also be used in order to determine the number of exchanges in the amount you have consumed. Use the following information to give you the Calories and the grams of carbohydrate, fat, and protein in each exchange. Multiplying the number of exchanges times these values will give you the total Calories, carbohydrate, fat, and protein in the food. Another good idea is to use the nutrition information on the foods' labels to record Calories, carbohydrate, fat and protein intake.

Exchange	Calories	Carbohydrate (Grams)	Fat (Grams)	Protein (Grams)
Milk (skim)	80	12	0	8
Meat (lean)	55	0	3	7
Bread	70	15	0	2
Fruit	40	10	0	0
Vegetable	25	5	0	2
Fat	45	0	5	0

When you have completed recording the data on the form, perform the following calculations.

1. Total number of exchanges: Calories per exchange: Calories:

   Milk _____ 80 _____

   Meat _____ 55 _____

   Bread _____ 70 _____

   Fruit _____ 40 _____

   Vegetable _____ 25 _____

   Fat _____ 45 _____

2. Total Calories: _____

3. Total grams of carbohydrate: _____ grams

4. Percent of carbohydrate in diet:

   grams   carbohydrate

   of carbohydrate _____ $\times$ 4 Calories = _____ Calories

   carbohydrate Calories $\div$ total Calories $\times$ 100 = _____ %

5. Total grams of fat: _____ grams

6. Percent of fat in diet:
grams of fat _____ × 9 Calories = _____ fat Calories
fat Calories ÷ total Calories × 100 = _____ %

7. Total grams of protein: _____ grams

8. Percent of protein in diet:
grams
of protein _____ × 4 Calories = _____ protein Calories
protein Calories ÷ total Calories × 100 = _____ %

After completing the Laboratory Inventory, you may ask yourself the following questions. Did I get *at least* 2–3 milk exchanges, 5–6 meat, 4 bread, 1–2 fruit, 3–4 vegetable, and 1–2 fat? Did I get about 60 percent of my Calories from carbohydrate? You may also wish to analyze the content for simple and complex carbohydrates, if you have that information available. Is the percentage of fat Calories less than 30 percent? Do I have about 10–12 percent or more of my Calories as protein? The answers to these questions may give you some insight into any needed dietary changes.

Doing the Laboratory Inventory is also good preparation for chapter 6. You may relate this information to Laboratory Inventories 6.3 and 6.4 relative to weight control.

The day of the week that you select should be typical of your average diet. A more representative account is a three-day analysis. For a college student, this might be a Monday, Thursday, and Saturday, representing two different class schedule days and one weekend day. Calculate each day separately to see if you are balancing the diet over a week's time.

Daily Food Intake

(1) Food	(2) Exchange List	(3) Amount	(4) Number of Exchanges	(5) Calories per Exchange	(6) Total Calories (4)$\times$(5)

Daily Food Intake

(7) Grams of Carbohydrate per Exchange	(8) Total Grams of Carbohydrate (4)×(7)	(9) Grams of Fat per Exchange	(10) Total Grams of Fat (4)×(9)	(11) Grams of Protein per Exchange	(12) Total Grams of Protein (4)×(11)

References

American Medical Association. *Nutrients in Processed Foods.* Acton, MA: Publishing Sciences Group, 1974.

Barrett, S., and Knight, G. *The Health Robbers.* Philadelphia: Stickley, 1976.

Borenstein, B. "Effect of Processing on the Nutritional Values of Foods." In *Modern Nutrition in Health and Disease,* edited by R. Goodhart and M. Shils. Philadelphia: Lea and Febiger, 1980.

Brody, J. *Jane Brody's Nutrition Book.* New York: W. W. Norton, 1980.

Burkitt, D. P., and Trowell, H. C. *Refined Carbohydrate Foods and Disease.* London: Academic Press, 1975.

Committee on Nutritional Misinformation, Food and Nutrition Board. *Vegetarian Diets.* Washington, DC: National Academy of Sciences, 1974.

Davis, T., et al. "Review of Studies of Vitamin and Mineral Nutrition in the United States (1950–1968)." *Journal of Nutrition Education* 1(suppl. 1):41–54 (1969).

Department of Health, Education and Welfare. "Third Special Report to the U.S. Congress on Alcohol and Health." In *NIAA Information and Feature Service,* DHEW Publication No. (ADM): 78–151 (November 1978).

Deutsch, R. *Realities of Nutrition.* Palo Alto, CA: Bull, 1976.

Felig, P. "Amino Acid Metabolism in Exercise." *Annals of The New York Academy of Sciences* 301:56–63 (1977).

Food and Nutrition Board, National Academy of Sciences—National Research Council. *Recommended Dietary Allowances.* Washington, DC: U.S. Government Printing Office, 1980.

Frieden, E. "The Chemical Elements of Life." In *Human Nutrition.* San Francisco: W. H. Freeman, 1978.

Goodhart, R. "Criteria of an Adequate Diet." In *Modern Nutrition in Health and Disease,* edited by R. Goodhart and M. Shils. Philadelphia: Lea and Febiger, 1980.

Goodhart, R., and Shils, M. (eds.) "The Vitamins." In *Modern Nutrition in Health and Disease.* Philadelphia: Lea and Febiger, 1980.

Grose, D. "Our Polluted Food—Fact or Fancy." *Royal Society of Health Journal* 97:193–96 (1977).

Halstead, C. "Nutritional Implications of Alcohol." In *Present Knowledge in Nutrition,* edited by D. Hegsted, et al. Washington, DC: The Nutrition Foundation, 1976.

Harper, A. "Dietary Goals—A Skeptical View." *American Journal of Clinical Nutrition* 31:310–21 (1978).

Hegsted, D. "Priorities in Nutrition in the United States." *Journal of the American Dietetic Association* 71:9–13 (1977).

Kannel, W. B. "Nutrition vs Atherosclerosis." In *The Medicine Called Nutrition,* edited by D. Mason and H. Guthrie. New York: Davis, Delaney and Arrow, 1979.

Kannel, W. B., et al. AHA Committee Report. "Risk Factors and Coronary Disease." *Circulation* 62:449A–455A (1980).

Kritchevsky, D. "An Update on Lipids, Lipoproteins and Fat Metabolism." In *The Medicine Called Nutrition,* edited by D. Mason and H. Guthrie. New York: Davis, Delaney and Arrow, 1979.

Lieber, C. "The Metabolism of Alcohol." *Scientific American* 234:25–33 (March 1976).

McLean, A. "Risk and Benefit in Food and Additives." *Proceedings of the Nutrition Society* 36:85–90 (1977).

Martin, A., and Tenenbaum, F. *Diet Against Disease.* Boston: Houghton Mifflin, 1980.

Munro, H., and Crim, M. "The Proteins and Amino Acids." In *Modern Nutrition in Health and Disease,* edited by R. Goodhart and M. Shils. Philadelphia: Lea and Febiger, 1980.

Null, G., and Null, S. *The New Vegetarian.* New York: Morrow, 1978.

"Nutrition and Vegetarianism." *Dairy Council Digest* 50:1–5 (January-February 1979).

Oser, B. "Chemical Additives in Foods." In *Modern Nutrition in Health and Disease,* edited by R. Goodhart and M. Shils. Philadelphia: Lea and Febiger, 1980.

Randall, H. "Water, Electrolytes, and Acid-Base Balance." In *Modern Nutrition in Health and Disease,* edited by R. Goodhart and M. Shils. Philadelphia: Lea and Febiger, 1980.

Reuben, D. *Everything You Always Wanted to Know about Nutrition.* New York: Simon and Schuster, 1978.

Scientific American. *Human Nutrition.* San Francisco: W. H. Freeman, 1978.

Scrimshaw, N., and Young, V. "The Requirements of Human Nutrition." In *Human Nutrition.* San Francisco: W. H. Freeman, 1978.

Shekelle, R. B., et al. "Diet, Serum Cholesterol and Death from Coronary Heart Disease. The Western Electric Study." *New England Journal of Medicine* 304:65–70 (January 1981).

Tatkon, M. *The Great Vitamin Hoax.* New York: Macmillan, 1968.

United States Department of Agriculture. *The Hassle-Free Guide to a Better Diet.* Leaflet No. 567. Washington, DC: U.S. Government Printing Office, 1980.

——— . *Nutrition Labeling: Tools for Its Use.* Agriculture Bulletin No. 382. Washington, DC: U.S. Government Printing Office, 1975.

United States Senate Select Committee on Nutrition and Human Needs. *Dietary Goals for the United States.* Washington, DC: U.S. Government Printing Office, 1977.

"The Vegetarian Approach to Eating." A position paper in the *Journal of the American Dietetic Association* 77:61–69 (1980).

"Vegetarian Diets." *American Journal of Clinical Nutrition* 32:1095 (1974).

White, P., and Mondeika, T. "Food Fads and Faddism." In *Modern Nutrition in Health and Disease,* edited by R. Goodhart and M. Shils. Philadelphia: Lea and Febiger, 1980.

White, P., and Selvey, N. *Let's Talk About Food.* Acton, MA: Publishing Sciences Group, 1974.

Williams, M. H. *Nutritional Aspects of Human Physical and Athletic Performance.* Springfield, IL: C. C. Thomas, 1976.

——— . *Nutrition For Fitness and Sport.* Dubuque, IA: Wm. C. Brown Publishers, 1983.

——— . "Vitamin, Iron and Calcium Supplementation: Effect on Human Physical Performance." In *Nutrition and Athletic Performance,* edited by W. Haskell, J. Whittam, and J. Skala. Palo Alto, CA: Bull, 1982.

6 Maintaining or Losing Body Weight

Key Terms

adult-onset obesity
basal metabolic rate (BMR)
behavior modification
caloric concept of weight control
Calorie
early-onset obesity
energy balance
essential fat
exercise metabolic rate (EMR)
height and weight charts

long-haul concept
metabolic rate
metabolism
negative energy balance
obesity
positive energy balance
resting metabolic rate (RMR)
storage fat

Key Concepts

Body composition may be subdivided into two major components: body fat and lean body mass. The latter is primarily bone and muscle tissue.

Although there are a number of sophisticated techniques for determining body fat percentage, the simpler, more practical tests are the best for use by the individual to monitor fat losses during a weight reduction program.

Although there are no methods that predict exactly what your ideal or desirable weight is, there are some normal ranges of body fat percentage, or weight, that appear to be related to better health.

The key to weight control is energy balance, or caloric balance; a negative energy balance results in body weight loss—a positive energy balance increases body weight.

Energy expenditure in humans represents the sum of the basal, resting, and exercise metabolic rates. The latter two are the most effective means for increasing energy output during a weight control program.

The recommended weight loss for adults is about 1–2 pounds per week, unless under the guidance of a physician.

To be effective, a diet for reducing or maintaining body weight should be low in Calories but high in nutrients; appeal to your taste; fit into your life-style; and be life-long.

The basic principles underlying an exercise program for weight control are the same as those for prevention of coronary heart disease; large muscle activities must be included at fairly intense levels, and duration and frequency are increasingly important.

Behavior modification techniques can be effective in helping to implement a diet-exercise program for weight control.

Weight losses during a diet or exercise program may not correspond exactly to caloric deficits, primarily because losses or gains in body water may mask actual body fat losses.

The best program for losing body fat, and improving body composition, is a combination of a well-balanced, low-Calorie diet with an aerobic exercise program.

Introduction

The human body is a remarkable food processor. Most adults can consume over a ton of food per year and still not gain or lose a pound of body weight. On the other hand, a large percentage of Americans do have problems in maintaining normal body weight. Experts at a recent national conference estimated that about one in every five Americans weighs 30 percent or more than their desirable body weight.

Obesity is an accumulation of fat beyond that considered to be normal for the age, sex, and body type of a given individual. As mentioned in chapter 2, it is one of the major health problems in the United States. Several health conditions (diabetes mellitus, high blood pressure, and high blood lipid levels) are known to be related to or due to obesity, while others (coronary heart disease, chronic lung disease, and emotional disorders) may be aggravated by it. Obesity is a complex medical problem for it may have a multitude of causes such as genetic background, hormonal imbalances, impaired metabolic rate, home environment, psychological disturbances, and level of physical activity.

One way to look at obesity is the time of onset. **Early-onset obesity,** as the term implies, occurs early in life, usually during the child's first year or during the beginning of adolescence. This may be the time when fat cells increase in number, resulting in a hyperplasia-type obesity. Genetic background, home environment, and physical inactivity may be important factors in the development of this type of obesity. Generally speaking, the obese child will be an obese adult. Hyperplasia-type obesity is difficult to treat. Fat cells have one major function—to convert what is eaten into fat and store it. The more fat cells an individual has, the greater the ability to accumulate fat.

Adult-onset obesity is usually caused by a different mechanism. The fat cells do not necessarily increase in number, however their size may increase to three-to-five-times normal. This type is called hypertrophic obesity. Adult-onset obesity is often referred to as creeping obesity, for it sneaks up on us, with low levels of physical activity an important factor in its development.

Extreme obesity may merit medical attention in order to reduce excess body fat. However, with proper knowledge and a strong desire to lose weight, almost anyone can design a diet-exercise program to achieve a desirable weight goal. The purpose of this chapter is to help provide that knowledge and some guidelines to help you lose weight, if that is one of your goals. The principles set forth in this chapter are also useful in helping you maintain your current desirable body weight, since in obesity, prevention is more effective than treatment. If you are now at a desirable body weight, plan to stay that way with a proper diet-exercise program.

Topics to be discussed in this chapter include the nature of body composition, how to determine your desirable weight, the basic principles of weight control, and the roles of diet, exercise, and behavior modification in maintaining or losing body weight.

Body Composition

We have all heard the expression "You are what you eat." In essence, this is true as our body takes the forty or so nutrients that we obtain in our food and rearranges them to form our body tissues. About 3–4 percent of your body is composed of minerals,

Figure 6.1 Adult-onset obesity is often referred to as creeping obesity, for it creeps up on us slowly. As little as 200 additional Calories per day above normal requirements would result in a gain of approximately 20 pounds of body fat in one year.

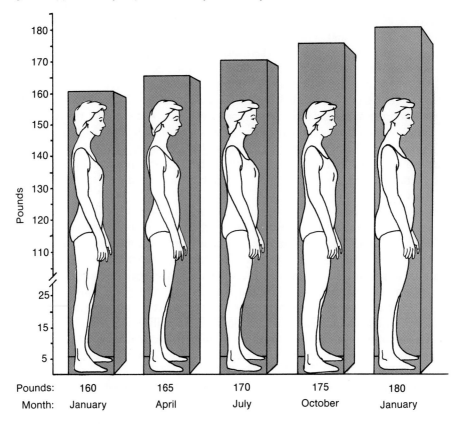

Pounds:	160	165	170	175	180
Month:	January	April	July	October	January

primarily the calcium and phosphorus in your bones. However, the vast majority of your body mass consists of four elements—carbon, oxygen, hydrogen, and nitrogen. These elements are the structural basis of your body stores of carbohydrates, protein, fat, and water. To understand body composition, and how one loses or gains body weight, you should understand how these substances are stored in the body.

Carbohydrate The body contains very little carbohydrate (about a pound) which is stored primarily in the muscles. However, about 3 pounds of water is stored with this carbohydrate.

Protein Protein is the major structural component of all body tissues. The muscle, heart, bone, liver, and other tissues have a high protein content.

Fat Body fat is of two types. **Essential fat** is necessary in the structure of various cells, and also for protection of some internal organs. It is also a major component of female breast tissue. **Storage fat** is simply a depot for excess energy; the main storage space is the adipose tissue cells just under the skin.

Table 6.1
Percentages of Body Weight Attributable to Body Fat and Lean Body Mass

	Adult Male		Adult Female	
Total Body Fat	15		26	
Essential fat		3		15
Storage fat		12		11
Lean Body Mass	85		74	
Muscle		43		36
Bone		15		12
Other tissues		27		26
	100	100	100	100

Figure 6.2 The majority of the body weight is water, while varying amounts of fat, protein, and carbohydrate make up the solid tissues. Body weight losses or gains may result from changes in any of these components.

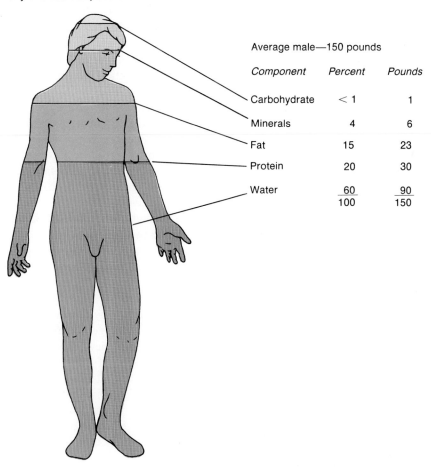

Average male—150 pounds

Component	Percent	Pounds
Carbohydrate	< 1	1
Minerals	4	6
Fat	15	23
Protein	20	30
Water	60	90
	100	150

Water The greatest percentage of the body's weight is water—approximately 60 percent of the weight of the average adult. Some water is found in all tissues; it is very high in some tissues (blood), and very low in others (bone). Water content in protein-type tissue, such as muscle, is high (about 72 percent), while it is low (about 10 percent) in fat-type tissue.

For the practical purposes of determining composition, the body may be regarded as being composed of two components, body fat and lean body mass. Body fat is the total amount of fat in the body. Lean body mass consists primarily of the muscles and bones, although in reality other body organs, such as the heart, liver, and kidneys, are part of the lean body mass. The values in table 6.1 represent approximate percentages of body weight partitioned as body fat and lean body mass.

Body composition may be influenced by a number of factors, such as age, sex, diet, and exercise. Age effects are significant during the developmental years, while muscle and other body tissues are being formed. Also, muscle mass may decrease during adulthood, due primarily to physical inactivity. There are some minor differences in body composition between boys and girls up to the age of puberty, but at this age the differences become fairly great. In general, beginning at puberty, the female deposits more fat, while the male develops more muscle tissue. Diet can affect body composition over the short haul, such as in acute water restriction and starvation, but its main effects are seen over the long haul. For example, chronic overeating may lead to increased body fat stores. Physical activity may also be very influential. A sound exercise program helps to build muscle and lose fat.

In the next section we look at how you can determine a desirable weight for yourself. But first, let us look briefly at the technique that is most commonly used to determine body composition. Since most of the storage fat is contained just under the skin, various skinfold measures have been used to predict body fat. The skinfold measures obtained are inserted into a formula to estimate the percent of body fat. Care must be taken to use a formula that is appropriate for your age and sex. Probably the best application of the skinfold technique is to use it periodically on yourself to see if you are losing body fat, particularly when you are on a weight loss program. Simply keep a record of the sum of skinfold thicknesses from selected body sites.

Since the skinfold technique is so practical to use, Laboratory Inventory 6.1 gives you an approximation of your body fat percentage. However, keep in mind that the percentage value may be only a rough approximation.

Simpler methods may also be used to determine if you are too fat. Probably the least complicated and most revealing is the mirror test as proposed by Jean Mayer, the internationally renowned authority on nutrition and obesity. He suggests that you look at yourself, nude, in a full length mirror using both a front and side view. This is usually all the evidence you need if you study yourself objectively. Most of us have a pretty good idea of how we would like our bodies to look, and this test offers us a guide to our desirable physical appearance, at least as far as body weight distribution is concerned. Exceptions to this suggestion are individuals who are obsessed with thinness and may suffer from a condition known as *anorexia nervosa*. Such individuals seem to believe they are always too fat, even though they are extremely thin. This topic is covered further in chapter 10.

Figure 6.3 A schematic drawing showing the skinfold of fat that is pinched up away from the underlying muscle tissue.
Source: Reprinted by permission of the American Alliance for Health, Physical Education, Recreation and Dance, 1900 Association Drive, Reston, VA 22091.

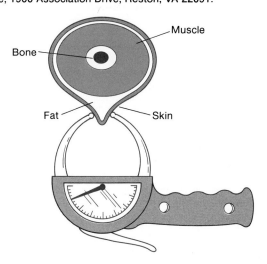

Desirable Body Weight

There does not appear to be any sound evidence to indicate exactly how much any given individual should weigh for optimal health. However, there are lower and upper range values for body fat or body weight that appear to be normal for most of the population. Those individuals who exceed these ranges may be subject to more health problems than they would have if they were in the normal range.

There are a number of ways to predict an optimal or desirable body weight. Some of these are presented in Laboratory Inventory 6.2 for your personal use. However, this section deals with two different, but related, approaches to determination of a desirable body weight. The first uses body fat percentage, and the second uses height-weight charts.

Body Fat Approach

If you have available to you a method of determining your body fat percentage, then this approach to determination of your desirable body weight is appropriate. Perusal of the literature reveals a number of recommended normal body fat percentage levels. The values presented in table 6.2 represent a consolidation of a number of studies, and may serve as a useful guide to you. You should attempt to get your body fat percentage at least to the "good" or "acceptable" level.

However, athletes may desire lower body fat levels. Some male athletes function effectively at 5–8 percent body fat, and some elite male marathon runners have been reported to have only 2–3 percent. Female athletes who compete in endurance sports competition are recommended to have no more than 10 percent body fat. If you compete in a sport where excess body fat may be detrimental to your performance, then

Table 6.2
Ratings of Body Fat Percentage Levels

Rating	Males (ages 18–30)	Females (ages18–30)
Excellent	6–10%	10–15%
Good	11–14%	16–19%
Acceptable	15–17%	20–24%
Too Fat	18–19%	25–29%
Obese	20% or over	30% or over

Keep in mind that these are approximate values. The *excellent* category for females may apply particularly to athletes who compete in events where excess body fat may be a disadvantage, such as gymnastics, ballet, and long-distance running.

it is important to keep the percent low, while still maintaining good strength and cardiovascular endurance levels. For the typical physically active male, the recommended level may be 10–12 percent; 14–16 percent is a sound level for the active female.

Once you have determined your body fat percentage (either by Laboratory Inventory 6.1 or another appropriate technique), consult Laboratory Inventory 6.2 (Method B) to determine your desirable body weight.

Height-Weight Table Approach

One of the most used, and often abused, methods of determining a desirable body weight has been the height-weight tables developed by life insurance companies. **Height and weight charts** are based on measurements obtained from large populations of people. The data obtained are then treated statistically, and the values that tend to cluster toward the midpoint (the mean or median) are considered to be normal, average, or desirable. Unfortunately, these tables reveal nothing to us of our body composition. Two individuals may be exactly the same height and weight, hence classified as having normal body weight, but the distribution of their body weight might be so different that one individual could possibly be considered obese while the other might be considered very muscular.

Nevertheless, even with this limitation, height-weight tables may be a practical guide to a desirable weight, especially if body frame size is part of the table. Tables 6.3 and 6.4 represent two of the more popular height-weight charts that have been developed by the Metropolitan Life Insurance Company. Body weight ranges are given for three body frames—small, medium, and large (determined by using the guide in table 6.5). Laboratory Inventory 6.2 (Method A) serves as a guide to determine an ideal weight with these tables.

Although the Metropolitan Life Insurance Company has recently released new height-weight tables for Americans, the data presented in tables 6.3 and 6.4 represent the 1959 figures. Why not use the most recent data? The new height-weight tables have been challenged by several major health organizations because the average body weights are higher than the 1959 figures (as much as 13 pounds for short men and 10 pounds for short women). The increases are less for medium-height adults and insignificant for tall individuals.

Table 6.3
Desirable Weights for Females Age Twenty-Five and Over

Height		Small Frame		Medium Frame		Large Frame	
(ft./in.)	(cm.)	(lb.)	(kg.)	(lb.)	(kg.)	(lb.)	(kg.)
5'10"	177.8	134–144	60.8–65.3	140–155	63.5–70.3	149–169	67.6–76.6
5'9"	175.3	130–140	59.0–63.5	136–151	61.7–68.5	145–164	65.8–74.4
5'8"	172.7	126–136	57.2–61.7	132–147	59.9–66.7	141–159	64.0–72.1
5'7"	170.2	122–131	55.3–59.4	128–143	58.1–64.9	137–154	62.1–69.9
5'6"	167.6	118–127	53.5–57.6	124–139	56.2–63.1	133–150	60.3–68.1
5'5"	165.1	114–123	51.7–55.8	120–135	54.4–61.2	129–146	58.5–66.2
5'4"	162.6	110–119	49.9–54.0	116–131	52.6–59.4	125–142	56.7–64.4
5'3"	160.0	107–115	48.5–52.2	112–126	50.8–57.2	121–138	54.9–62.6
5'2"	157.5	104–112	47.2–50.8	109–122	49.4–55.3	117–134	53.1–60.8
5'1"	154.9	101–109	45.8–49.4	106–118	48.1–53.5	114–130	51.7–59.0
5'0"	152.4	98–106	44.4–48.1	103–115	46.7–52.2	111–127	50.3–57.6
4'11"	149.8	95–103	43.1–46.7	100–112	45.4–50.8	108–124	49.0–56.2
4'10"	147.3	92–100	41.7–45.4	97–109	44.0–49.4	105–121	47.6–54.9
4'9"	144.7	90–97	40.8–44.0	94–106	42.6–48.1	102–118	46.3–53.5

For women between eighteen and twenty-five, subtract one pound for each year under twenty-five. Height measured without shoes.

Source: Used with permission of the Metropolitan Life Insurance Company.

Table 6.4
Desirable Weights for Males Age Twenty-Five and Over

Height		Small Frame		Medium Frame		Large Frame	
(ft./in.)	(cm.)	(lb.)	(kg.)	(lb.)	(kg.)	(lb.)	(kg.)
6'3"	190.5	157–168	71.2–76.2	165–183	74.9–83.0	175–197	79.4–89.3
6'2"	188.0	153–164	69.4–74.4	160–178	72.6–80.8	171–192	77.6–87.1
6'1"	185.4	149–160	67.6–72.6	155–173	70.3–78.5	166–187	75.3–84.8
6'0"	182.9	145–155	65.8–70.3	151–168	68.5–76.2	161–182	73.0–82.6
5'11"	180.3	141–151	64.0–68.5	147–163	66.7–74.0	157–177	71.2–80.3
5'10"	177.8	137–147	62.1–66.7	143–158	64.9–71.7	152–172	69.0–78.0
5'9"	175.3	133–143	60.3–64.9	139–153	63.1–69.4	148–167	67.1–75.3
5'8"	172.7	129–138	58.5–62.6	135–149	61.2–67.6	144–163	65.3–74.0
5'7"	170.2	125–134	56.7–60.8	131–145	59.4–65.8	140–159	63.5–72.1
5'6"	167.6	121–130	54.9–59.0	127–140	57.6–63.5	135–154	61.2–69.9
5'5"	165.1	117–126	53.1–57.2	123–136	55.8–61.7	131–149	59.4–67.6
5'4"	162.6	114–122	51.7–55.3	120–132	54.4–59.9	128–145	58.1–65.8
5'3"	160.0	111–119	50.3–54.0	117–129	53.1–58.5	125–141	56.7–64.0
5'2"	157.5	108–116	49.0–52.6	114–126	51.7–57.2	122–137	55.3–62.1
5'1"	154.9	105–113	47.6–51.3	111–122	50.3–55.3	119–134	54.0–60.8

Height measured without shoes.

Source: Used with permission of the Metropolitan Life Insurance Company.

Table 6.5
Approximation of Body Frame Size

Extend your arm and bend the forearm upward at a 90 degree angle. Keep fingers straight and turn the inside of your wrist toward your body. If you have a caliper, use it to measure the space between the two prominent bones on either side of your elbow. Without a caliper, place thumb and index finger of your other hand on these two bones. Measure the space between your fingers against a ruler or tape measure. Compare it with the accompanying tables that list elbow measurements for medium-framed men and women. Measurements lower than those listed indicate that you have a small frame. Higher measurements indicate a large frame.

Height (ft./in.)	Elbow Breadth (in.)
Men (1″ heels)	
5′2″–5′3″	2½″–2⅞″
5′4″–5′7″	2⅝″–2⅞″
5′8″–5′11″	2¾″–3″
6′0″–6′3″	2¾″–3⅛″
6′4″	2⅞″–3¼″
Women (1″ heels)	
4′10″–4′11″	2¼″–2½″
5′0″ –5′3″	2¼″–2½″
5′4″ –5′7″	2⅜″–2⅝″
5′8″ –5′11″	2⅜″–2⅝″
6′0″	2½″–2¾″

Source: Used with permission of the Metropolitan Life Insurance Company.

The data in the new tables represent those weights at which Americans now between the ages of twenty-five and twenty-nine can expect to live the longest. However, certain factors may have contributed to the increase in the weight values since 1959. First, the change by many Americans to a healthier life-style, and improvements in medical technology have led to better prevention and treatment of conditions such as coronary heart disease and diabetes—both of which are associated with obesity. Second, there is an increasing death rate among heavy smokers, who are usually underweight. Thus, the weights in the new charts may not be the most healthful.

The American Heart Association has recommended that Americans continue to use the 1959 version, and even the Metropolitan Life Insurance Company no longer refers to the new tables as ideal or desirable weights. Moreover, the new charts do not appear to reflect ideal weights as far as physical appearance is concerned.

Basic Principles of Weight Control

The vast majority of individuals who are interested in body weight control are really interested in body *fat* control. Body fat is nature's primary way of storing energy in the human body for future use. In essence, body fat control is human energy control. In order for you to maintain your current body weight, you must be in **energy balance.** You must expend as much energy through your daily activities as you consume in your daily diet.

Figure 6.4 Weight control is based upon energy balance. Too much food input or too little exercise output can result in a positive energy balance or weight gain. Decreased food intake or increased physical activity can result in a negative caloric balance or weight loss.

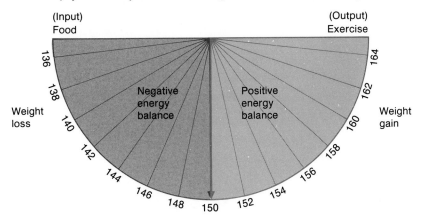

In other words, energy output must equal energy input. During the growth and development years of childhood and adolescence, energy input predominates slightly, creating a positive energy balance and growth of body mass. As the adolescent enters young adulthood, the major growth processes are just about complete and energy input and output must equalize. An individual loses weight if output predominates—a condition of **negative energy balance.** If the input is greater, a **positive energy balance** exists, and the individual gains weight. For example, the input of an extra doughnut (125 Calories) per day, if not balanced by an increased energy expenditure of 125 Calories, can lead to an increase of about 13 pounds of body weight in a year. Thus, the key principle to all weight control programs is proper energy balance.

The Calorie

Although there are a number of ways to express energy, the most common term is the *Calorie*. The Calorie is used as the unit for measuring energy requirements in the 1980 RDA; it is the way we express the energy content of the foods we eat; and it is one means to express the energy expenditure of physical activity. Thus, energy balance and caloric balance are synonymous.

A calorie is a measure of heat. One small calorie represents the amount of heat needed to raise the temperature of 1 gram of water 1 degree Celsius; it is sometimes called the *gram calorie*. A large **Calorie,** or kilocalorie, is equal to 1000 small calories. It is the amount of heat needed to raise 1 kilogram of water (1 liter) 1 degree Celsius. In human nutrition, the kilocalorie is the main expression of energy. It is usually abbreviated as kcal, kc, C, or capitalized as Calorie. Throughout this book, Calorie refers to the kilocalorie.

According to the principles underlying the First Law of Thermodynamics, energy may be equated from one form to another. Thus, the Calorie, which represents heat energy, may be equated to other forms, such as the mechanical energy utilized during work (as in exercise). This concept is expanded later in this chapter when we discuss the role of exercise in weight control, but first let us look at how the human body expends energy through its metabolic activities.

Metabolism

Human **metabolism** represents the sum total of all physical and chemical changes that take place within the body. The transformation of food to energy, the formation of new compounds such as hormones and enzymes, the growth of bone and muscle tissue, the destruction of body tissues, and a host of other physiological processes are parts of the metabolic process.

Metabolism involves two fundamental processes, anabolism and catabolism. Anabolism is a building-up process, or constructive metabolism. Complex body components, such as muscle tissue, are synthesized from the basic nutrients. Catabolism is the tearing-down process, or destructive metabolism. This involves the disintegration of body compounds, such as fat, into energy. Metabolism is life. It represents human energy. The **metabolic rate** reflects how rapidly the body is using its energy stores. This rate can vary tremendously depending upon a number of factors—the most influential one is exercise.

For our purpose the metabolic rate may be conveniently subdivided into three components, the basal metabolic rate, the resting metabolic rate, and the exercise metabolic rate.

The **basal metabolic rate (BMR)** represents the energy necessary for basic life functions. Other than during sleep, it is the lowest level of energy expenditure. The determination of the BMR is a clinical procedure conducted in a laboratory or hospital setting. In the average individual approximately 50–60 percent of the total daily energy expenditure is accounted for by the BMR.

There are several ways to estimate the BMR. Whichever method is used, keep in mind that the value obtained is an estimate. In order to get a truly accurate value, a standard BMR test is needed. However, the formula in table 6.6 may give you a good approximation of your daily BMR.

The **resting metabolic rate (RMR)** is slightly higher than the BMR. It represents the BMR plus any additional energy expenditure associated with digestion of food, sitting, reading, standing, or other such very sedentary activities. In most sedentary individuals, the RMR governs total daily energy expenditure.

The **exercise metabolic rate (EMR)** represents the energy expenditure during physical exercise, which may be ten to twenty times greater than the RMR. The EMR may be a key factor to weight control.

Caloric Concept of Weight Control

The **caloric concept of weight control** is relatively simple. If you take in more Calories than you expend, you gain weight. If you expend more than you take in, you lose weight. To maintain your body weight, caloric input and output must be equal. As far as we know, human energy systems are governed by the same laws of physics that rule all

Table 6.6
Estimation of the Daily Basal Metabolic Rate

Adult Male	Adult Female
BMR estimate = 1 Calorie/kg body weight/hour	BMR estimate = 0.9 Calorie/kg body weight/hour
Example:	Example:
154 pound male	121 pound woman
154 pounds ÷ 2.2 = 70 kg	121 pounds ÷ 2.2 = 55 kg
70 kg × 1 Calorie = 70 Calories/hour	55 kg × 0.9 Calories = 49.5 Calories/hour
70 × 24 hours = 1680 Calories/day	49.5 × 24 hours = 1188 Calories/day
Rounded BMR estimate = 1700 Calories/day	Rounded BMR estimate = 1200 Calories/day

Figure 6.5   Total Daily Caloric Expenditure for an Average-Sized Female (121 Pounds). BMR represents basal metabolic rate; RMR is the resting metabolic rate; and EMR is the exercise metabolic rate. EMR could be increased considerably through an expanded exercise program.

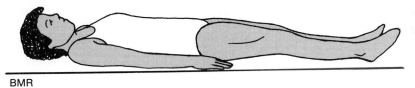

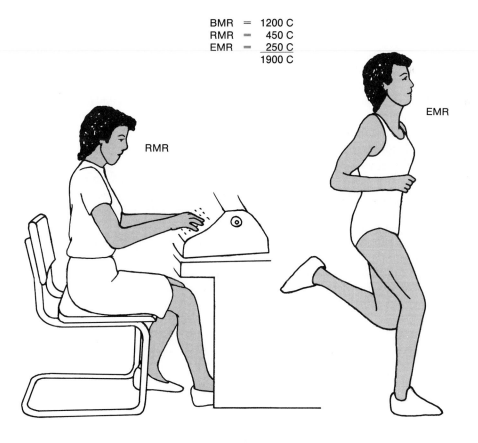

BMR

BMR = 1200 C
RMR =   450 C
EMR =   250 C
         1900 C

RMR

EMR

energy transformations. The First Law of Thermodynamics is as pertinent to us in the conservation and expenditure of our energy sources as it is to any other machine. Since a Calorie is a unit of energy, and since energy can neither be created nor destroyed, those Calories that we consume must either be expended in some way or conserved in the body. No substantial evidence is available to disprove the caloric theory. It is still the physical basis for body weight control.

Keep in mind however that total body weight is made up of different components—those notable in weight control programs are body water, protein, and fat stores. Changes in these components may bring about body weight fluctuations that would appear to be contrary to the caloric concept. You may lose 5 pounds in an hour, but it will be water weight. Starvation techniques may lead to rapid weight losses, but a good proportion of the weight loss will be in body protein stores, such as muscle mass, and water weight. In programs to lose body weight, we usually desire to lose excess body fat. Certain dietary and exercise techniques may help to maximize fat losses, while they minimize protein losses. The metabolism of human energy sources is complex. Although the caloric theory is valid relative to body weight control, one must be aware that weight changes will not always be in line with caloric input and output, and that weight losses may not be due to body fat loss alone. These concepts are explored later in this chapter.

Since the caloric concept is a sound basis for weight control, you may ask the question, "How many Calories do I need daily in order to maintain my body weight?" This depends upon a number of factors, notably age, body weight, sex, and physical activity levels. The caloric requirement per kg of body weight is very high during the early years of life when the child is developing and adding large amounts of body tissue. The Calorie/kg requirement decreases throughout the years from birth to old age. Body weight influences the total amount of daily Calories you need, but not the Calorie/kg level. The large individual simply needs more total Calories to maintain body weight. Up to the age of eleven or twelve, the caloric needs of boys and girls are similar in terms of Calories/kg body weight. After puberty, however, males need more Calories/kg, probably due to their greater percentage of muscle tissue in comparison to females. Individual variations in BMR may either increase or decrease daily caloric needs, depending on whether the BMR is above or below normal. Physical activity levels above resting may have a very significant impact upon caloric needs, in some cases adding 1000–1500 or more Calories to the daily energy requirement. All of these factors make it difficult to make an exact recommendation relative to daily caloric needs, but some guidelines are available.

Table 6.7 presents some figures from the American Heart Association relative to the approximate daily caloric intake that will help the average adult maintain body weight. For example, a sedentary individual who weighs 170 pounds needs approximately 2380 Calories per day (170 × 14) simply to maintain body weight. If you want

Table 6.7
Approximate Daily Caloric Intake Needed to Maintain Desirable Body Weight

Activity Level	Calories per Pound
1. Very sedentary (movement restricted, such as patient confined to house)	13
2. Sedentary (most Americans, office job, light work)	14
3. Moderate activity (weekend recreation)	15
4. Very active (meet ACSM standards for vigorous exercise three times/week)	16
5. Competitive athlete (daily vigorous activity in high-energy sport)	17+

to lose or gain weight, the caloric intake must be adjusted accordingly. Keep in mind that these figures are approximations, and your actual daily caloric needs may vary somewhat. However, they do offer you a ballpark estimate of your daily caloric needs, and may be a useful guideline to start your weight control program.

If you decide to lose weight without the guidance of a physician, the recommended maximal value for adults is 2 pounds/week. Since there are 3500 Calories in a pound of body fat, this necessitates a deficit of 7000 Calories for the week, or 1000 Calories/day. For growing children, the general recommendation is only about 1 pound/week, or a daily 500 Calorie deficit. Weight losses may not parallel the caloric deficit incurred during the early stages of a weight reduction program. Hence the 2 pound limit may be adjusted during that time period.

Laboratory Inventory 6.3 presents a method to determine the caloric deficit needed to lose excess body fat.

The Role of Diet in Weight Control

As you are probably aware, there are literally hundreds of different diet plans available that are designed to help you lose body weight. Hardly a month goes by without a new miracle diet being revealed in a leading magazine, and some type of diet book always seems to be on the best-seller list. Many of these diets are based upon sound nutritional principles, but others are not and may even lead to serious health problems in some individuals. Space does not permit an analysis of the various diet plans available on the market today, so the interested reader should consult the current edition of *Rating the Diets* by the editors of *Consumer Guide*. However, if you know some basic principles, you should be able to evaluate the value of most diet plans yourself.

Research with dieters has shown that any weight reduction diet, in order to be effective, should adhere to the following principles:

1. It should be low in Calories, and yet supply all nutrients essential to normal body functions.
2. It should contain foods that appeal to your taste and help to prevent hunger sensations between meals.

3. It should be easily adaptable to your current life-style and readily obtainable whether you eat most of your meals at home or you dine out frequently.

4. It should be a lifelong diet, one that will satisfy the previous three principles, once you attain your desired weight.

As for the diet itself, there are a variety of suggestions that may be helpful in the battle against Calories.

1. The key principle is to select low-Calorie, high-nutrient foods from the Exchange Lists. Avoid refined, processed foods as much as possible, and include more natural, unrefined products in your diet.

2. Milk products are excellent sources of protein, but may contain excess Calories unless the fat is removed. Use skim milk, low-fat cottage cheese, low-fat yogurt, and nonfat dried milk, instead of their high-fat counterparts like whole milk, sour cream, and powdered creamers.

3. Meat products are also sources of protein and many other nutrients, but also may contain excess fat Calories. Use leaner cuts of meat, and also trim away excess fat; broil or bake your meats. Fish, chicken, and eggs are excellent low-Calorie substitutes.

4. Fruits and vegetables provide many of the necessary vitamins and minerals. They provide bulk to the diet and a sensation of fullness, without excessive amounts of Calories. Low-Calorie items like carrots, radishes, and celery are highly nutritious snacks for munching.

5. Grain products are also high in vitamins and minerals. Use whole grain breads, cereals, brown rice, oatmeal, beans, and bran products for dietary fiber.

6. Fluid intake should remain high, especially on high-protein diets, as water is necessary to eliminate protein waste products from the body. Water is the recommended fluid, although diet drinks and unsweetened coffee and tea may be used.

7. Salt intake should be limited to that which occurs naturally in our foods. Try to use dry herbs, spices, and other non-salt seasonings as substitutes to flavor your food.

8. Avoid high-Calorie foods like salad dressings, butter, margarine, and cooking oil. Substitute low-Calorie dietary versions instead.

9. Avoid alcohol as much as possible. It is high in Calories and has zero nutrient value. One gram of alcohol is equal to 7 Calories—almost twice that of protein and carbohydrate.

10. Instead of two or three large meals a day, eat five or six smaller ones. Research has shown that this may help in the fight against obesity by helping to control sensations of hunger between meals.

11. Another approach is to cut the size of the portion you eat. Cook only half of an 8-ounce steak, rather than the whole piece.
12. Learn what foods are low in Calories in each of the Exchange Lists and incorporate those that are palatable to you in your diet. The key to a lifelong weight maintenance diet is your knowledge of sound nutritional principles and the application of this knowledge to the design of your personal diet.

Your Personal Diet

The key to your personal diet is nutrient density, or the selection of low-Calorie, high-nutrient foods. As mentioned previously, low-Calorie foods must be selected wisely. For our purposes here the Exchange List system is used as the means to select low-Calorie foods. In ascending order, the caloric content of one serving from each of the six groups is as follows:

1 vegetable exchange	= 25 Calories
1 fruit exchange	= 40 Calories
1 fat exchange	= 45 Calories
1 meat exchange	= 55 Calories
1 bread exchange	= 70 Calories
1 milk exchange	= 80 Calories

The Food Exchange Lists may be found in appendix B. Study these lists carefully to get an appreciation for the amount of Calories in the foods you eat. Knowledge of the Exchange Lists enables you to substitute one low-Calorie food for another in your daily menu. As you become familiar with the caloric content of various foods it becomes easier to select those that are low in Calories, but high in nutrient value—and to avoid those foods that are just the opposite. Pay particular attention to the fat exchanges and foods that include fat exchanges, such as whole milk products and high-fat meats. It requires a little effort in the beginning phases of a diet to learn the Calories in a given quantity of a certain food exchange, but once learned and incorporated into your life-style, it is a valuable asset to possess when trying to lose weight. Knowledge, however, is not the total answer; your behavior should reflect your knowledge. For example, you may know that regular milk contains 70–80 more Calories per glass than skim milk, but if you cannot develop a taste for skim milk, the advantage of your knowledge is lost.

Table 6.8 presents a suggested meal plan adapted from a model developed by the Committee on Dietetics of the Mayo Clinic. The total caloric values are close approximations for a three meal pattern. If you decide to include snacks such as a fruit or vegetable in your diet, then remove it from one of the main meals. The beverages, other than milk, should contain no Calories. Although only four meal plans are listed (800, 1000, 1200, and 1400 Calories) you may calculate almost any amount of Calories you need by using a little simple addition or multiplication. For example, if you wanted a 2200 Calorie diet, you could add the 1000 and 1200 Calorie exchanges. However, you need not increase the salad or beverage allocations.

Table 6.8
Daily Meal Plan Based on the Food Exchange List

	800 Calorie	1000 Calorie	1200 Calorie	1400 Calorie
Breakfast				
Milk	1	1	1	1
Meat	1	1	1	2
Fruit	1	1	1	1
Bread	1	1	1	1
Fat	0	1	1	1
Beverage	1	1	1	1
Lunch				
Milk	1	1	1	1
Meat	2	2	3	3
Fruit	1	1	1	1
Vegetable	1	1	1	1
Salad	1	1	1	1
Bread	0	1	1	2
Fat	0	0	1	1
Beverage	1	1	1	1
Dinner				
Milk	1	1	1	1
Meat	3	3	3	4
Fruit	1	1	1	1
Vegetable	1	1	1	1
Salad	1	1	1	1
Bread	0	1	2	2
Fat	0	0	1	1
Beverage	1	1	1	1

Key points:

1. Caloric values:

Milk exchange	= 80
Meat exchange	= 55
Fruit exchange	= 40
Vegetable exchange	= 25
Bread exchange	= 70
Fat exchange	= 45
Beverage	= 0
Salad	= 20

2. See appendix B for a listing of foods in each exchange. Note the following:
   a. Foods other than milk, such as yogurt, are included in the milk exchange.
   b. The meat list includes foods such as eggs, cheese, fish, poultry, and low-fat products, like beans and peas.
   c. Some starchy vegetables are included in the bread list.

3. Foods should not be fried or prepared in fat unless you count the added fat as a fat exchange. Broil or bake foods instead.
4. Low-Calorie vegetables like lettuce and radishes should be used in the salads. Use only small amounts of very low-Calorie salad dressing.
5. Beverages should contain no Calories.

Figure 6.6 Knowledge of the various food exchanges and their caloric values can be very helpful in planning a diet. With a little effort, you can learn to estimate the caloric value of most basic foods.

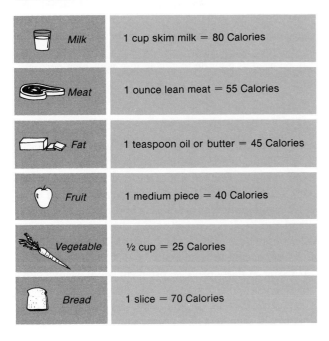

Milk	1 cup skim milk = 80 Calories
Meat	1 ounce lean meat = 55 Calories
Fat	1 teaspoon oil or butter = 45 Calories
Fruit	1 medium piece = 40 Calories
Vegetable	½ cup = 25 Calories
Bread	1 slice = 70 Calories

After you have determined the number of Calories you need daily in order to lose 2 pounds of body weight per week, then select the appropriate diet plan from table 6.8. In order to help implement your diet plan and keep track of the food exchanges you eat on a daily basis, you should design a 3″ × 5″ card similar to the model below for the number of food exchanges in your daily diet. As you consume an exchange at each meal, simply cross if off on the card. Make a new card for each day. The model shown is for 2200 Calories (1000 plus 1200 Calorie plans).

Daily Meal Plan		**2200 Calories**
Milk exchange	(6)	1 2 3 4 5 6
Meat exchange	(13)	1 2 3 4 5 6 7 8 9 10 11 12 13
Fruit exchange	(6)	1 2 3 4 5 6
Vegetable exchange	(4)	1 2 3 4
Salad	(2)	1 2
Bread exchange	(7)	1 2 3 4 5 6 7
Fat exchange	(4)	1 2 3 4
Beverage	(3)	1 2 3

Keep in mind that this is not a rigid diet plan. You may do some slight interchanging between the various exchanges as the total number of Calories in the diet increases. For example, you could possibly delete three meat exchanges (165 Calories) in the model and substitute two bread and one vegetable (165 Calories). Memorizing the caloric value of each exchange and knowing the types of foods in each will help you develop a diet plan suited to your needs and tastes.

Laboratory Inventory 6.4 may be used as a guide to developing your own personal diet plan.

The Role of Exercise in Weight Control

Humans are meticulously designed for physical activity, yet our modern mechanical age has eliminated many of the opportunities we once had to incorporate moderate physical activity as a natural part of our lives. The regulation of food intake was never designed, through the evolutionary process, to adapt to the highly mechanized conditions in today's society. Hence, the combination of overeating and inactivity has led to increasing levels of overweight and obesity. It is generally recognized that prevention of obesity, or excess body weight, is more effective than treatment. Most people do not become overweight overnight, but rather accumulate an extra 75–150 Calories per day that, over time, leads to excess fat tissue. A daily exercise program could easily counteract the effect of these additional Calories. Dr. Jean Mayer, an international authority on weight control, has reported that no single factor is more frequently responsible for the development of obesity than lack of physical exercise. A large body of knowledge substantiates the point that exercise can help to reduce and control body weight. The purpose of this section is to explore the different mechanisms whereby increased levels of physical activity may help you lose body fat.

Exercise and the Metabolic Rate

As you may recall, we can look at the metabolic rate in three ways: the basal metabolic rate (BMR), the resting metabolic rate (RMR), and the exercise metabolic rate (EMR). Increasing the level of any of these metabolic rate components helps to expend Calories. The BMR may be changed slightly through an exercise program, but increasing the RMR and EMR are the primary mechanisms to weight loss through exercise.

Of all the factors that influence the BMR, the change in body composition may be one way we may help to alter it. Decreasing the amount of body fat and increasing lean body mass (muscle tissue) may increase the BMR. This effect may be due to the increased activity levels of muscle tissue as compared to fat tissue, or the increased ratio of body surface area to body weight.

The RMR may be increased or decreased, depending on your average daily activities. Sitting burns up fewer Calories than standing; standing burns up less than walking, and so on. Simply changing the nature of your daily sedentary activities, like walking to the store rather than driving, and climbing the stairs to your class or office, may increase the RMR. Unfortunately, most of us are inclined to save our energy during most daily activities and, unless we make a conscious effort to change them,

Figure 6.7 It is very easy to consume 200 additional Calories per day, which can lead to an increase of about 2 pounds of body fat per month. However, increased physical activity may help to expend these Calories.

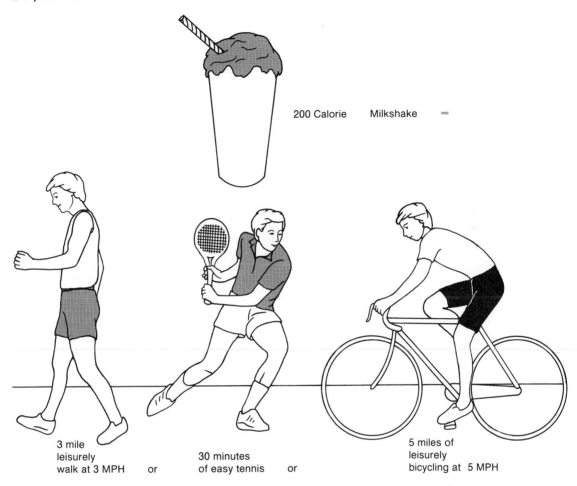

200 Calorie   Milkshake   =

3 mile leisurely walk at 3 MPH   or   30 minutes of easy tennis   or   5 miles of leisurely bicycling at 5 MPH

the RMR remains relatively constant as a percentage of our daily energy expenditure. Some research has reported that the RMR accounts for about 30 percent of our caloric expenditure above the BMR. Thus, for a BMR of 1500 Calories, the RMR would add 30 percent of that to the daily caloric needs. Thus, the daily caloric needs would be 1500 + (.30 × 1500) = 1950 Calories. Simply increasing the RMR in this example from 450 to 500—an increase of 50 Calories per day—could account for over 5 pounds of body fat in one year.

Increasing the EMR, however, is the most effective means to increase our daily caloric expenditure and should be a major component of a weight control program. For example, while the average person may expend only about 60–70 Calories per hour during rest, this value may approach 1000 Calories per hour during a sustained, high level activity, such as running, swimming, or bicycling. Fat is mobilized from the body's fat cells in order to supply energy to the muscle cells. Hence, body fat stores are reduced.

Figure 6.8 Exercise helps to release fat (free fatty acids) from the adipose tissues. The fat then travels by way of the bloodstream to the muscles where the free fatty acids are oxidized to provide the energy for exercise. Thus, exercise is an effective means to reduce body fat.

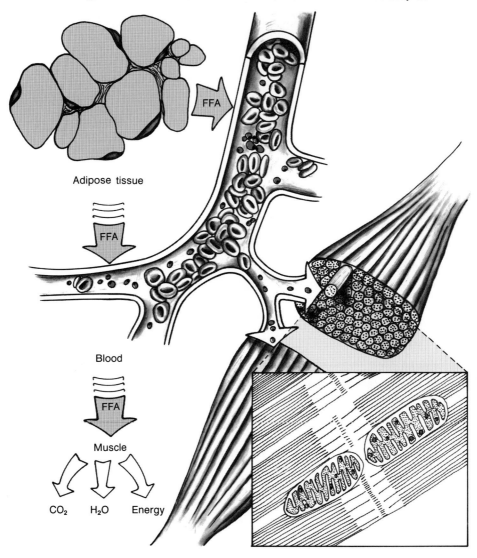

Adipose tissue

FFA

Blood

FFA

Muscle

CO_2 H_2O Energy

The most important factor affecting the EMR is the intensity or speed of the exercise. In order to move faster, your muscles must contract more rapidly and, hence, consume proportionately more energy. However, other factors may affect the total caloric expenditure during exercise. First, the nature of the activity is critical; swimming a mile expends more Calories than running the same distance; and running a mile costs more than bicycling. Second, the efficiency of movement in some activities modifies the number of Calories expended; a beginning swimmer wastes a lot of energy while one who is more efficient may swim with less effort, hence saving Calories. Third, the individual with a greater body weight burns more Calories for any given amount of work where the body has to be moved, as in walking, jogging, or running. It simply costs more energy to move a heavier load. Now we do not recommend that you become less skilled or gain body weight in order to burn more Calories during exercise. In fact, the opposite is true—try to become more efficient so that the exercise task may become more enjoyable.

Exercise Programs

As you are probably well aware, there are a number of different exercise programs available to lose body weight. Perusal of the daily newspaper reveals numerous advertisements for weight reduction programs sponsored by various commercial physical fitness businesses. Weight training with sophisticated equipment, slimnastics exercises, aerobic dancing, and special exercise apparatus are a few of the approaches often advertised as the best means to lose body fat fast. The truth is that you do not need any special apparatus or any specially designed program. The design of an exercise program to lose body fat is based upon the same principles underlying an aerobic exercise program as discussed in chapter 4. An aerobic exercise program to lose body fat should involve large muscle groups, should be rhythmic and continuous in motion, should be enjoyable, and should be properly designed relative to exercise intensity, and, especially, to duration and frequency.

Intensity

The higher the intensity of the exercise, the more Calories you expend. Per unit of time, walking uses less Calories than jogging, which uses less Calories than fast running. Simply put, it costs you more energy to move your body weight at a faster pace. However, there is an optimal intensity level for each person depending on how long the exercise will last. You can run at a very high intensity for 200 yards, but you certainly could not maintain that same fast pace for 2 miles. Intensity and duration are interrelated.

In order to facilitate the determination of the energy cost (in Calories) of a wide variety of physical activities, appendix F has been developed. It is a composite table of a wide variety of individual reports in the literature. When using this appendix, keep the following points in mind.

1. The figures are approximate and include the resting metabolic rate. Thus, the total cost of the exercise includes not only the energy expended by the exercise itself, but also the amount you would have used anyway during the same period of time. Suppose you ran for 1 hour and the calculated energy cost was 800 Calories. During that same time at rest you may have expended 75 Calories, so the net cost of the exercise is only 725 Calories.

2. The figures in the table are only for the time you are performing the activity. For example, in an hour of basketball you may only exercise strenuously for 35–40 minutes, as you may take time-outs and rest during foul shots. In general, record only the amount of time that you are actually moving during the activity.

3. The figures may give you some guidelines to total energy expenditure, but actual caloric costs might vary somewhat due to such factors as your skill level, environmental factors (running against the wind or up hills), and so forth.

4. Not all body weights could be listed, but you may approximate by going to the closest weight listed.

5. There may be small differences between men and women, but not enough to make a marked difference in the total caloric value for most exercises.

Appendix F is a useful means to determine which types of activities may be of the appropriate intensity for your weight control program. Listing those activities with higher caloric expenditure per minute may suggest several that you could blend into your life-style. Also, refer to chapter 4 for exercises that expend large amounts of Calories.

Duration

Probably the most important factor in total energy expenditure is the duration of the exercise. In swimming, bicycling, running, or walking, distance is the key. For example, running a mile costs the average-sized individual about 100 Calories. Five miles would approximate 500 Calories. Running 1 mile a day would take over 1 month to lose 1 pound of fat, whereas 5 miles a day would shorten the time span to about 1 week. Thus, if the purpose of the exercise program is to lose weight, the individual should stress the duration concept.

One of the key points about the duration concept is the notion of distance traveled rather than time. For example, an hour of tennis and an hour of running are both good exercises. However, the runner expends considerably more Calories due to the fact that the activity is continuous. The tennis player has a number of rest periods in which the energy expenditure is lower. Consequently, at the end of an hour's activity, the runner may have expended two to three times more Calories than the tennis player.

A major reason many adults do not use exercise as a weight loss mechanism is that their level of physical fitness is so low that they cannot sustain a moderate level of exercise intensity for very long. However, you should keep in mind that, as you continue to train, your body will begin to adapt so that in time your exercise period may be prolonged.

Many individuals have a major misconception of the duration concept that may deter them from initiating an exercise program for weight control. They believe that exercise is a poor means to lose body weight because it expends so few Calories. For example, they have heard that one has to jog about 35 miles to lose a pound of body fat. Well, since the average person uses approximately 100 Calories per mile, and since 1 pound of body fat contains about 3500 Calories, there is some truth to that statement. However, you must look at the **long-haul concept** of weight control. Jogging about 2 miles a day expends about 6000 Calories in a month, accounting for almost 2 pounds of body fat. Over a year, the weight loss may be substantial.

Figure 6.9 To lose body fat by exercising, you must look at the long-haul concept of weight control. The average-weight individual needs to jog about 35 miles to burn off one pound of body fat. This would be nearly impossible for most of us to do in one day. At 2 miles per day, however, it could be done in about 2½ weeks—and at 5 miles per day, in only one week. Be aware that an exercise program takes time to reduce excess body fat, but it is a very effective approach.

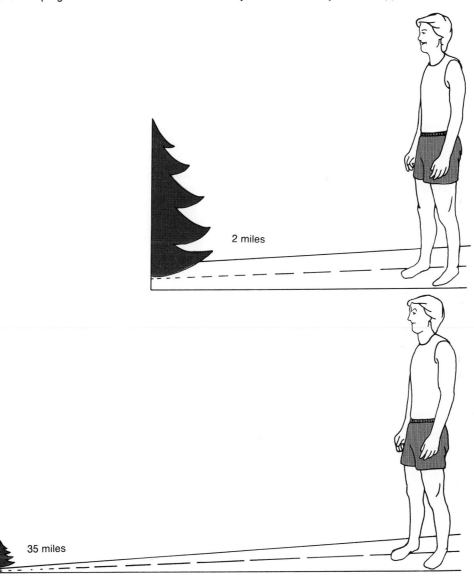

2 miles

35 miles

Frequency

Frequency of exercise complements duration and intensity. Frequency of exercise refers to how often each week you participate. As would appear obvious, the more often you exercise, the greater the total weekly caloric expenditure. In general, three to four times per week is satisfactory, provided duration and intensity are adequate, but six to seven times would just about double your caloric output. A daily exercise program is recommended.

Walking, Running, Swimming, and Bicycling

In general, activities that use the large muscle groups of the body, and are performed in a continuous manner expend the greatest amount of Calories. Intensity and duration are the two key determinants of total energy expenditure. Activities in which you are able to exercise continuously at a fairly high intensity for a prolonged period of time maximize your caloric loss. Although this may encompass a wide variety of different physical activities, those which recently have become increasingly popular include walking, jogging, running, swimming, and bicycling. A few general comments are in order relative to these common modes of exercising.

As a general rule, the caloric cost of running a given distance does not depend on the speed. It will take you a longer time to cover the distance at a slower speed, but the total caloric cost will be similar to that expended at a faster speed. However, walking is more economical than running and, hence, you generally expend fewer Calories for a given distance walking than you do running. This does not hold true, however, if you walk vigorously at a high speed. At high walking speeds, you may expend more energy than if you jogged at the same speed. Fast, vigorous walking, known as aerobic walking, can be an effective means to expend Calories. Due to water resistance, swimming takes more energy to cover a given distance than does walking or running. Bicycling takes less energy per distance unit.

You may calculate the approximate caloric expenditure for running a given distance by either of the following formulas:

Caloric cost = 1 C/kg body weight/kilometer
Caloric cost = .73 C/pound body weight/mile

If you are an average-sized male of about 154 pounds (70 kg), or an average-sized female of about 121 pounds (55 kg), you burn about the following amounts of Calories for either a kilometer or a mile.

	Average Male	**Average Female**
Kilometer	70 Calories	55 Calories
Mile	112 Calories	88 Calories

Slow leisurely walking uses about half this number of Calories per mile. Swimming uses approximately four times this amount, bicycling about one-third. High speed swimming and bicycling increase the caloric cost due to increased water and air resistance, respectively.

Spot Reducing

Whether or not you can reduce fat from a specific body site (e.g. stomach, thighs, or back of the arm), is a controversial question. *Spot reducing* uses local exercises such as sit-ups for the abdominal area, in an attempt to deplete local fat depots. Several studies support the use of spot reducing, while several others show it to be ineffective. The current viewpoint suggests that reduction of fat is most likely to occur from fat deposits throughout the body, not from specific areas, regardless of the exercise format. Although both large muscle activities and local isolated muscle exercises may both be beneficial in reducing fat stores, the former is recommended because the total caloric expenditure is larger.

The Role of Behavior Modification in Weight Control

Changing dietary and exercise habits often involves a significant change in behavior. Many different **behavior modification** techniques, ranging from the bizarre to the pragmatic, are utilized in attempts to modify eating and exercise behavior. In general these techniques center around the elimination of cues that stimulate eating, the substitution of some other activity for eating, or the development of self-discipline. Only the major highlights of behavior modification techniques are presented below. For the interested student, John Ferguson's book *Habits, Not Diets: The Real Way to Weight Control* provides a more detailed discussion. Also, organizations such as Weight Watchers, Overeaters Anonymous, and TOPS (Take Off Pounds Sensibly) use behavior modification techniques as a major means to help you lose weight.

Although we may be unaware of it, many cues in our life-style trigger an eating response. Keeping a diary of your eating behavior may give you some insight relative to situations in which you normally eat. Not all weight control experts recommend that you keep a diary of your daily activities, but some suggest it will help you to identify behavioral patterns that contribute to overeating and extra body weight. The following are some of the factors that might be recorded each time you eat, along with a brief explanation of their possible importance.

1. Type of food and amount. This may be related to the other factors. For example, do you eat a specific type of food during your snacks?
2. Meal or snack. You may find yourself snacking four or five times a day.
3. Time of day. Do you eat at regular hours or have a full meal just before retiring at night?
4. Degree of hunger. How hungry were you when you ate—very hungry or not hungry at all? You may be snacking when not hungry.
5. Activity. What were you doing while eating? You may find that TV watching and eating snack foods are related.
6. Location. Where do you eat? The office cafeteria may be the place you eat a high-Calorie meal.
7. Persons involved. Who do you eat with? Do you eat more when alone or with others? Being with certain people may trigger overeating.
8. Emotional feelings. How do you feel when eating? You might eat more when depressed than when happy.

Recording this information should make you aware of the circumstances under which you tend to overeat. This awareness may be useful to help implement behavioral changes that make dieting easier to do.

The following suggestions to eliminate cues for eating, or to change your style of eating, may be helpful adjuncts to the low-Calorie diet described in a previous section.

1. Do not keep high-Calorie, low-nutrient snacks in the house.
2. Keep food out of sight. Put it in sealed containers or cupboards. A bowl of peanuts sitting on a table is hard to bypass without taking a handful.
3. Do keep low-Calorie snacks, such as carrots and celery, available.
4. Make a food shopping list and stick to it. Plan on buying low-Calorie foods.
5. Do not do food shopping when you are hungry.
6. Serve smaller portions of food.
7. Do not put serving dishes on the table. It is too easy to take a second helping.
8. Have a designated eating space such as the kitchen table. Do not eat anywhere in the house except there.
9. Eat slowly. Chew your food thoroughly to avoid rapid eating. Enjoy what you eat.
10. Do not do anything else, such as reading or watching television, while eating.

Substitute behaviors can help reduce eating. If you feel yourself getting hungry, do something physical, like taking a brief walk. If possible, exercise before eating a meal, as it may help to curb your appetite. Get involved in various activities that will keep you active with other people and away from a sedentary night routine.

When breaking any well-established habit, self-discipline, or will power, is the key. We are constantly bombarded with food stimuli from TV, from other advertising media, and from our family and friends that makes it difficult to adhere to a weight reduction diet. You must be convinced that reduced body weight will enhance your self-concept, and you must establish this as a high priority in your life. If you do, the will power to refuse unnecessary food intake and to stay involved in an aerobic exercise program should be a natural consequence.

Special Considerations in Weight Control

The preceding sections in this chapter offer a number of suggestions to help you lose body fat, primarily by a decrease in energy intake through dieting, and an increase in energy expenditure through exercise. However, your body weight losses may often be different than what you expect them to be. Thus it is important for you to understand what may be happening in your body so you do not become discouraged during periods of time when you are not losing body weight but are still dieting and exercising. This last section deals with predicting your body weight losses, the variation in the rate of weight loss during different phases of your program, and a comparison of the values of dieting versus exercise.

Table 6.9
Approximate Number of Days Required to Lose Body Fat for a Given Caloric Deficit

Daily Caloric Deficit	To Lose 5 Pounds	To Lose 10 Pounds	To Lose 15 Pounds	To Lose 20 Pounds	To Lose 25 Pounds
100	175	350	525	700	875
200	87	175	262	350	438
300	58	116	175	232	292
400	44	88	131	176	219
500	35	70	105	140	175
600	29	58	87	116	146
700	25	50	75	100	125
800	22	44	66	88	109
900	19	39	58	78	97
1000	17	35	52	70	88
1250	14	28	42	56	70
1500	12	23	35	46	58

Prediction of Weight Loss

The human body is compartmentalized into body fat and lean body mass. Because of this fact, it is difficult to predict exactly how much body weight one will lose on any given diet, but an approximate value may be obtained. Remember, weight loss may reflect decreases in body fat, body water, or muscle mass.

For our purposes, we will use the value of 3500 Calories to represent 1 pound of body fat, or body weight, loss. In order to lose 1 pound of body fat, you must create a 3500 Calorie deficit. Thus you must be aware of both your caloric intake and your caloric expenditure. The caloric intake reflects your dietary restrictions, while your caloric expenditure involves your basal metabolic rate and your normal daily activities, including exercise. Laboratory Inventory 6.3 presents some guidelines for you to create a deficit of 1000 Calories per day, but this may be adjusted to other levels, such as 500, 700, 1200, and so forth.

Table 6.9 illustrates the importance of the caloric deficit in determining the rapidity of weight loss by dieting. The higher the deficit, the faster you lose weight, although you should recall that no more than 2 pounds per week should be lost without medical supervision. Also, if you want to maintain a constant caloric deficit you will have to decrease your caloric intake as you lose body weight. This point is discussed further in the following section.

Although these prediction methods are good for the long run, daily body weight changes may not coincide with daily caloric deficits. The rate of weight loss may vary considerably during different stages of your program.

Rate of Body Weight Losses

The rate at which you lose weight may vary somewhat during different phases of your weight control program, and may be partially dependent on the method you use to lose weight—diet or exercise.

Dieting and Rate of Weight Loss

If you start a diet with a significant caloric deficit, say 1000 Calories/day, it would normally take you about 3½ days to lose 1 pound of body fat. However, body weight loss would be more rapid than this during the first several days, possibly totalling as much as 3–4 pounds. A large percentage of this weight loss would be due to a decrease in body carbohydrate and water stores. When you restrict your food intake, the body would then draw on its reserves to meet its energy needs. These reserves consist of both fat and carbohydrate stores, but much of the carbohydrate, stored as liver and muscle glycogen, could be used up in a day or so. Since each gram of glycogen is stored with about 3 grams of water, a significant weight loss could occur. For example, 300 grams of glycogen, along with 900 grams of water stored with it, would account for a loss of 1200 grams, or 1.2 kg; this would equal over 2½ pounds alone. About 70 percent of the weight loss during the first few days of a reduced Calorie diet is due to body water losses. About 25 percent comes from body fat stores and 5 percent from protein tissue. It is important to keep in mind that rather large fluctuations in daily body weight (2–3 pounds) are not due to rapid changes in body fat or lean body mass; these fluctuations are due primarily to body water changes.

Since water has no Calories, caloric loss during the first phase of your weight control program does not need to total 3500 in order to lose 1 pound of weight. You may lose 1 pound of body weight with a deficit of only about 1200 Calories, since 70 percent of the weight loss is water. The 1200 Calories are mostly from fat, with a small amount of protein. However, by the end of the second week of dieting, water loss may account for only about 20 percent of body weight loss; 1 pound of weight loss will now cost you approximately 2800 Calories. At the end of the third week, water losses are minimal. The energy deficit needed to lose 1 pound of body weight is now 3500 Calories. In essence, as you continue your diet, weight losses cost you more Calories, since less body water is being lost. At the end of 3 weeks you can still be losing weight, but at a much slower rate than during the early stages.

Another factor also slows down the rate of weight loss. As you lose weight, you need fewer Calories to maintain your new body weight. Let's take an example. Suppose you weigh 200 pounds and from table 6.7 you see that you need 15 Calories/pound body weight to maintain your weight. At 200 pounds this represents 3000 Calories/day (200 × 15). However, if your weight drops to 180 pounds after dieting for 2 months, you would need only 2700 Calories, a difference of 300 Calories per day.

If you want to continue to have a standard caloric deficit, then you will have to adjust your caloric intake as you lose weight. Suppose at 200 pounds you wanted to have a daily caloric deficit of 1000 Calories. Your diet should then contain about 2000 Calories/day (3000 − 1000). However, once you are down to 180 pounds, your diet should now include only 1700 Calories/day (2700 − 1000). If you did not adjust your diet from 2000 Calories, then the daily deficit would only be 700 Calories/day, not the standard 1000 you wanted. Weight loss would continue, but at a slower rate.

You should realize that the rate of weight loss decreases as a natural consequence of your diet, but the weight you are losing at that point is primarily body fat. To keep a standard caloric deficit may also require an additional reduction in caloric intake as you progress on your diet. Knowledge of these factors may help you through the latter stages of a diet designed to attain a set weight goal.

It should also be noted at this point that fasting, starvation, or very low-Calorie diets may cause the body to adapt to the reduced Calorie intake by lowering its basal metabolic rate, thus partially defeating the purpose of such drastic diet plans. This may also be true with any low-Calorie diet program where muscle tissue is part of the weight loss. Moreover, fasting diets may predispose the individual to a host of medical problems, including hypoglycemia, anemia, and decreased heart muscle tissue.

Exercise and Rate of Weight Loss

Many individuals are disappointed during the early stage of an exercise program because they do not lose weight very rapidly. Unless they understand what is happening in their body, the results on the scale may convince them that exercise is not an effective means to reduce weight, and they may quit exercising altogether. Let's look at several reasons why an individual may not lose weight during the early stages of a weight reduction program, and also why it becomes more difficult after some weight loss has occurred.

When a sedentary individual begins a daily exercise program, the body reacts to the exercise stress and produces changes so it can more easily handle the demands of exercise. The muscles may increase in size. Certain structures within the muscle cell that process oxygen (along with numerous enzymes involved in oxygen use) increase in quantity. Energy substances in the cell increase, particularly glycogen, which binds water. The connective tissue toughens and thickens. The total blood volume may increase. At the same time, body fat stores begin to diminish somewhat as fat is used as a source of energy for exercise. Overall, there is an increase in the lean body mass and body water, and a decrease in body fat. These changes may counterbalance each other and the individual may not lose any weight. However, although little or no weight is lost during these early phases, the body composition changes are favorable. Body fat is being lost.

Once these adaptive changes have occurred (usually in about a month), body weight should decrease in relationship to the amount of Calories spent through exercise. Keep in mind that weight loss is slow on an exercise program, but if you can build up to an exercise energy expenditure of about 300 Calories per day, then about 3 pounds per month will be exercised away.

After several months you may begin to notice that your body weight has stabilized, even though you continue to exercise and have not reached your weight goal. Part of the reason may be due to your lower body weight. If you look at appendix F you can see that the less you weigh, the fewer Calories you burn for any given exercise. If you have been doing the same amount of exercise all along, you may now be at the body weight where your energy output is matched by your energy input in food, and your body weight has stabilized. In addition you may become more skilled, and hence more efficient, in your physical activity. Less Calories may then be expended for any given amount of time. However, this is usually only true of activities that involve a skill factor. It can be highly significant in swimming, but not as great in jogging.

In summary, your body weight may not change during the early stages of an exercise program; it may then begin to drop during a second stage, and then plateau at the third stage. If you are aware of these possible stages, your adherence to an exercise

Figure 6.10 Body weight may not change much during the beginning phases of an aerobic exercise program. However, body composition may change. The exercise stimulates an increase in muscle tissue, blood volume, and muscle glycogen stores, which tends to increase weight. Body fat is reduced, but the increases in the other components can balance out the fat losses with no net loss of body weight. Eventually, body weight begins to drop as the exercise program is continued.

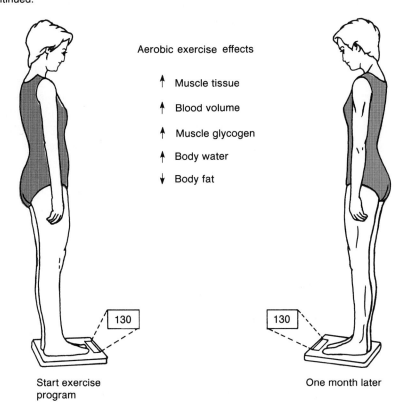

Aerobic exercise effects

↑ Muscle tissue

↑ Blood volume

↑ Muscle glycogen

↑ Body water

↓ Body fat

130

130

Start exercise program

One month later

program may be enhanced. Also, during the third stage, if you desire to lose more weight by exercise, the amount of exercise must be increased.

One last point should be made before leaving this section. A very rapid weight loss may occur during exercise. Some individuals have lost as much as 10–12 pounds in an hour or so. As you probably suspect, this weight loss may be attributed to body water losses. This is particularly evident while exercising in warm or hot weather. The weight loss is temporary; under normal food and water intake the body water content will return to normal within a day. In the heat of summer you may occasionally see individuals training with heavy sweat clothes or a rubberized suit. The reason often given is to lose more body weight. They will lose more body weight, but again it will be body water, which will be regained as soon as they drink fluids. In this regard the technique is worthless. Moreover, it may predispose the individual to unusually high heat stress, which may cause severe medical problems.

Figure 6.11 The most effective weight reduction program involves both dieting and exercise. Mild caloric restriction and an aerobic exercise program can be combined effectively to lose 2 pounds per week.

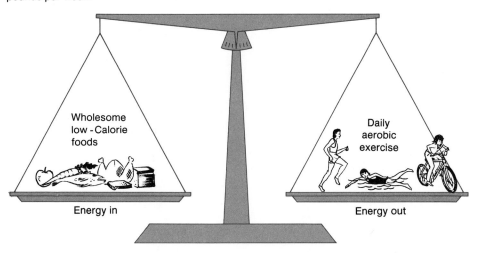

Dieting versus Exercise for Weight Control

By now you may be wondering which is better for weight control—diet or exercise. Both methods may be effective when used separately, but the recommended approach is to use a combination of dieting and exercise. A recent review by the American College of Sports Medicine strongly indicates that optimal body composition changes occur with a combination of caloric restriction (through a well-balanced diet) and an aerobic exercise program. The major highlights of this review are presented in appendix C.

A dietary reduction of 500 Calories per day, along with an exercise energy expenditure of 500 Calories per day, could lead to approximately 2 pounds of weight loss per week—about the maximal amount recommended unless under medical supervision. The removal of 500 Calories from the diet could be done immediately, but it may take a month or more before you may be able to exercise enough to use 500 Calories daily. By following the principles for developing an aerobic exercise program as outlined in chapter 4, you should be able to reach that exercise level safely.

Creating a caloric deficit through dieting contributes to a negative caloric balance, and may help produce a rapid weight loss during the early stages of the program. However, some of this weight loss will be lean body mass, such as muscle tissue. Exercise helps to develop and maintain the lean body mass that otherwise might be lost on a diet program. Moreover, exercise mobilizes free fatty acids from the adipose tissue, and produces greater proportions of body fat loss than dieting will.

Exercise may complement dieting in other ways. For example, exercise may be used to curb the appetite at an appropriate time. Exercise raises the body temperature and stimulates the secretion of several hormones (notably adrenalin) in the body—both of these conditions, it has been hypothesized, depress the appetite. If you exercise before a meal, your food intake may be reduced considerably. Try it and see if it works for you. If you have the facilities available, a good 30 minutes of exercise may be an effective substitute for a large lunch. You may lose Calories two ways, expending them through exercise and replacing the large lunch with a low-Calorie nutritious snack.

Changing your diet by reducing Calories, saturated fats, and cholesterol—and eating more nutritious foods, along with initiating and continuing a good endurance exercise program are considered to be two of the most important components of a Positive Health Life-style. These two life-style changes complement each other nicely both for helping you maintain a proper body weight, and in the prevention of other health problems noted previously.

Once you have reached the body weight level you want, a proper exercise program will help to keep you there. If you like to eat, but do not want excess body fat, exercise is the key.

A. Skinfold Caliper Technique

In order to make accurate measurements, it is best to use skinfold calipers that have pressure built into the instrument itself. However, some of the newer, less expensive, plastic models may also be effective.

1. Take a full fold of fat between the thumb and index finger, being sure to separate the fat from the underlying muscle. Measurements must include only the skinfold, not clothing such as leotards, shirts, etc.
2. Hold the skin firmly and place the contact surface of the calipers at the base of the fold about one-half inch below your fingers.
3. Release the grip on the calipers slowly so that full pressure is exerted at the base of the fold. Continue to hold the skin.
4. Take recordings to the nearest half millimeter after the needle comes to a full stop. Duplicate the measurements until two consecutive measurements agree within one-half millimeter.

B. Skinfold Sites

Females

1. Suprailiac. The skinfold is grasped at an angle of 45 degrees just above the iliac crest at the side of the body. See figure 6.12.
2. Triceps. The skinfold is grasped on the back of the upper arm, midway between the tip of the shoulder and the tip of the elbow. See figure 6.13.

Males

1. Thigh. The skinfold is grasped at the front of the thigh, halfway between the front point of the hip bone and the knee cap. See figure 6.14.
2. Subscapular. The skinfold is taken just below the lower angle of the scapula, at about a 45 degree angle from the spinal column. See figure 6.13.

C. Calculation of Body Density

The skinfold measurements, in millimeters, are entered in the formula below in order to calculate the body density.

Females (from formula of Sloan, Burt, and Blyth)

Body density $= 1.0764 - 0.00081$ (suprailiac) $- 0.00088$ (triceps)

Males (from formula of Sloan)

Body density $= 1.1043 - 0.001327$ (thigh) $- 0.001310$ (subscapular)

D. Calculation of Body Fat (from Brozek, Grande, Anderson, and Keys)

For both males and females:

$$\text{Percent body fat} = \left[\frac{457.0}{\text{Body density}} \right] - 414.2$$

E. Calculation of Pounds of Body Fat

$$\frac{\text{Body weight in pounds} \times \text{Percent body weight}}{100}$$

F. Personal Data
   Females:

   1. **Site**   **Thickness**
      Suprailiac   _____ mm
      Triceps   _____ mm
   2. Body Density

      $1.0764 - 0.00081$ (suprailiac) $- 0.00088$ (triceps) = _____
   3. Percent Body Fat

      $$\left[\frac{457.0}{\text{Body density}} \right] - 414.2 = \text{_____}$$

   4. Pounds of Body Fat

      $$\frac{\text{Body weight} \times \text{Percent body fat}}{100} = \text{_____}$$

   Males:

   1. **Site**   **Thickness**
      Thigh   _____ mm
      Subscapular   _____ mm
   2. Body Density

      $1.1043 - 0.001327$ (thigh) $- 0.001310$ (subscapular) = _____
   3. Percent Body Fat

      $$\left[\frac{457.0}{\text{Body density}} \right] - 414.2 = \text{_____}$$

   4. Pounds of Body Fat

      $$\frac{\text{Body weight} \times \text{Percent body fat}}{100} = \text{_____}$$

Figure 6.12   The Suprailiac Skinfold

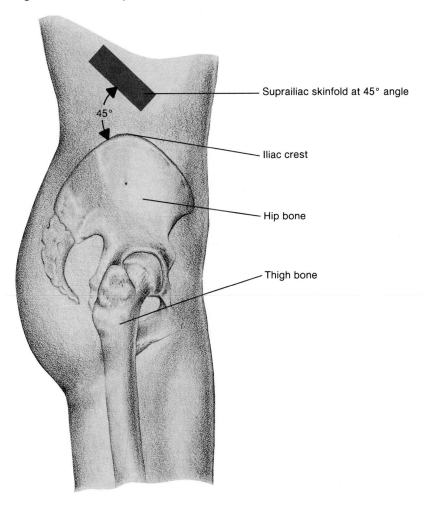

Suprailiac skinfold at 45° angle

45°

Iliac crest

Hip bone

Thigh bone

Figure 6.13 The Triceps and Subscapular Skinfolds

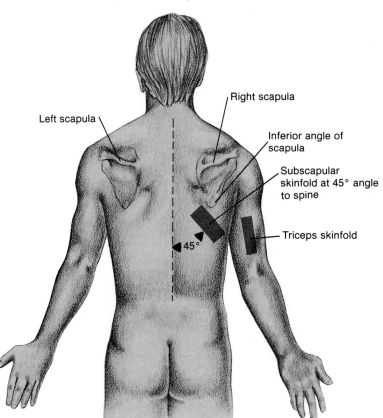

Left scapula

Right scapula

Inferior angle of scapula

Subscapular skinfold at 45° angle to spine

45°

Triceps skinfold

Figure 6.14 The Thigh Skinfold

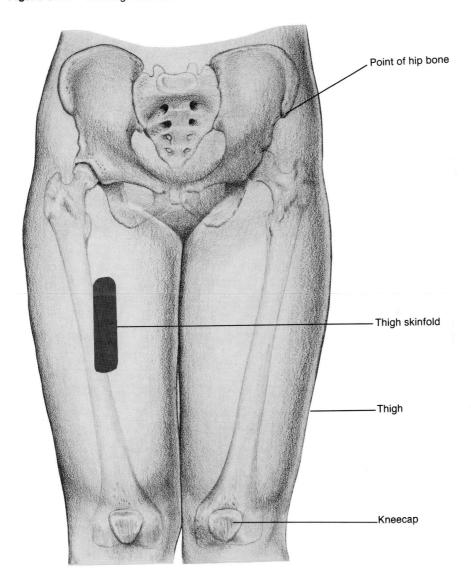

Point of hip bone

Thigh skinfold

Thigh

Kneecap

There are a number of different techniques utilized to determine a desirable body weight. The following two methods may offer you an estimate of an appropriate body weight. Method A is based on height-weight charts. Method B is based on body fat percentages.

Method A

1. Measure your height in 1 inch shoes.
2. Measure your elbow width and determine your frame size from table 6.5.
   _____ Elbow width   _____ Frame size
3. Consult table 6.3 or 6.4 to determine your desirable weight range. The midpoint is halfway into the range.
   _____ Height
   _____ Frame size
   _____ Desirable weight range
   _____ Midpoint of range
4. Obtain your current weight (as close to nude weight as feasible).
   _____ Current body weight
5. Determination of desirable weight. You should attempt to reach the midpoint or lower end of the range.

   Current body weight − Desirable weight = Pounds of fat to lose

   Your data:

Current body weight	− Midpoint of range	= Pounds of fat to lose
_____	− _____	= _____
Current body weight	− Low end of range	= Pounds of fat to lose
_____	− _____	= _____

Method B

Use the following formula to calculate your desired body weight. You will need to have your body fat percentage determined by Laboratory Inventory 6.1 or another appropriate technique. You will also need to determine the body fat percentage you desire. See table 6.2 for guidelines.

To use the formula to calculate your desired body weight, you need to know the following information. The formula is keyed to the letters for each.

CBW (Current body weight in pounds)
CBF% (Current body fat percent)
DBF% (Desired body fat percent)
DBW (Desired body weight)

You may get CBF% from Laboratory Inventory 6.1 or another appropriate method. DBF% should be selected from table 6.2.

Formula:

$$DBW - (DBW \times DBF\%) = CBW - (CBW \times CBF\%)$$

Example:

CBW = 195

CBF% = 22

DBF% = 14

DBW = X (to be solved)

$X - (X \times .14) = 195 - (195 \times .22)$

$X - .14X = 195 - (43)$

$.86X = 152$

$X = 152/.86$

$X = 176$

DBW = 176 pounds, or a loss of 19 pounds of body fat.

Your data:

CBW =

CBF% =

DBF% =

DBW = X

$X - (X \times . \underline{\hspace{1cm}}) = \underline{\hspace{1cm}} - (\underline{\hspace{1cm}} \times . \underline{\hspace{1cm}})$

$X - . \underline{\hspace{1cm}} X = \underline{\hspace{1cm}} - (\underline{\hspace{1cm}})$

$. \underline{\hspace{1cm}} X = \underline{\hspace{1cm}}$

$X = \underline{\hspace{1cm}} / . \underline{\hspace{1cm}}$

$X = \underline{\hspace{1cm}}$

1. Calculate the number of daily Calories needed to maintain current body weight. Find your activity level in table 6.7 and calculate the following:

(Calories per pound body weight)	×	(Body weight in pounds)	=	Number of Calories to maintain body weight
_____	×	_____	=	_____

2. Since 2 pounds of body fat equals 7000 Calories, and there are 7 days in the week, you must achieve a daily dietary caloric deficit of 1000 Calories (7000 ÷ 7).

Number of daily Calories to maintain body weight	−	Daily dietary deficit	=	Number of daily Calories to lose 2 pounds per week
_____	−	1000	=	_____

3. Calculate daily average number of exercise Calories in 1 week in your planned aerobic program. See appendix F for appropriate exercise Calories. Divide the total exercise Calories expended by 7 to get your daily average.

Day	Exercise	Calories Expended
Monday	_____	_____
Tuesday	_____	_____
Wednesday	_____	_____
Thursday	_____	_____
Friday	_____	_____
Saturday	_____	_____
Sunday	_____	_____

Total Calories expended _____

Daily average number of exercise Calories expended = _____

4. Add the average daily exercise Calories to the daily dietary Calories without exercise to calculate the total number of Calories you may consume and still lose 2 pounds of body fat per week.

Number of daily Calories to lose 2 pounds per week	+	Average daily exercise Calories	=	Total number of daily dietary Calories you may consume
_____	+	_____	=	_____

5. Plot your weight losses on the accompanying graph. Keep in mind that actual weight losses may not parallel caloric deficits due to reasons noted in this chapter.

Note: May be adjusted to lose less weight per week. A 3500 Calorie deficit per week is the equivalent of 1 pound of body weight. See table 6.9 for daily caloric deficits and number of days to lose a given amount of weight.

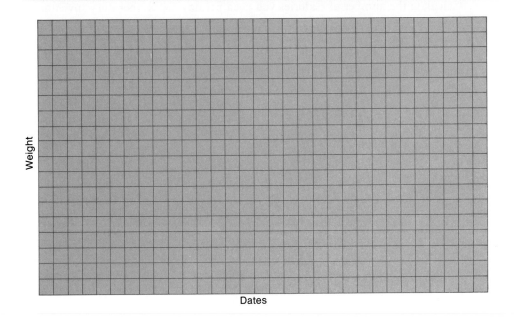

Weight

Dates

1. Calculate the number of Calories you need per day. See Laboratory Inventory 6.3 for guidelines.
2. Use table 6.8 to determine how many servings you need from each food group. For example, if you want 2400 Calories per day, you can multiply the number of servings in the 800 Calorie diet by a factor of 3, or those in the 1200 Calorie diet by 2. The results will not be identical but will provide you with adequate nutrition.
3. Multiply the number of servings by the Calories per serving in order to get the total Calories. Add the total Calories column to get total daily intake.
4. Select appropriate foods from the Exchange Lists in appendix B.

Personal Diet:

Calories ＿＿＿＿＿＿＿＿

	Number of Servings	Calories Per Serving	Total Calories	Foods Selected
Breakfast				
Milk		80		
Meat		55		
Fruit		40		
Vegetable		25		
Bread		70		
Fat		45		
Beverage		0		
Lunch				
Milk		80		
Meat		55		
Fruit		40		
Vegetable		25		
Bread		70		
Fat		45		
Beverage		0		
Dinner				
Milk		80		
Meat		55		
Fruit		40		
Vegetable		25		
Bread		70		
Fat		45		
Beverage		0		
Total Calories			＿＿＿＿＿＿	

References

Adler, J., and Gosnell, M. "What It Means to Be Fat." *Newsweek* 100:84–90 (December 1982).

Allsen, P., et al. *Fitness for Life.* Dubuque, IA: Wm. C. Brown Publishers, 1980.

American College of Sports Medicine. "Proper and Improper Weight Loss Programs." *Medicine and Science in Sports and Exercise* 15:ix-xiii (1983).

American Dietetic Association. *Exchange Lists for Meal Planning.* Chicago: American Dietetic Association and American Diabetes Association, 1976.

Angel, A. "Pathophysiologic Changes in Obesity." *Canadian Medical Association Journal* 119:1401 (1978).

Atkinson, R. "Nutrition vs. Obesity." In *The Medicine Called Nutrition,* edited by D. Mason and H. Guthrie. New York: Davis, Delaney, and Arrow, 1979.

Banister, E., and Brown, S. "The Relative Energy Requirements of Physical Activity." In *Exercise Physiology,* edited by H. Falls. New York: Academic Press, 1968.

Berland, T. *Diets '81: Rating the Diets.* Skokie, IL: Publications International, 1981.

Blair, S.; Blair, A.; Pate, R.; Howe, H.; Rosenberg, M.; and Parker, G. "Interactions among Dietary Pattern, Physical Activity and Skinfold Thickness." *Research Quarterly for Exercise and Sport* 52:505–11 (1981).

Bray, G. "The Energetics of Obesity." *Medicine and Science in Sports and Exercise* 15:32–40 (1983).

Brozek, J.; Grande, F.; Anderson, J.; and Keys, A. "Densitometric Analysis of Body Composition. Revision of Some Quantitative Assumptions." *Annals of the New York Academy of Sciences* 110:131–40 (1963).

Christakis, G., and Plumb, R. *Obesity.* New York: The Nutrition Foundation, n.d.

Clarke, H. "Exercise and Fat Reduction." *Physical Fitness Research Digest* 5:1–27 (April 1975).

Cureton, K.; Hensley, L.; and Tiburzi, A. "Body Fatness and Performance Differences between Men and Women." *Research Quarterly* 50:333–40 (1979).

Dahlkoetter, J.; Callahan, E.; and Linton, J. "Obesity and the Unbalanced Energy Equation: Exercise versus Eating Habit Change." *Journal of Consulting and Clinical Psychology* 47:898–905 (1979).

Dean, R., and Garabedian, A. "Obesity and Level of Activity." *Perceptual Motor Skills* 49:690 (1979).

Dennison, D. "How Many Calories Should You Eat per Day?" *Health Education* 13:53 (1982).

Deutsch, R. *Realities of Nutrition.* Palo Alto, CA: Bull Publishing, 1976.

deVries, H., and Gray, D. "Aftereffects of Exercise upon Resting Metabolic Rate." *Research Quarterly* 34:314–21 (1963).

Durnin, J., and Passmore, R. *Energy, Work and Leisure.* London: Heinemann, 1967.

Durnin, J., et al. "How Much Food Does Man Require?" *Nature* 242:418 (April 1973).

Epstein, L., and Wing, R. "Aerobic Exercise and Weight." *Addictive Behavior* 5:371–88 (1980).

"Exercise, Nutrition and Caloric Sources of Energy." *Nutrition Reviews* 28:180–84 (1970).

Fellingham, G., et al. "Caloric Cost of Walking and Running." *Medicine and Science in Sports* 10:132–36 (1978).

Ferguson, J. *Habits, Not Diets.* Palo Alto, CA: Bull Publishing, 1976.

Food and Nutrition Board. National Research Council. *Recommended Dietary Allowances.* Washington, DC: National Academy of Sciences, 1980.

Franklin, B., and Rubenfire, M. "Losing Weight through Exercise." *Journal of the American Medical Association* 244:377–79 (1980).

Godin, G., and Shephard, R. "Body Weight and the Energy Cost of Activity." *Archives of Environmental Health* 27:289–93 (1973).

Golding, L., and Holmes, K. "The Validation of Estimating Percent Body Fat in Vivo from Body Density." *Medicine and Science in Sports and Exercise* 14:159 (1982).

Hamilton, E., and Whitney, E. *Nutrition Concepts and Controversies.* St. Paul, MN: West, 1979.

Holloszy, J. "Biochemical Adaptation to Exercise. Aerobic Metabolism." In *Exercise and Sport Science Reviews,* edited by J. Wilmore. New York: Academic Press, 1973.

Howley, E., and Glover, M. "The Caloric Costs of Running and Walking One Mile for Men and Women." *Medicine and Science in Sports* 6:235–37 (1974).

Jackson, A., and Pollock, M. "Generalized Equations for Predicting Body Density in Men." *British Journal of Nutrition* 40:497–504 (November 1978).

Jackson, A., et al. "Generalized Equations for Predicting Body Fat in Women." *Medicine and Science in Sports* 12:175–81 (1980).

Jankowski, L., and Foss, M. "The Energy Intake of Sedentary Men after Moderate Exercise." *Medicine and Science in Sports* 4:11–13 (1972).

Jordan, H., et al. "Managing Obesity: Why Diet is Not Enough." *Postgraduate Medicine* 59:185 (1976).

Katch, F., and McArdle, W. *Nutrition, Weight Control and Exercise.* Boston: Houghton Mifflin, 1977.

Keren, G.; Epstein, Y.; Magazanik, A.; and Sohar, E. "The Energy Cost of Walking and Running with and without a Backpack Load." *European Journal of Applied Physiology* 46:317–24 (1981).

Konishi, F. *Exercise Equivalents of Foods.* Carbondale, IL: Southern Illinois University Press, 1973.

Lohman, T. "Skinfolds and Body Density and Their Relation to Body Fatness: A Review." *Human Biology* 53:181–225 (1981).

Mayer, J. "Obesity." In *Modern Nutrition in Health and Disease,* edited by R. Goodhart and M. Shils. Philadelphia: Lea and Febiger, 1980.

———. *Overweight: Causes, Cost and Control.* Englewood Cliffs, NJ: Prentice-Hall, 1968.

———. "Physiology of Hunger and Satiety." In *Modern Nutrition in Health and Disease,* edited by R. Goodhart and M. Shils. Philadelphia: W.B. Saunders, 1980.

Mayo Clinic Committee on Dietetics. *Mayo Clinic Diet Manual.* Philadelphia: W.B. Saunders, 1971.

McArdle, W., and Katch, F. *Exercise Physiology.* Philadelphia: Lea and Febiger, 1981.

Metropolitan Life Insurance Company. *How to Control Your Weight.* New York: Metropolitan Life Insurance Company, 1958.

Moore, M. "New Height-Weight Tables Gain Pounds, Lose Status." *The Physician and Sportsmedicine* 11:25 (May 1983).

Oscai, L. "The Role of Exercise in Weight Control." In *Exercise and Sport Sciences Reviews,* edited by J. Wilmore. New York: Academic Press, 1973.

Passmore, R., and Durnin, J. "Human Energy Expenditure." *Physiological Reviews* 35:801–40 (1955).

Pavlou, K.; Steffee, W.; Lerman, R.; et al. "Effects of Diet and Exercise on the Nature of Weight Loss and Related Physiological Parameters." *Medicine and Science in Sports and Exercise* 15:148 (1983).

Rago, K. "Exercise: A Misused Factor in Weight Control." *Journal of School Health* 49:459–62 (1979).

Schauf, G. "Is the Caloric Theory Valid?" *Nutrition Today* 14:29–31 (January/February 1979).

Seligman, J., and Shapiro, D. "Why You Can't Lose Weight." *Newsweek* 96:109 (December 1980).

Sloan, A. "Estimation of Body Fat in Young Men." *Journal of Applied Physiology* 23:311 (1967).

Sloan, A.; Burt, J.; and Blyth, C. "Estimation of Body Fat in Young Women." *Journal of Applied Physiology* 17:967–70 (1962).

Sours, H., et al. "Sudden Death Associated with Very Low Calorie Weight Reduction Regimens." *American Journal of Clinical Nutrition* 34:453 (1981).

Stare, F., and Whelan, F. *Eat OK, Feel OK.* Quincy, MA: Christopher, 1978.

Stern, J. "Genetic Influence in the Development of Obesity: Focus on Food Intake." *International Journal of Obesity* 4:304–309 (1980).

United States Department of Agriculture. *Food and Your Weight.* (HG74). Washington, DC: Superintendent of Documents, 1977.

Williams, M. H. *Nutritional Aspects of Human Physical and Athletic Performance.* Springfield, IL: C.C. Thomas, 1976.

Wilmore, J. "Body Composition in Sport and Exercise: Directions for Future Research." *Medicine and Science in Sports and Exercise* 15:21–31 (1983).

Wilson, G. "Behavior Modification and the Treatment of Obesity." In *Obesity,* edited by A. Stunkard. Philadelphia: W.B. Saunders, 1980.

Zuti, W. "A Comparison of Weight Reduction Methods that Use Diet and Exercise." In *Abstracts of Research Papers, 1973 National Convention, Minneapolis.* Washington, DC: AAHPER, 1973.

7 Gaining Body Weight and Strength

Key Terms

hernia
muscle fiber splitting
muscle fibers
muscular hypertrophy

myofibrils
progressive resistance exercise (PRE)
tendon
Valsalva phenomenon

Key Concepts

Gains in body weight should not be undertaken at the expense of other components of a Positive Health Life-style, such as sound nutrition and an aerobic exercise program.

Gains in body weight should be in the form of increased lean body mass, such as muscle—not in increased amounts of body fat. A gain of 1–2 pounds per week is a sound goal.

The dietary changes needed to gain 1 pound of muscle tissue per week are relatively small, an increase of approximately 400 Calories and 14 grams of protein per day above the normal RDA.

A weight training program that exercises all of the major muscle groups in the body is the best technique to gain lean body mass.

Although weight training generally is not recognized as an acceptable means for training the cardiovascular system, the increased strength levels and decreased body fat may help to reduce the stress on the heart during exercise.

Weight training increases muscle size by various mechanisms. The most important appears to be an increased amount of connective tissue and an increase in the size and number of myofibrils in the muscle cell.

The two major principles underlying all weight training programs are the overload principle and the progressive resistance exercise principle, although others (such as specificity, exercise sequence, and recuperation) are important.

Weight training may be contraindicated for individuals with certain health problems, such as hernia, high blood pressure, coronary heart disease, and low back pain.

As long as the major principles underlying a weight training program are followed, the various methods of training, such as free weights or machines, appear to be equally effective in producing body weight gains.

Although weight training is regarded as a relatively safe exercise program, the beginner should be aware of proper breathing techniques, the use of spotters, safe use of equipment, and proper lifting techniques for each exercise.

Introduction

When the term weight control is mentioned we normally think about losing weight and, as was noted in the last chapter, there are some very important health reasons that many Americans should lose some of the excess body weight they may be carrying. On the other hand, there are many individuals today who are attempting to gain body weight. With the exception of a few medical conditions, there do not appear to be any direct health benefits attributed to body weight gains. However, many individuals desire to increase their body weight in order to improve their appearance or athletic performance. Also, improvements in these areas may help foster an enhanced body image and/or self-concept that may improve the psychological health of the individual. Although a weight gaining program may be an important means to improve psychological well-being in some individuals, it should not be in opposition to the basic principles of a Positive Health Life-style.

The energy balance equation, as you may recall from chapter 6, is the basis for weight control. A negative caloric balance results in a weight loss, preferably a loss of body fat and not lean body mass. A positive caloric balance results in a weight gain. In order to improve your appearance or athletic performance and still be in accord with a Positive Health Life-style, the weight gain should be lean body mass and not body fat. As diet and exercise are the two mechanisms to create a weight loss, they are also the main means to increase body weight. However, in the case of weight gain the diet must be designed to increase caloric intake without excessive amounts of fat and cholesterol, and the exercise program should be designed to increase the muscle mass.

Before we look at dietary and exercise principles to gain body weight, the cause of being underweight in the first place should be determined. A physician should be consulted to rule out nutritional problems caused by organic diseases, hormonal imbalance, inadequate absorption of nutrients, or psychological factors. Being extremely underweight may be considered to be a symptom of malnutrition or undernutrition. It is important to determine the cause before prescribing a treatment. Our concern is with the individual who does not have any of these problems, medical or otherwise, but who simply is lean and desires to increase muscle mass.

If you decide to initiate a weight gaining program, the following information should be helpful. A reasonable goal should be established within a certain time period. In general, a gain of about 1–2 pounds per week is a sound approach, once you have acquired some basic strength through a month of weight training.

Dietary Considerations

Before you initiate changes in your diet to gain weight you should review chapter 5. The basic principles of nutrition are as relevant to those attempting to gain weight as they are to those who desire to maintain or lose weight. The major adjustments to the diet include an increased caloric intake and assurance that you are obtaining adequate amounts of dietary protein.

Figure 7.1 In order to add a pound of muscle tissue per week, you need to consume approximately 400 additional Calories and 14 grams of additional protein per day. A weight training program is an essential part of a muscle building program. One glass of skim milk, three slices of whole wheat bread, and a medium egg provide the necessary Calories and about 20 grams of protein.

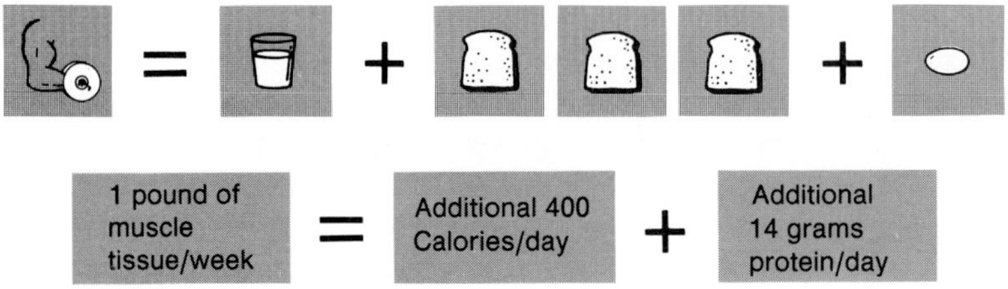

Increased Caloric Intake

The key to gaining weight is to create a positive energy balance; if you accumulate an additional 3500 Calories, then about 1 pound of body fat will be formed. But you are not interested in increasing body fat content, you are interested in increasing your muscle mass. Muscle tissue consists of about 70 percent water, 22 percent protein, and the remainder fat and carbohydrate. The total caloric value of muscle tissue is only about 700–800 per pound, but extra energy is needed to help synthesize the muscle tissue. It is not known exactly how many additional Calories are necessary to form 1 pound of muscle tissue in human beings, nor is it known in what form these Calories have to be consumed. However, the literature suggests that approximately 2500–3000 additional Calories and about 100 additional grams of protein are necessary to synthesize 1 pound of body protein. This averages out to an additional 400 Calories and 14 grams of protein per day in order to gain a pound of muscle tissue per week. Doubling this amount results in the recommended maximal weight gain of 2 pounds per week. See Laboratory Inventory 7.1 for a guide to daily caloric intake.

In order to increase your caloric intake, you should follow the basic recommendations for food selection from the Exchange Lists as presented in the last two chapters and then simply increase the amount of food you eat. A good suggestion is to calculate your caloric needs from Laboratory Inventory 7.1 and then consult table 6.8 for the number of servings from each Exchange List. For example, if you need 3600 Calories per day, simply triple the number of exchanges from the 1200 Calorie diet. This will provide you with the additional Calories you need, yet give you a balanced diet across the food groups.

In addition to the basic nutrition principles presented in chapter 5 relative to selecting a balanced diet, the following suggestions may be helpful for those trying to gain weight.

1. Decrease the intake of bulky foods that are filling, yet contain few Calories, such as bran products, low-Calorie vegetables, and foods with high water content.

2. Increase the intake of foods that are high in both nutrient and caloric content. Lean meats and poultry, whole milk, high-caloric vegetables like corn, peas, and potatoes, high-caloric liquids (orange juice), dried fruit (dates), and similar types of foods are recommended.

Table 7.1
A High-Calorie Diet Based upon the Exchange List Concept

Exchange		Calories
	Breakfast	
Milk	8 ounces whole milk	150
Meat	1 poached egg	80
Bread	2 pieces whole wheat toast	140
Fruit	8 ounces of orange juice	110
Fat	2 pats margarine	90
Other	1 tablespoon jelly	50
		620
	Mid-Morning Snack	
Fruit	8 ounces apricot nectar	140
Bread	2 pieces whole wheat bread	140
Meat	1 tablespoon peanut butter	95
		375
	Lunch	
Milk	8 ounces whole milk	150
Meat	5 ounces lean sandwich meat	350
Bread	2 slices whole wheat bread	140
	3 granola cookies	150
Fruit	1 banana	80
Vegetable	1 large order French fries	300
Fat	1 tablespoon mayonnaise	100
		1270
	Dinner	
Milk	8 ounces whole milk	150
Meat	5 ounces chicken breast	300
Bread	2 dinner rolls	170
Fruit	1 piece apple pie	350
Vegetable	1 cup peas	160
	1 sweet potato, candied	300
Fat	2 pats margarine	90
		1520
	Evening Snack	
Fruit	½ cup dried peaches	215
Total		**4000**

3. Although the amount of saturated fat and simple sugars normally increases in this type of diet, try to keep the intake of these types of foods to a minimum. Use vegetable fats and oils rather than animal fat. For example, substitute polyunsaturated margarine for butter.

4. Eat three balanced meals per day, supplemented with two to three snacks. Some of the high-Calorie, high-nutrient liquid meals on the market make good snacks. Although convenient, they are relatively expensive.

5. There are many foods that are high in Calories and nutrients, yet the costs may vary considerably. Gaining weight may be expensive, but wise selection of high-energy content foods may help keep food costs down.

Table 7.1 presents an example of a high-Calorie diet plan based upon the Exchange List concept. It consists of three main meals and two snacks, and totals approximately 4000 Calories. Alternate foods may be substituted from the food Exchange Lists presented in appendix B.

This suggested diet provides the necessary nutrients, Calories, and protein essential to increased development of body mass and yet less than 30 percent of the Calories are derived from fat. The total number of Calories can be adjusted to meet individual needs as calculated in Laboratory Inventory 7.1.

From a health standpoint probably the most important consideration in developing a high-Calorie diet is to keep the fat content as low as is feasible, particularly saturated fats. If there is a history of heart disease in the family, or if an individual is known to have high blood lipid levels, a high-fat diet could be potentially harmful. The high-fat content, even though primarily vegetable fat, could aggravate lipid metabolism in the body and possibly contribute in some way to the problems associated with coronary heart disease (CHD). Selection of high-protein, low-fat foods and high-Calorie fruits, vegetables, and grain products will help to reduce this problem often associated with high-caloric diets.

Adequate Dietary Protein Intake

If you do decide to go on a weight gaining program, will you need to increase the amount of protein in your diet? If you are currently eating a typical American diet, the answer is probably no. Let us look at the mathematics underlying this response, using an average-sized male as our example. The RDA for protein is 0.8 grams per kilogram of body weight per day. For a 70 kg male (154 pounds) this would be 56 grams of protein per day (0.8 $\times$ 70). The average American diet, however, contains about 100 grams of protein, which is more than sufficient to meet the RDA.

Let us look at some mathematics to determine how much protein is needed for someone undertaking a weight gaining program to add 1 pound of muscle tissue per week. One pound of muscle is equal to 454 grams, but only about 22 percent of this tissue, or about 100 grams (454 $\times$ .22), is protein; the remainder is primarily water (with a small amount of lipids and carbohydrates). If we divide 100 grams by 7 days, we would need approximately 14 grams of protein per day above our normal protein requirements, if we are in protein balance. In our previous example for a 70 kg male, the RDA is only 56 grams of protein per day, so the additional 14 grams increase it to a total of 70 grams. As you can see, if you are eating the typical American diet containing about 100 grams of protein per day, you are consuming more than is necessary to support muscle growth. It should also be noted that even the RDA of 56 grams includes a safety factor, and is probably more protein than is necessary to meet minimal daily requirements.

Incidentally, 14 grams of protein can be obtained in such small amounts of food as 2 glasses of milk, or about 2 ounces of meat, fish, cheese, or poultry. Selection of a wide variety of foods from the food groups should ensure more than adequate protein intake to meet the demands of a weight gaining program. For example, in table 6.8, the protein content in the 1000 Calorie diet totals approximately 70 grams. The 4000

Calorie diet in table 7.1 contains nearly 150 grams of protein. A diet with about 60 percent carbohydrate, less than 30 percent fat, and 12–15 percent protein provides adequate protein for muscle building programs. Expensive protein supplements designed specifically for weight gaining are not necessary.

Exercise Considerations

In the previous chapter we suggest that exercise can be a very effective means to lose excess body weight, particularly body fat. Now we suggest that you exercise in order to gain body weight. Are these suggestions in disagreement? Not necessarily, for it depends upon the mode of exercise you do. Aerobic exercises, as discussed in chapters 4 and 6, may be designed to help you lose body weight by expending rather large amounts of Calories. Your body composition will also change as a result of an aerobic exercise program, for you will lose body fat and experience a slight gain in lean body mass, especially in the legs.

On the other hand, weight training programs, particularly if used in conjunction with a high-Calorie diet, may be designed to produce increases in body weight through increased muscle mass and some loss of body fat. Although exercise does cost Calories, the amount expended during weight training is relatively small. In any weight training workout, the amount of time actually spent lifting the weights is not great enough to use substantial amounts of Calories. For example, in an hour workout, only about 10–15 minutes may be involved in actual exercise, the remainder being recovery between exercises. Although weight training can be a high-intensity exercise, the duration is usually too short, which limits the number of Calories used (usually in the range of 200–250 per workout).

Although the principles underlying the development of an aerobic training program and a weight training program are similar, the purposes of each are rather different. Besides the differences relative to weight control, an aerobic program is designed to improve the efficiency of the cardiovascular system, with some major resultant health benefits. The major purposes of most weight training programs are increased muscle size and strength. Although it is generally accepted that weight training programs do not improve the efficiency or health of the cardiovascular system, there may be some health-related benefits of such a program. Increased muscular strength and endurance levels reduce the stress of many work tasks, such as lifting heavy objects, and may result in less stress on the heart. Weight training programs have been shown to alter body composition, primarily by increasing lean body mass and decreasing total body fat and percent body fat—changes that are believed to be healthful. Weight training may also help increase flexibility, if done properly. The health-related value of increased flexibility is discussed in the next chapter. Moreover, the gain in body weight and muscular development may have important psychological health implications for some individuals.

Although weight training may elicit some health benefits, it still does not offer the major benefit of an aerobic program. Thus, you should continue to exercise aerobically even when you are attempting to gain body weight through weight training. The health-related benefits of an aerobic exercise program for the cardiovascular system should

Figure 7.2 All modes of exercise increase caloric expenditure. However, an hour of weight training expends only about one-third to one-fourth as many Calories as vigorous aerobic activity.

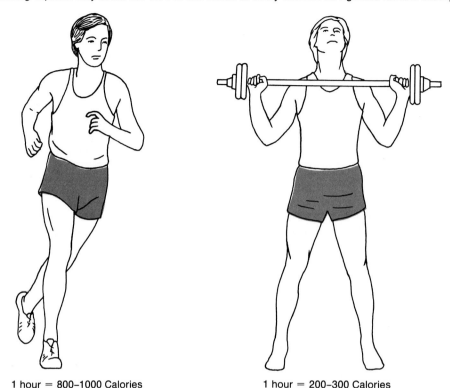

1 hour = 800–1000 Calories   1 hour = 200–300 Calories

not be neglected. These aerobic exercise programs do consume more Calories, so you would have to balance the caloric expenditure with increased food intake. However, the expenditure does not need to be excessive in order to get a training effect. For example, running 3 miles a day for 4 days each week provides you with an adequate training effect for your heart. The combined energy expenditure of weight training and aerobic exercise would only average about 300 Calories per day when based on a 7 day week. This 300 Calorie expenditure could be replaced easily by consuming a 300 Calorie snack.

Muscle Hypertrophy

For our purposes, the major result of a weight training program is **muscular hypertrophy,** which simply means increased muscle size. The principles underlying the design of a program to increase muscle size are discussed in the next section, but let us first look at the theorized mechanisms of muscle hypertrophy.

Figure 7.3 represents a cross section through various parts of a muscle. The entire muscle, such as the biceps, is composed of bundles of muscle tissue. The bundles are composed of a number of **muscle fibers,** which are the actual muscle cells. The muscle

Figure 7.3 Muscle Structure. The whole muscle is composed of separate bundles of individual muscle fibers. Each fiber is composed of numerous myofibrils, each of which contains the thin protein filaments, arranged so that they can slide by each other to cause muscle shortening or lengthening. Various layers of connective tissue surround the muscle fibers, bundles, and whole muscles, which eventually bind together to form the tendon.
Source: From Hole, John W., Jr., *Human Anatomy and Physiology*, 3d. ed. © 1978, 1981, 1984. Wm. C. Brown Publishers, Dubuque, Iowa. All Rights Reserved. Reprinted by Permission.

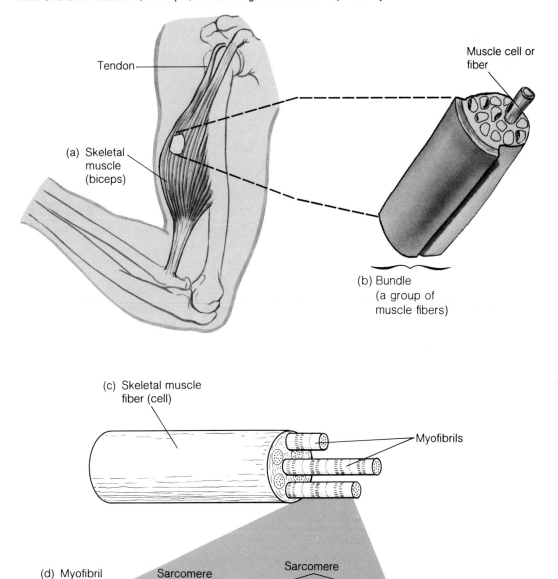

fiber is composed of **myofibrils,** which are the contractile units within the muscle fiber. Finally, the myofibrils are composed of thin protein filaments that interact during contraction and slide by each other. The whole muscle—the bundles and the muscle fibers—are all covered by connective tissue that binds them together. The connective tissue blends together and forms the **tendon,** which attaches to the bones, such as the biceps tendon that can be felt in the front bend of the elbow.

Weight training exercises induce muscular hypertrophy in several possible ways. First, the muscle cells and myofibrils may simply increase their size by incorporating more protein. Second, the myofibrils may increase in number. Third, the amount of connective tissue may increase and thicken. And fourth, the muscle fibers may increase in number, a result called **muscle fiber splitting** (hyperplasia). Although all of these are proposed mechanisms to explain muscular hypertrophy, the first three are fairly well-established, while hyperplasia is the subject of continued research.

Whatever the actual mechanism, weight training in conjunction with increased caloric intake may be an effective means to increase muscle size and lean body mass, and hence, to gain body weight.

Principles of Weight Training

The principles relative to weight training include overload, progressive resistance, specificity, exercise sequence, and recuperation.

The Overload Principle

The overload principle is the most important principle in all weight training programs. The use of weights places a stress on the muscle cell that is greater than it usually meets in normal activities. This overload stress stimulates the muscle to grow—to become stronger—in order to more effectively overcome the increased resistance imposed by the weights. There are basically two ways you may overload the muscle. One is to increase the amount of resistance, or weight, that you use, and the other is to increase the number of repetitions you do.

The Principle of Progressive Resistance Exercise (PRE)

As the muscle continues to get stronger during your training program, you must increase the amount of resistance, the overload, in order to continue to get the proper stimulus for muscle growth. This is known as **progressive resistance exercise (PRE)** and is another basic principle of weight training. Weight lifting is usually done in sets and repetitions. Although there is no single best combination of sets and repetitions, usually 2 or 3 sets with 5–10 repetitions provides an adequate stimulus for muscle growth. A recommended combination for beginners is 3 sets with 5 repetitions in each set. The first step for each individual exercise is to determine the maximum amount of weight that you can lift for 5 repetitions. If you can do more than 5 repetitions, the weight is too light and you need to add more poundage. During the succeeding weeks, as you get stronger you will be able to lift the original weight more easily. When you

Figure 7.4 The principle of progressive resistance exercise (PRE) simply means that, as you get stronger, you need to progressively increase the resistance in order to continue to gain strength and muscle.

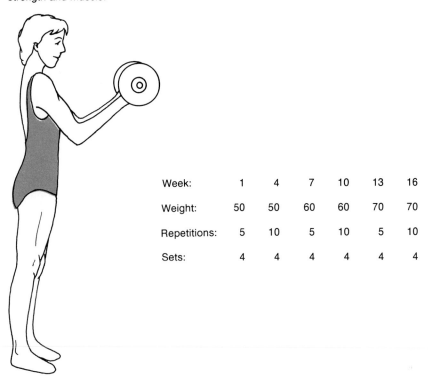

Week:	1	4	7	10	13	16
Weight:	50	50	60	60	70	70
Repetitions:	5	10	5	10	5	10
Sets:	4	4	4	4	4	4

can perform 10 repetitions, add more weight to force you back down to 5 repetitions; this is the progressive resistance principle. Over several months time, the weight will probably need to be increased several times as you continue to get stronger.

The Principle of Specificity

Specificity of training is a broad principle with many implications for weight training, including specificity for various sports movements, strength gains, endurance gains, and body weight gains. For our purposes, we simply note that in order for a particular muscle or muscle group to increase in size, the weight training program must be specifically designed for that purpose.

The Principle of Exercise Sequence

Your exercise routine should be based upon the principle of exercise sequence. This means that if you have ten exercises in your routine, they should be arranged in a logical order so that fatigue does not limit your lifting ability. For example, the first exercise in a sequence of ten might stress the biceps muscle, the second the abdominals, the third the quadriceps of the thigh, and so forth. After you perform one set of each of the ten exercises, you then do a complete second set, followed by the third set. Another popular option is to do three sets of the same exercise, with a rest between each set; then do three sets of the second exercise, and so on.

The Principle of Recuperation

Weight training, if done properly to achieve the greatest gains, imposes a rather severe stress on the muscles, requiring a period of recovery. For beginners, weight training should generally be done about 3 days a week, with a rest or recuperation day in between. Following this recuperation principle should allow sufficient time for muscle growth and also help to prevent undue muscular fatigue.

These general principles should serve as guidelines during the beginning phase of your weight training program, and should be used to guide your progress during the first 3 months of the basic weight training program discussed in the next section.

Preliminary Considerations

Before we actually list the specific exercises of your weight training program, let's look at several factors you should keep in mind prior to and during the program.

Contraindications to Weight Training

There are several health conditions that may be aggravated by weight training, due primarily to the increased pressures that occur within the body when lifting heavy weights. Individuals with a **hernia** (a weakness in the abdominal wall) should refrain from strenuous weight lifting; the increased pressure may cause a rupture. Blood pressure may increase rapidly when straining to lift weights, so those with high blood pressure may be exposed to an increased risk of blood vessel rupture. Lifting with the arms and straining exercises increase the work of the heart and thus may be contraindicated for individuals who have coronary heart disease. Low back problems may also be aggravated by improper weight lifting techniques. Although most healthy young individuals may initiate a weight training program without worry, if you have any of these health problems, you should refrain from this type of activity or first consult your physician for recommendations.

Methods of Training

There are various methods to train with weights: isometric, isotonic, and isokinetic. Moreover, there are a number of different types of apparatus available, such as Nautilus®, Universal Gym®, Cybex®, Hydra-Gym®, and others, that are designed to use one or more of these different methods. A number of research studies have been conducted to determine which of these methods is best, particularly in relation to strength and power gains. The results of many of these studies are contradictory, particularly when isotonic and isokinetic programs are compared. However, at the present time, it is probably safe to say that isotonic and isokinetic programs are comparable in their ability to produce gains in muscle size and strength. Other than possible safety considerations, the use of specialized machines and weight training devices does not appear to have any advantage over the use of free weights, such as barbells and dumbbells. All methods may be effective provided the basic principles of weight training, particularly the overload principle, are followed. The major advantage to free weights is that they are relatively inexpensive compared to the machines.

Safety Concerns

Weight training is generally regarded as a relatively safe sport, particularly if these guidelines are followed.

1. Learn to breathe steadily during the most strenuous part of the exercise. This helps to prevent the large increase in abdominal pressure that may cause a hernia. Moreover, it also helps to prevent a "black out" that may occur while straining to lift a heavy object and holding your breath. This is the **Valsalva phenomenon** that results from decreased blood flow to the brain due to a reduced return of blood to the heart caused by the increased pressure in the chest. Breathing in while lifting the weight and breathing out while lowering it is the recommended system.
2. Use spotters to help you control the weight when doing certain exercises that may be dangerous, such as in the bench press.
3. Place lock collars on the ends of the bar when using free weights so the plates do not fall off and cause injury to the feet. The use of machines, such as Nautilus® and Universal Gym®, eliminates this safety hazard.
4. Beginners should learn the technique of a given exercise using light weights so they do not strain themselves if an improper technique is used. When the proper technique is mastered, the weights may be increased.
5. Avoid exercises that may cause or aggravate low back problems. In essence, try to prevent a forward motion of the lower back area. Figure 7.5 illustrates some positions to be avoided. See chapter 8 for elaboration.
6. Lower weights slowly. If you lower them rapidly, your muscles have to contract rapidly in an eccentric fashion as you approach the starting position. This necessitates the development of a large amount of force that may tear some connective tissue and cause muscular soreness.

Goals

As discussed earlier, a sound goal for weight gains is 1–2 pounds of muscle tissue per week. Laboratory Inventory 7.1 is helpful in determining the number of Calories you should consume to increase your body weight at this rate. This Laboratory Inventory takes into account the Calories expended during aerobic exercise and the weight training program itself.

Girth and skinfold measurements are also recommended so that weight gain is ascertained as muscle tissue and not body fat.

Figure 7.5 Avoid exercises or body positions that place excessive stress on the low back region. Poor form in exercises like the bench press (a) and the curl (b) exaggerates the lumbar curve. Be sure to keep the lower back as flat as possible. Exercises similar to the bentover row (c) place tremendous forces on the lower back because the weight or resistance is so far in front of the body.

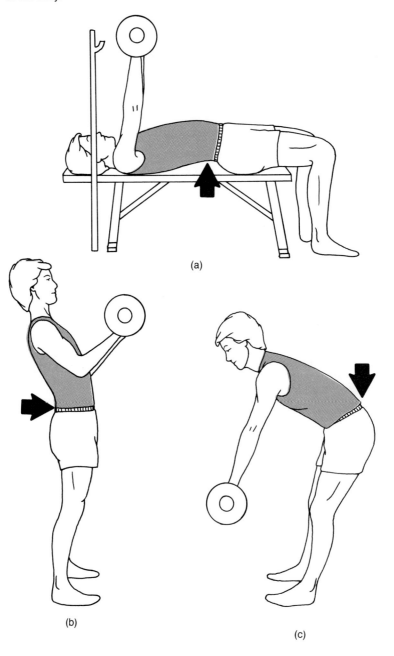

(a)

(b)

(c)

Figure 7.6 Body builders use a variety of techniques to maximize individual muscle development.

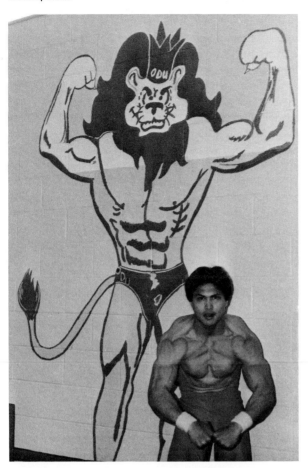

Program Design for Body Building

An acceptable technique to gain body weight is the bulk-up method. This method involves the use of 6–8 exercises that stress the major muscle groups of the body (4–5 sets of each exercise are done). The PRE concept is used, starting with a weight you can handle for 5 repetitions, progressively increasing the repetitions to 10. After you reach 10 repetitions, increase the weight until you must come back to 5 repetitions.

The bulk-up method should be used for several months to increase your weight. You may then wish to shape that bulk, a technique that body builders call razoring or cutting up. This technique uses a wide variety of exercises done with lighter weights but with many repetitions at high speed. Once you have achieved your desired weight, you may alternate the bulk-up and razoring techniques to maintain your weight and shape.

A Basic Weight Training Program
for Weight Gains and Strength

In this section you find one exercise for each of the major body areas. Since barbells and dumbbells appear to be the most common means of doing weight training, this is the method utilized. However, as mentioned previously, other apparatus such as the Nautilus®, Universal Gym®, and others can also be used effectively to gain weight and strength. Most of the exercises described here using barbells or dumbbells have similar counterparts on these other apparatus.

Note that muscles seldom operate alone, and most weight training exercises stress more than one muscle group. Thus you should keep in mind that, although an exercise may be listed specifically for the chest muscle, for example, it may also stress the arm and shoulder muscles. The exercises described in this section generally stress more than one body area, although their main effect is on the area noted.

These eight exercises stress most of the major muscle groups in the body, and thus provide an adequate stimulus for gaining body weight and strength through an increase in muscle mass. Literally hundreds of different weight training exercises and techniques to train are available, so if you become interested in diversifying your program (such as using the razoring technique) it is suggested that you consult a book specific to weight training. Several may be found in the reference list at the end of this chapter.

The beginner should adhere to the following procedure using the basic weight training program.

1. Learn the proper technique for each exercise with a light weight, possibly only the bar itself, for 2 weeks. Do 10–12 repetitions of each exercise to develop form. Do not strain during this initial learning phase.
2. For each exercise, determine the maximum weight that you can lift for 5 repetitions after the 2 week learning phase.
3. Do 1 set of the 8 exercises in the sequence as listed on page 221.
4. Since the exercise sequence is designed to stress different muscle groups in order, not much recuperation is necessary between exercises—possibly only 30 seconds or so.
5. Do 4–5 complete sets. You may wish to rest 2–3 minutes between sets.
6. Exercise 3 days per week and, in each succeeding day try to do as many repetitions as possible for each exercise in each set. When you can do 10 repetitions each after a month or so, add more weight to the bars so you can do only 5 repetitions.
7. Repeat Step 6 as you progressively increase your strength.

Figure 7.7   The Bench Press. The pectoralis major muscle group in the chest is the primary muscle group developed by the bench press, but the deltoid in the shoulder and the triceps at the back of the arm are also developed.

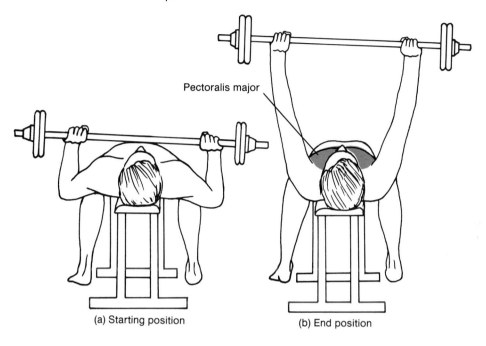

Pectoralis major

(a) Starting position   (b) End position

Chest

Figure 7.7

Exercise	Bench press
Chest Muscles	Pectoralis major
Other Muscles	Deltoid, triceps
Sets	4–5
Repetitions	5–10, PRE concept
Safety	Have spotter stand behind bar to assist as fatigue sets in.
Equipment	Bench with support for weight, or two spotters to hand weight to you
Description	Lie supine on bench. Use wide grip for chest development. Secure bar and lower *slowly* to chest. Press bar to full extension straight up. Do not arch back.

Figure 7.8A The Lat Machine Pulldown. The lat machine pulldown primarily trains the latissimus dorsi in the back and side of the upper body, but the biceps on the front of the upper arm and the pectoralis major in the chest are also developed.

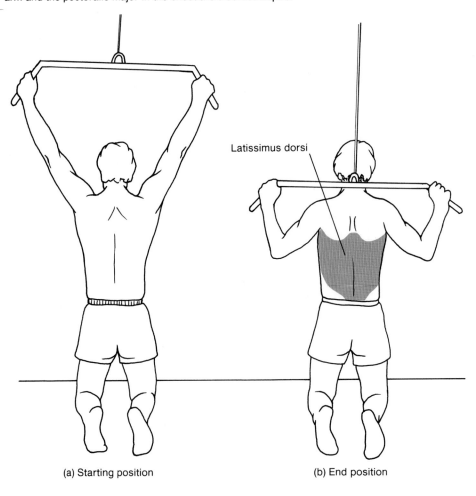

Latissimus dorsi

(a) Starting position   (b) End position

Back	Figures 7.8A and 7.8B
Exercise	Lat machine pull down
Back Muscles	Latissimus dorsi
Other Muscles	Biceps, pectoralis major
Sets	4–5
Repetitions	5–10, PRE concept
Safety	A very safe exercise
Equipment	Lat machine
Description	From seated or kneeling position take a wide grip on the bar overhead at arm's length. Pull bar down until it reaches back of the neck. Return slowly to starting position.

Note: If a lat machine is not available, the bent arm pullover may be substituted.

Figure 7.8B The Bent-arm Pullover. The bent-arm pullover also trains the latissimus dorsi and develops the pectoralis major.

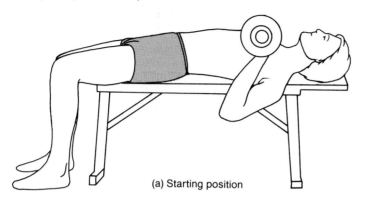

(a) Starting position

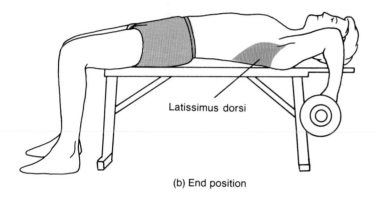

Latissimus dorsi

(b) End position

Alternate Exercise	Bent-arm pullover
Back Muscles	Latissimus dorsi
Other Muscles	Pectoralis major
Sets	4–5
Repetitions	5–10, PRE concept
Safety	Do not arch back. Start with light weights when learning the technique.
Equipment	Bench
Description	Lie supine on bench, entire back in contact with the bench, feet on the bench, knees bent. Weight is on chest with elbows bent. Swing weight over head, just brushing hair, and lower as far as possible without taking back off the bench. Keeping elbows in, return the weight to the chest.

Figure 7.9 The Half-Squat or Parallel Squat. The half-squat develops the quadriceps muscle group on the front of the thigh, as well as the hamstrings on the back of the thigh.

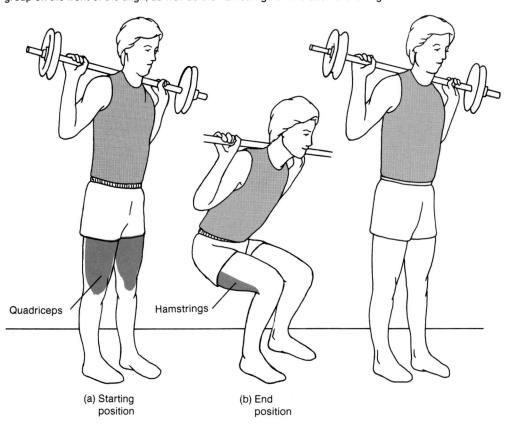

Quadriceps   Hamstrings

(a) Starting   (b) End
    position   position

Thigh

Figure 7.9

Exercise	Half-squat or parallel squat
Thigh Muscles	Quadriceps (front), hamstrings (back)
Other Muscles	Gluteus maximus
Sets	4–5
Repetitions	5–10, PRE concept
Safety	Have two spotters to assist if using free weights. Keep back straight. Drop weight behind you if you lose balance. Do not squat more than halfway down.
Equipment	Squat rack if available. Pad the bar with towels if necessary.
Description	In standing position, take bar from squat rack or spotters and rest on the shoulders behind the head. Squat until thighs are parallel to ground or until buttocks touch a chair at this parallel position. Do not squat beyond half way. Keep back as straight as possible. Return to standing position.

Figure 7.10 Standing Lateral Raise. The standing lateral raise primarily develops the deltoid muscle in the shoulder, but the trapezius in the upper back and neck area is also trained.

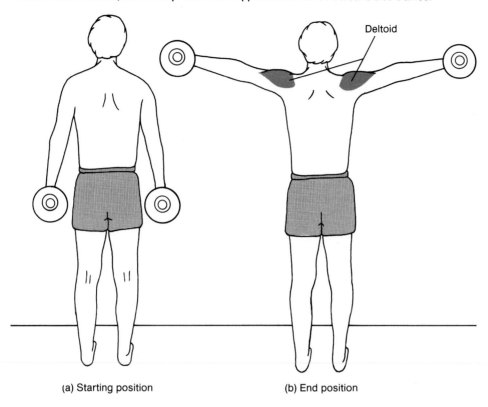

Deltoid

(a) Starting position   (b) End position

Shoulders

Figure 7.10

Exercise	Standing lateral raise
Shoulder Muscles	Deltoid
Other Muscles	Trapezius
Sets	4–5
Repetitions	5–10, PRE concept
Safety	Do not arch back.
Equipment	Dumbbells
Description	Stand with dumbbells in hands at sides. With palms down raise straight arms sideways to shoulder level. Do not bend elbows. Return slowly to starting position.

Figure 7.11 Heel Raise. The heel raise mainly develops the two major calf muscles—the gastrocnemius and the soleus.

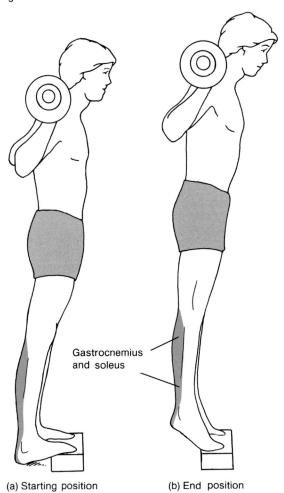

Gastrocnemius
and soleus

(a) Starting position   (b) End position

Calf   Figure 7.11

Exercise	Heel raises
Calf Muscles	Gastrocnemius, soleus
Other Muscles	Deep calf muscles
Sets	4–5
Repetitions	5–10, PRE concept
Safety	Have two spotters if you use free weights.
Equipment	Squat rack, if available. Pad the bar with a towel if necessary.
Description	Place bar on back of shoulders as in squat exercise. Raise up on your toes as high as possible, and then return to standing position. Place the toes on a board so heels can drop down lower than normal. Point toes in, out, and straight ahead during different sets in order to work the muscles from different angles.

Figure 7.12 The Standing Curl. The standing curl strengthens the biceps muscle in the front of the upper arm as well as several other muscles in that region that bend the elbow.

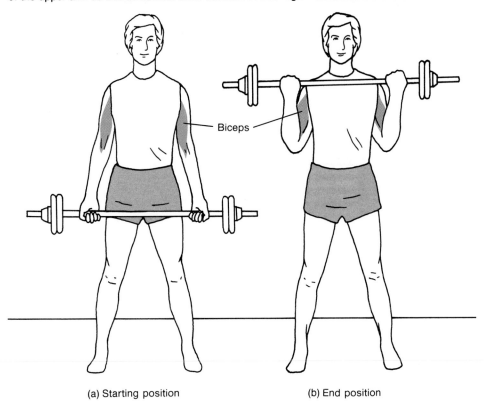

Biceps

(a) Starting position   (b) End position

Front of arm   Figure 7.12

Exercise	Standing curl
Arm Muscle	Biceps
Other Muscles	Several elbow flexors
Sets	4–5
Repetitions	5–10, PRE concept
Safety	Do not arch back. Place back against wall to control arching motion.
Equipment	Curl bar if available
Description	Stand with weight held in front of body, palms forward. Place back against wall. Bend the elbows and bring the weight to the chest. Lower it slowly.

Figure 7.13 The Seated Overhead Press. The seated overhead press primarily develops the triceps muscle on the back of the upper arm, but also trains the trapezius in the upper back and neck.

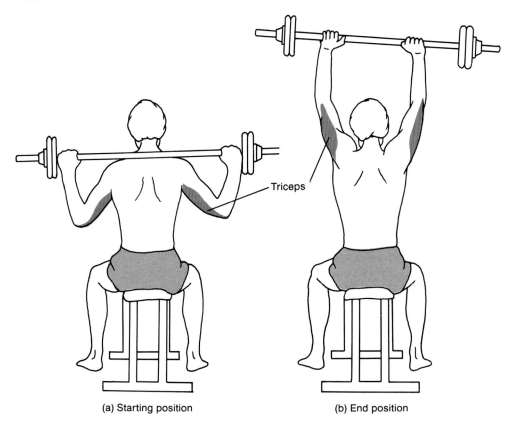

Triceps

(a) Starting position   (b) End position

Back of arm   Figure 7.13

Exercise	Seated overhead press
Arm Muscle	Triceps
Other Muscles	Trapezius
Sets	4–5
Repetitions	5–10, PRE concept
Safety	Do not arch back excessively. Have spotter available as fatigue sets in.
Equipment	Bench or chair
Description	Sit on bench with weight held behind the head near the neck. Hands should be close together, elbows bent. Straighten elbows and press weight over head to arm's length. Lower weight slowly to starting position.

Figure 7.14 The Sit-Up. The sit-up trains the rectus abdominis, as well as the oblique abdominis muscles.

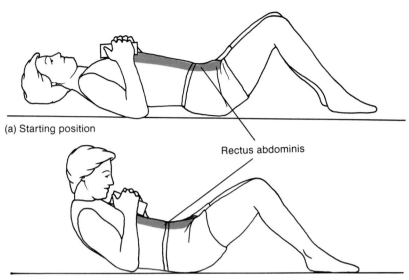

(a) Starting position

Rectus abdominis

(b) End position

Abdominal area   Figure 7.14

Exercise	Sit-ups
Abdominal Muscles	Rectus abdominis
Other Muscles	Oblique abdominis muscles
Sets	4–5
Repetitions	5–10, PRE concept
Safety	Develop sufficient abdominal strength before using weights with this exercise. Do not arch back when exercising.
Equipment	Free weight plates; incline sit-up bench if available.
Description	Lie on back, knees bent up with heels close to buttocks, hands should hold weights on chest. Sit up about half way. Return to starting position slowly.

Note: This exercise may be done without weights, but with an increased number of repetitions. See chapter 8 for more information on the sit-up exercise.

The sequence of exercises should be:
1. Bench press—chest muscles
2. Lat machine pull down or bent-arm pullover—back muscles
3. Half squat—thigh muscles
4. Standing lateral raise—shoulder muscles
5. Heel raise—calf muscles
6. Standing curl—front upper arm muscles
7. Seated overhead press—back upper arm muscles
8. Sit-up—abdominal muscles

A weekly record form, similar to the one in table 7.2, should be used to keep track of your progress.

Table 7.2
Weekly Weight Training Record, Basic Eight Exercises

	Chest (Bench Press)		Back (Lats Exercise)		Thigh (Half Squat)		Shoulder (Lateral Raise)		Calf (Heel Raise)		Front Arm (Curls)		Back Arm (Seated Press)		Abdominal Area (Sit-ups)	
	Wt	Reps	Wt	Reps	Wt	Reps	Wt	Reps	Wt	Reps	Wt	Reps	Wt	Reps	Wt	Reps
Date _____																
Set 1																
Set 2																
Set 3																
Set 4																
Set 5																
Date _____																
Set 1																
Set 2																
Set 3																
Set 4																
Set 5																
Date _____																
Set 1																
Set 2																
Set 3																
Set 4																
Set 5																
Date _____																
Set 1																
Set 2																
Set 3																
Set 4																
Set 5																

The keys to gaining weight, primarily muscle mass, are to create a positive caloric balance through increased caloric intake, and to use a weight training program for most of the major muscle groups in the body. Use the following as a guide to increasing your caloric intake while assuring that the weight gain is muscle tissue and not body fat.

1. From table 6.7, determine how many Calories you need daily simply to maintain body weight.

2. Plan to expend about 300 Calories per day exercising. Three days per week should involve a weight training program as described in this chapter. Each session will take about an hour. Four days per week should involve aerobic activities lasting approximately 20–30 minutes. Each of these types of activities will expend approximately 300 Calories daily, when based on a 7 day week.

3. Consume an additional 400–500 Calories per day if you want to add 1 pound per week; and about 800–1000 Calories per day if you want to add 2 pounds per week.

4. Total the Calories from Steps 1 to 3 to determine your recommended daily caloric intake. Then refer to table 6.8 to design your own diet plan.

5. Use a good cloth or steel tape to take body measurements. Be sure you take them at the same points about once a week. Those body parts measured should include the neck, upper arm, chest, abdomen, thigh, and calf. This is to insure that body weight gains are proportionately distributed. You should look for good gains in the chest and limbs; the abdominal girth increase should be kept low because that is where the fat will increase the most. If you have skinfold calipers, then various skinfold measures can also be used to check on body fat levels. See Laboratory Inventory 6.1 for the skinfold technique.

Personal data:

1. Number of Calories to maintain body weight _____

2. Daily exercise Calories ___+300___

3. Add 400–500 Calories for 1 pound gain per week; 800–1000 for 2 pounds per week _____

4. Recommended daily caloric intake (Total Steps 1 to 3) _____

5. Body measurements

	Date ___	Date ___	Date ___	Date ___	Date ___
Girths:					
Neck	___	___	___	___	___
Upper arm	___	___	___	___	___
Chest	___	___	___	___	___
Abdomen	___	___	___	___	___
Thigh	___	___	___	___	___
Calf	___	___	___	___	___
Skinfolds:					
Triceps	___	___	___	___	___
Abdominal	___	___	___	___	___
Subscapular	___	___	___	___	___

References

Berger, R. *Conditioning for Men.* Boston: Allyn and Bacon, 1973.

Clarke, H. H. "Development of Muscular Strength and Endurance." *Physical Fitness Research Digest* 4:1–17 (January 1974).

Consolazio, C. F., et al. "Protein Metabolism during Intensive Physical Training in the Young Adult." *American Journal of Clinical Nutrition* 28:29–35 (1975).

Costill, D.; Coyle, E.; Fink, W.; Lesmes, G.; and Witzmann, F. "Adaptations in Skeletal Muscle following Strength Training." *Journal of Applied Physiology* 46:96–99 (1979).

Darden, E., and Schendel, H. "Dietary Protein and Muscle Building." *Scholastic Coach* 40:70 (March 1971).

Etheridge, G., and Thomas, T. "Physiological and Biochemical Changes of Human Skeletal Muscle Induced by Different Strength Training Programs." *Medicine and Science in Sports and Exercise* 14:141 (1982).

Falls, H.; Baylor, A.; and Dishman, R. *Essentials of Fitness.* Philadelphia: Saunders College Publishing, 1980.

Fox, E., and Mathews, D. *The Physiological Basis of Physical Education and Athletics.* Philadelphia: Saunders College Publishing, 1981.

Gettman, L.; Ayres, J.; Pollock, M.; Durstine, L.; and Grantham, W. "Strength Training and Jogging." *Archives of Physical and Medical Rehabilitation* 60:115–20 (1979).

Gettman, L.; Ward, P.; and Hagan, R. "A Comparison of Combined Running and Weight Training with Circuit Weight Training." *Medicine and Science in Sports and Exercise* 14:229–34 (1982).

Gregory, L. "Some Observations on Strength Training and Assessment." *Journal of Sports Medicine and Physical Fitness* 21:130–37 (1981).

Hickson, J.; Wilmore, J.; Constable, S.; and Buono, M. "Characterization of Standardized Weight Training Exercise." *Medicine and Science in Sports and Exercise* 14:169 (1982).

Hooks, G. *Weight Training in Athletics and Physical Education.* Englewood Cliffs, NJ: Prentice-Hall, 1974.

Kondalenko, V.; Sergeeva, Y.; and Ivanitskaya, V. "Electron Microscopic Study of Signs of Skeletal Muscle Fiber Hyperplasia in Athletes." *Arkhiv anatomii gistologii i Embriologii* 80:66–70 (June 1981).

Lamb, D. R. "Anabolic Steroids." In *Ergogenic Aids in Sport,* edited by M. H. Williams. Champaign, IL: Human Kinetic Publishers, 1983.

Larson, L. "Physical Training Effects on Muscle Morphology in Sedentary Males at Different Ages." *Medicine and Science in Sports and Exercise* 14:203–6 (1982).

Liverman, R., and Groden, C. "Metabolic Analysis of High Intensity Weight Training." *Medicine and Science in Sports and Exercise* 14:169 (1982).

Marable, N., et al. "Urinary Nitrogen Excretion as Influenced by a Muscle-Building Program and Protein Intake Variation." *Nutrition Reports International* 19:795–805 (1979).

McArdle, W., and Foglia, G. "Energy Cost and Cardiorespiratory Stress of Isometric and Weight Training Exercises." *Journal of Sports Medicine and Physical Fitness* 9:23 (1969).

O'Shea, J. *Scientific Principles and Methods of Strength Fitness.* Reading, MA: Addison-Wesley, 1976.

Pipes, T. "Strength Training Modes: What's the Difference." *Scholastic Coach* 46:96 (May-June 1977).

President's Council on Physical Fitness and Sports. *Weight Training for Strength and Power.* Washington, DC: General Printing Office.

Rasch, P. "The Present Status of Negative (Eccentric) Exercise: A Review." *American Corrective Therapy Journal* 28:77 (May-June 1974).

————. *Weight Training.* Dubuque, IA: Wm. C. Brown Publishers, 1975.

Sale, D., and MacDougall, D. "Specificity in Strength Training: A Review for the Coach and Athlete." *Canadian Journal of Applied Sports Sciences* 6:87–92 (1981).

Smith, N. "Gaining and Losing Weight in Athletics." *Journal of the American Medical Association* 236:149 (July 1976).

Stone, M., et al. "Physiological Effects of a Short-Term Resistive Training Program on Middle-Aged Untrained Men." *National Strength Coaches Association Journal* 4:16–20 (October-November 1982).

Weltman, A., and Stamford, B. "Strength Training: Free Weights vs. Machines." *The Physician and Sportsmedicine* 10:197 (November 1982).

Westcott, W. L. *Strength Fitness.* Boston: Allyn and Bacon, 1982.

Williams, M. H. *Dietary Protein for Athletes: A Review.* Montreal: International Federation of Bodybuilders, 1981.

Wilmore, J. "Alterations in Strength, Body Composition and Anthropmetric Measurements Consequent to a 10 Week Weight Training Program." *Medicine and Science in Sports* 6:133–38 (1974).

Wilmore, J., et al. "Energy Cost of Circuit Weight Training." *Medicine and Science in Sports* 10:79 (1978).

Wright, J.; Patton, J.; Vogel, J.; Mello, R.; Hayford, R.; deMoya, R.; and Stauffer, R. "Aerobic Power and Body Composition after 10 Weeks of Circuit Weight Training Using Various Work:Rest Ratios." *Medicine and Science in Sports and Exercise* 14:170 (1982).

Flexibility, Abdominal Strength, and Low Back Pain

Key Terms

ballistic
curl-up
dynamic flexibility
flexibility
hamstrings
hip flexion
low back pain syndrome
lumbar lordosis

psoas major
rectus abdominis
rectus femoris
round shoulders
sacroiliac
soft tissues
spinal flexion
static flexibility

Key Concepts

Most low back problems occur because the back has not been physically conditioned for the amount of stress people put on it.

The keys to prevent low back problems are to avoid positions or movements that may subject the back to injury, to increase flexibility of the muscles in the low back region, and to increase strength of the abdominal musculature.

The soft tissues of the body, such as muscles, tendons, ligaments, and connective tissue, contain elastic fibers that can be stretched in order to improve flexibility.

Although both static stretching and ballistic stretching techniques may improve flexibility, the static stretching technique is recommended because the slow movement is less likely to cause an injury.

In order to improve flexibility the muscle must be overloaded (stretched beyond its normal range of motion) and held in this position for about 15–60 seconds 3 times a day.

The key to flexibility exercises for the low back area is to flatten out the forward curve in the lumbar area—as it would appear if you curled yourself up into a ball.

Joggers and runners may benefit from flexibility exercises for several body areas—the low back region, the hamstrings, the calf muscles or Achilles tendon, and the groin muscles.

To strengthen the abdominal muscles, you need to do exercises that either flex the spine or rotate the pelvic bone backwards.

Improper abdominal exercises may actually contribute to the development of low back problems, rather than helping them.

Introduction

One of the most common chronic health problems in the United States is the **low back pain syndrome,** a chronic pain or ache in the low back region. Low back problems are the most common complaint in Workmen's Compensation cases and account for billions of dollars yearly in compensation and medical expenses for American industry. There are a number of different causes of low back pain, including structural deformities and direct trauma to the spinal column. However, some recent research suggests that most back problems are not due to structural deformities, but rather from seemingly insignificant activities like bending over to pick up a pencil or some light object. The medical director of this research project suggests that most back problems occur because the back has not been physically conditioned for the amount of work people put on it. Thus, a sedentary life-style may predispose the back musculature and ligaments to weakness so any physical activity, such as lifting objects, chopping wood, or even starting a jogging program, may result in the low back pain syndrome. You may wish to review chapter 2 for further discussion of low back pain.

There have been some attempts to identify those individuals who may be susceptible to back injury and low back pain. Tight musculature in the back and hip region may predispose you to low back pain. A general assessment procedure for tight musculature in these areas is found in Laboratory Inventory 8.1.

Most of us will injure our backs for one reason or another sometime in our lives and be victims of the low back pain syndrome. Fortunately, in most cases, especially in the young, a few days of rest may relieve the pain completely. However, other cases may become chronic and require medical services, including physical therapy and drugs for pain relief.

Although low back pain may strike anyone at anytime, and may be caused by a wide variety of reasons, there appear to be a number of recommendations that may help prevent its onset. These recommendations are grouped into three general categories: (1) avoidance of body positions and movements that may subject the back to injury, (2) exercises to increase flexibility of various muscle groups in the back and hip region, and (3) exercises to increase the strength of the abdominal musculature. A brief review of the first category is presented in the next section, while exercise programs for flexibility and abdominal strength constitute most of the rest of this chapter. Flexibility exercises are advocated primarily for the low back region, but exercises to increase flexibility in other regions of the body are also noted.

Body Positions and Movements to Avoid

As mentioned in chapters 2 and 7, the major body positions to avoid are those in which the lower region of the back curves forward excessively. This type of position is known as **lumbar lordosis,** or hollow back, and is depicted in figure 8.1. The pelvic bone inclines downward in the front of the body, the abdominal musculature becomes stretched, and the lower back musculature in the lumbar region becomes shortened and tight.

We should recognize the fact that we cannot avoid this position altogether. Indeed, the body does have a natural forward curve in the lumbar region. Moreover, this body position may be an inherent part of some athletic movements and may be practiced as

Figure 8.1 Lumbar Lordosis. Lumbar lordosis, or hollow back, is a position in which the normal curve in the lower portion of the back increases toward the front of the body. Any type of movement that causes increased curvature in the lumbar spine region (arrow) may be a causative factor of low back pain. This type of position may be common in many sports.

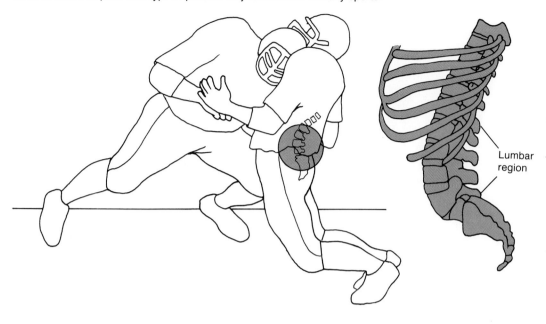

Lumbar region

Figure 8.2 Methods of Lifting. The stoop style (*a*) should be avoided. A modified squat style (*b*) is preferred, keeping the back as straight as possible.

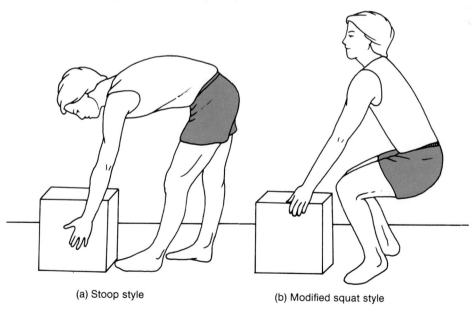

(a) Stoop style   (b) Modified squat style

Figure 8.3 Lifting Techniques. Position *a* represents an improper lifting technique that may stress the ligaments and muscles of the back, putting excessive stress on the lower lumbar region. The total resistance is equal to the product of the weight (*W*) times the weight arm (*WA*), which is the perpendicular distance from the weight to the lower lumbar joints. Position *b* minimizes the weight arm and thus decreases the total resistance that needs to be overcome.

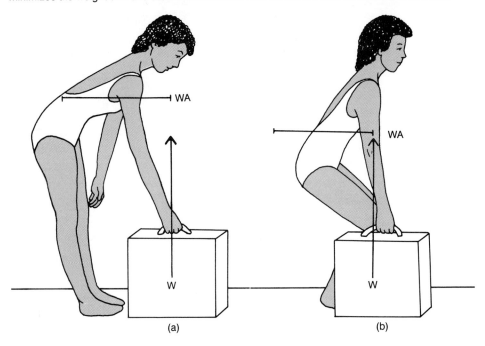

(a) (b)

such (for example, in certain gymnastic stunts). However, the primary concern for most of us is to avoid excessive curvature in this region when lifting heavy loads or doing certain exercises.

Various movements also seem to cause back injury in many individuals. Clinical research supports the following suggestions as possible means to avoid back injury.

1. Do not bend over quickly to touch your toes or pick up an object while your knees are straight. This action may create tremendous pressure in the lumbar region, primarily when stopping rapidly as you touch your toes, and again when you begin to straighten up.
2. You should keep your back relatively straight and bend at the hip and knees when lifting objects. Use your leg muscles to lift. It is not necessary to go to a full squat position, but you should avoid the stoop position as much as possible. Use a modified squat style as shown in figure 8.2.
3. When lifting objects, keep them as close to the body as possible. The farther away the object is in front of you, the greater the stress on the lower back when lifting. See figure 8.3 for the rationale.
4. Do not attempt to lift or carry objects that are too heavy for you. A sudden shift of the weight may place an excessive stress on the lower back area.

Flexibility

At several previous points in this text it is suggested that improved flexibility may be part of a Positive Health Life-style, so at this point we should define flexibility and explain how it may be improved.

In essence, **flexibility** is simply the range of motion that the bones may go through at the various joints in your body. Flexibility is specific to each joint, and is primarily limited by the nature or structure of the joint. For example, the elbow joint is constructed like a hinge. You may bend the forearm forward fairly freely, but it becomes locked when you extend it to its limit. Thus, the hinge structure of the elbow joint limits the range of motion to about 150 degrees. Moreover, the hinged joint allows movement only forward and backward. On the other hand, joints such as the shoulder are constructed like a ball and socket that allows movement in all directions and permits a full circular movement of 360 degrees.

If flexibility were limited only by the structure of the joint, we would not be able to improve it through a flexibility program because we cannot change the basic joint structure. However, other body tissues, called **soft tissues,** also limit flexibility. These tissues include the muscles and the sheaths of tissue that surround them, the connective tissue (tendons and ligaments), and the skin. These tissues possess varying amounts of elastic fibers that permit them to change their lengths—to shorten or lengthen. Thus, as we move our bodies, the elasticity, or flexibility, of these soft tissues usually allows for a normal range of motion. However, if the body assumes a certain position for a prolonged period of time, then the soft tissues will adjust to that position. An example is illustrated in figure 8.4, which depicts a condition of round shoulders caused by habitual slouching of the shoulders. The soft tissues in the chest area have become rather shortened and tight, whereas those in the upper back region have become lengthened. Fortunately, a proper exercise program can help to increase the flexibility of those soft tissues that have become shortened.

The major thrust of the flexibility exercise program presented in this chapter is to help prevent or relieve low back pain. However, improved flexibility may be helpful for other reasons. Postural problems that are caused by shortened soft tissues (such as round shoulders mentioned previously) may be ameliorated. Athletes who participate in sports in which a great deal of flexibility is required may need to increase flexibility to the maximum possible. A good example of maximum flexibility is the cheerleader or gymnast doing a split. Some suggest that improved flexibility may also help to prevent injuries, particularly in certain sports where joint movements may be forced beyond the normal range of motion. A strength and flexibility program should be developed specifically for sports in which this might occur. Moreover, the current thinking among many, but not all, medical advisors is that flexibility exercises are important in preventing some of the common running injuries. Since aerobic exercise, such as jogging or running, is advocated in this book as a major component of the Positive Health Life-style, it is important to include here some flexibility exercises commonly recommended for joggers and runners.

The flexibility exercise programs presented later in this chapter are designed for three different purposes: to help prevent or relieve low back pain, to improve posture (correct round shoulders), and to stretch soft tissues that are commonly injured in runners.

Figure 8.4 Round Shoulders. Round shoulders are accompanied by a stretching of the muscles in the upper back region and a tightening, or shortening, of those in the chest area.

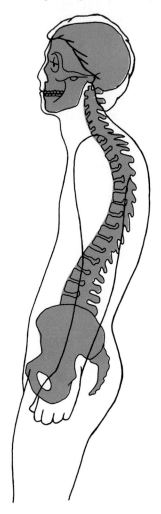

Principles of Flexibility Exercises

Flexibility may be subdivided into two different types: static and dynamic. Flexibility exercise programs have been patterned after each type. **Static flexibility** represents the range of motion that you may achieve through a slow steady stretch to the limits of joint movement. This approach uses slow stretching exercises. **Dynamic flexibility** is characterized by the range of motion obtained when moving a body part rapidly to its limits. **Ballistic,** or rapid bouncing, stretching exercises are used in a dynamic flexibility program.

Most flexibility exercises may be done using both static and ballistic techniques. For example, from a standing position you could bend over slowly, touch your fingers to the floor and hold this position (remain static) for a period of time. On the other hand, you could move rapidly to touch the floor, straighten up rapidly, and repeat this ballistic exercise several times. Although research has shown that both types of exercise programs will equally improve flexibility, there appears to be a trend away from the ballistic exercises and toward the static type. The major reason for this is that ballistic exercises may greatly exceed the normal range of motion, and tear the muscle tissue or connective tissue. For example, as you bounce down to touch your toes as described, the soft tissues in the lower back are stretched rapidly; at the end of the movement, the muscles contract to stop your back from flexing too far forward. The stress created may exceed the elasticity of the soft tissues in the lower back, and may damage the discs in the spinal column as well. The result may be a disabling back injury or muscle soreness. This does not mean that all individuals should refrain from all ballistic flexibility exercises. Many athletes, for example, may include these exercises in their training regimen. However, before doing ballistic exercises the individual should warm-up with static exercises for the same body areas.

Static stretching exercise programs appear to be the safest way to improve flexibility. In order to improve your flexibility, however, you must adhere to the same principles underlying the development of other fitness components, such as aerobic endurance and strength. In essence, the principles of specificity and overload—with the emphases on intensity, duration, and frequency—are the bases for your flexibility program.

The following specific guidelines should be followed for a beginning static stretching program:

1. For intensity, the muscle must be stretched, or overloaded, beyond its normal range of motion. A good general rule is to stretch until you feel mild to moderate pain or discomfort. You should not stretch to a point of excessive pain, for this may cause an injury in itself. Be very cautious when stretching the muscles in the low back area.
2. For duration, hold this static position for about 15–60 seconds. Repeat three times. In the beginning, stretch for 15 seconds and use the principle of progression to increase it to 60 seconds. When you can hold a set position for 60 seconds, stretch a little further and hold the new position for 15 seconds. Continue with the progression principle.
3. For frequency, you may do flexibility exercises on a daily basis if you desire, but at least 3–4 days per week appear to be necessary for flexibility improvement to occur.
4. For specificity, select those exercises designed to improve flexibility in a specific body area. Try to do several exercises for each area of interest.
5. Avoid excessive stretching of injured muscles, because the condition may be aggravated.
6. Use Laboratory Inventory 8.1 to evaluate your progress for improving flexibility in the low back area.

Figure 8.5   Backward Pelvic Tilt Exercise. Lie on back with knees bent and feet flat on floor. Tighten the abdominal muscles and other muscles necessary to flatten the lower back against the floor. This exercise may also be done standing against a wall or sitting in a chair. Hold static position for 15 to 60 seconds. Repeat three times.

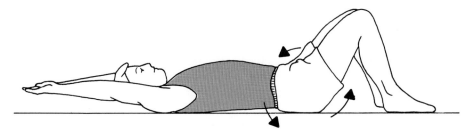

Figure 8.6   Forward Bend. Sit down on the floor with knees straight as in *a*. Bend forward *slowly*, reaching as far as you can until you experience mild pain. This exercise may also be done from a standing position as in *b, but may put more stress on the back*. Hold static position for 15 to 60 seconds. Repeat three times.

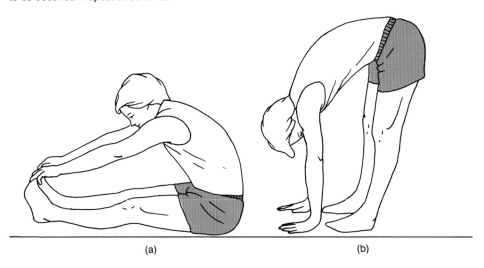

(a)   (b)

Flexibility Exercises for the Low Back Area

The key to flexibility exercises for the low back area is to flatten out the forward curve in the lumbar region. By rotating the hips backward, the lumbar curve will tend to flatten. This is known as a backward pelvic tilt and should be a part of all flexibility and abdominal exercises for the low back area (see fig. 8.5). A good example of this, and also a good exercise, is to stand with your back against a wall, then suck in your stomach and roll your hips backward in order to straighten your entire back against the wall. This type of exercise tends to stretch the tight muscles in the lower back region and those muscles that tend to pull the hips forward.

Figure 8.7 Single or Double Knee to Chest. Lie with back on the floor, knees bent, and feet flat on the floor. In single knee exercise (*a*), draw one knee to the chest and pull it in tightly with the arms. In double knee exercise (*b*), draw both knees in. Pull in tightly for 15 to 60 seconds. Repeat three times each for single knee, or total of three times for double knee exercise.

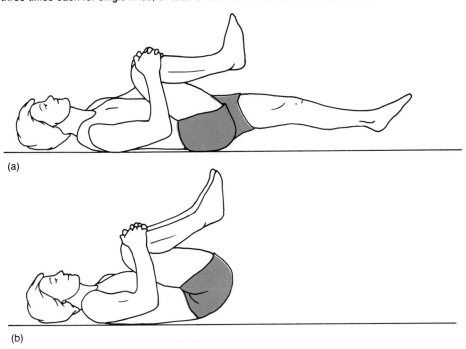

(a)

(b)

When doing flexibility exercises for the low back area you should be especially cautious. Although a mild degree of pain is normally needed to improve flexibility of the muscle groups in this area, it should be the type of pain associated with muscle stretching. If you experience any other type of pain, such as a sharp pain, discontinue that exercise. For those who do suffer from low back pain, select those exercises that will flatten your back, and also those that you find help relieve the pain when you are in the stretched position. Figures 8.5, 8.6, and 8.7 illustrate some useful exercises for low back pain.

Flexibility Exercises for Round Shoulders

In the condition of **round shoulders,** the muscular forces in the chest and upper back are out of balance. The chest muscles are shortened and stronger while those in the back are lengthened and weaker, thus allowing the shoulders to be pulled forward somewhat. Exercises to help correct this condition should be designed to increase the length or flexibility of the chest muscles and strengthen the back muscles. Several exercises for round shoulders are depicted in figures 8.8 and 8.9.

Figure 8.8 Doorway Stretch. Stand in a doorway with arms outstretched and placed against wall on one side of the doorway. Lean forward gradually until tension and mild pain is experienced in muscles of the chest. Hold static position for 15 to 60 seconds. Repeat three times.

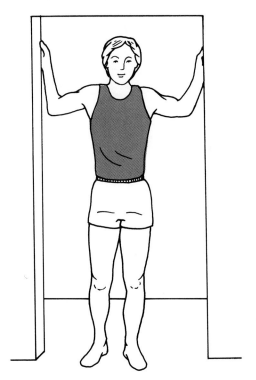

Flexibility Exercises for Joggers and Runners

Joggers and runners often may develop some minor aches and pains, or minor injuries, in various parts of their bodies, particularly during the beginning stages of a jogging program or when they overdo it. Those who are strong advocates of flexibility exercises for joggers and runners suggest that these minor injuries may be prevented by a proper flexibility exercise program. On the other hand, there are those individuals who note that flexibility training has not been shown to prevent injuries because no evidence is available to support this claim. Nevertheless, the theory that a more flexible muscle may be less susceptible to injury appears to be sound. At the least, since improved flexibility should not be harmful, joggers and runners may want to do flexibility exercises for four body areas.

First, the low back area may be prone to injury through improper running form or overuse. The exercises suggested for relief or prevention of low back pain presented earlier in this chapter are highly recommended for joggers and runners.

Figure 8.9 Isometric Chest Stretcher. In standing or sitting position, raise arms sideways to shoulder level with elbows bent and hands near the chest. Try to move your elbows back sideways as far as possible by pulling your shoulder blades together. Hold static position for 15 to 60 seconds. Repeat three times.

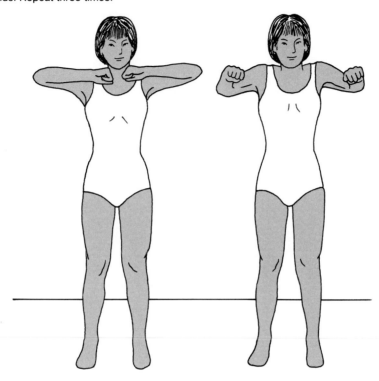

Second, the **hamstrings,** a muscle group at the back of the thigh, should also be stretched. Some of the exercises for the low back pain, such as those in figures 8.6 and 8.7 help improve hamstring flexibility. A more strenuous exercise for hamstring flexibility is depicted in figure 8.10.

Third, the calf muscles in the back of the lower leg should be stretched to prevent possible problems with the Achilles tendon, which is one of the more common injuries among joggers and runners. An example of such an exercise is presented in figure 8.11.

The fourth area to stretch is the groin, the muscles on the inside of the thigh that often tighten up in runners. Figure 8.12 illustrates an exercise for stretching the adductor muscles in the groin.

Figure 8.10 Hurdle Stretch. Place one leg out straight on some type of support. Bend forward at the waist and try to place your head as close to your leg as possible. Keep knee straight. Flatten back upward to also help stretch low back area. Hold forward position for 15 to 60 seconds. Repeat three times for each leg.

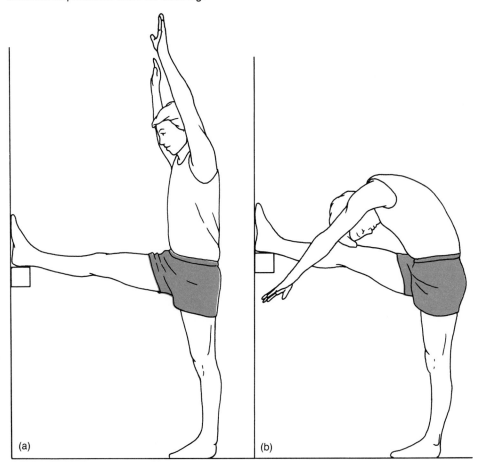

(a)

(b)

Figure 8.11 Achilles' Stretcher. Place the balls of the feet on a solid object like a book or a stair step and then lower the heel below the top surface about two inches. Hold static position for 15 to 60 seconds. Repeat three times.

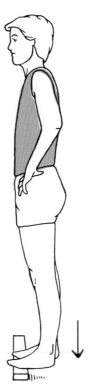

Figure 8.12 Groin Stretcher. Sit on the floor with knees bent and feet turned so that the soles of both feet are together. Bring feet as close to crotch as possible. While in this position, push down on knees until mild pain is experienced in the groin muscles. Hold this position for 15 to 60 seconds. Repeat three times.

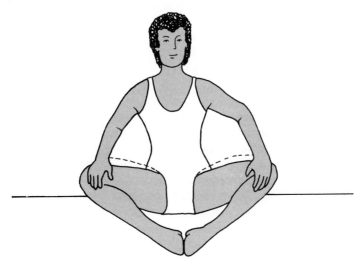

Figure 8.13 Spinal flexion occurs primarily in the spine itself, with little to no movement at the hip joint. A forward curvature in the spine is flexion, and the lumbar curve tends to flatten out or reverse its direction.

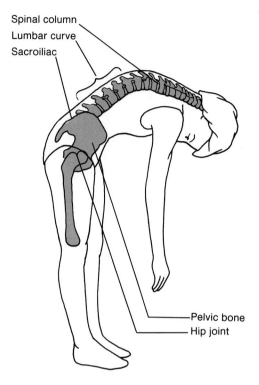

Spinal column
Lumbar curve
Sacroiliac

Pelvic bone
Hip joint

Abdominal Strength

While stretching exercises to improve the flexibility of the lumbar region are very important in the prevention of low back pain, so too are exercises to strengthen the abdominal musculature. There is a wide variety of exercises that are utilized to help improve abdominal strength, but some of these exercises may actually predispose an individual to low back problems rather than help prevent them. In order to understand why, let us look at the movements that occur in some of these exercises and at the primary muscles that are involved.

For our discussion, it is important to understand the difference between flexion of the spine and flexion of the hip. **Spinal flexion** occurs only between the vertebrae in the spinal column. If you lie flat on the floor on your back and then begin to curl your head, neck and shoulders forward while keeping your lower back flat against the floor, you are doing primarily spinal flexion. This movement is often called the **curl-up**, and we shall refer to it later. It is important to realize that no movement occurs where the spine joins the pelvis. This is an immovable joint called the **sacroiliac** joint where the sacrum (part of the spine) fuses with the iliac bones of the pelvis.

Figure 8.14 Hip flexion occurs at the joint between the pelvic bone and the thigh bone. Both *a* and *b* are examples of hip flexion.

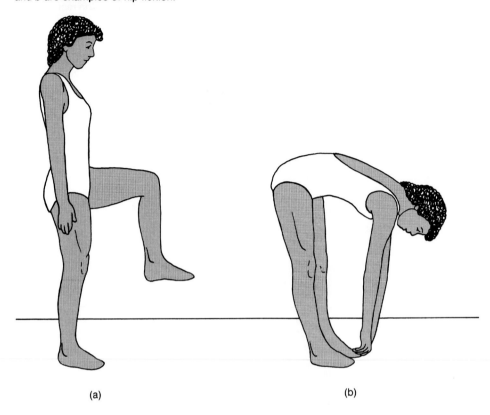

(a)   (b)

Hip flexion occurs only at the hip joint, which is the joint between the pelvic bone and the thigh bone. If you stand and lift one leg forward, you are doing hip flexion. Also, if you keep your back straight and bend over to touch your toes, you are doing hip flexion. In some exercises, you may do both spinal flexion and hip flexion. For example, spinal flexion occurs in the early phase of a full sit-up, but after about 30 degrees, hip flexion takes over. It is also important to realize that, although the pelvic bone usually moves in order to facilitate spine and thigh movements, it may also be moved independently. For example, if you stand with your back against a wall and simply pull in your stomach to flatten your back against the wall, you are primarily moving the pelvic bone.

The muscles we are primarily interested in are the abdominals, particularly the **rectus abdominis.** The rectus abdominis is illustrated in figure 7.14. As the rectus abdominis contracts, it causes one of two movements. First, it pulls on the ribs, which, because the ribs are attached to the spine, causes spinal flexion. Second, it pulls up on the lower part of the pelvic bone, thus tilting it backward and helping to flatten out the lower back. Thus, exercises that highlight spinal flexion, or backward pelvic tilt, help to strengthen the abdominal muscles.

Figure 8.15 The Effect of the Psoas Major on the Spine. The psoas major is shown in *a*. In the straight leg position, *b,* the psoas major may pull forward on the lower spine area, thus increasing the lumbar lordosis. This is particularly true if the abdominal muscles are weak. The rectus femoris can also pull forward on the pelvis and increase the lumbar lordosis.

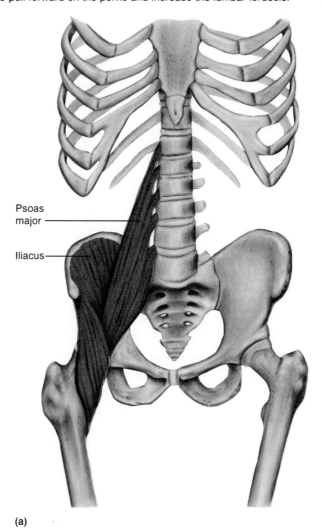

Psoas major

Iliacus

(a)

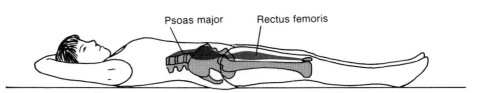

Psoas major   Rectus femoris

(b)

Figure 8.16 The Bent-knee Position. By bending the knees while on the back, thus flexing the hips, the psoas major and rectus femoris are shortened somewhat and have a lesser tendency to accentuate the curve in the low back area. Putting the feet flat on the floor with the knees bent achieves the same effect.

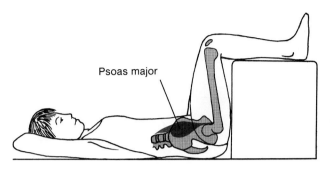

Psoas major

Several muscles that cause hip flexion may also act on the spine or pelvis. A deep muscle, the **psoas major,** is primarily a hip flexor, but as you can see in figure 8.15, it may also pull forward on the lumbar spine area. The **rectus femoris** (see fig. 7.9), the main muscle in the front of the thigh, is also a hip flexor, but it can also pull forward on the pelvic bone. The actions of both of these muscles may cause an increased curve in the lumbar area, which is exactly the opposite of the purpose of abdominal exercises. Thus, exercises that increase this forward curve should be avoided as much as possible.

One good way to help avoid the adverse effects of the psoas major and rectus femoris muscles is simply to flex the hips in the starting position for abdominal exercises. Figure 8.16 illustrates one possible method. In this position the psoas major and rectus femoris are shortened somewhat so they are not in a position to increase the lumbar curve.

Research has shown that the curl-up exercise is very effective for increasing abdominal strength, and is least likely to create increased pressure in the lumbar area, which could cause low back problems. The curl-up should be performed to the point where only the shoulder blades are lifted off the floor. The basic position is shown in figure 8.17a. As you develop greater abdominal strength, you may add weights as illustrated in figure 8.17b.

The bent-knee sit-up (figure 8.18) is also a good abdominal exercise. The backward pelvic tilt in figure 8.5 is also helpful, and can be done while standing or sitting, as well as lying down.

A number of other exercises may be used to develop abdominal strength, but you should avoid those that cause an increased lumbar curve as shown in figure 8.19. It is important to incorporate the backward pelvic tilt in all exercises. Always try to keep the lower part of the back flat against the supporting surface, an action that will insure that the abdominal muscles are being exercised.

Figure 8.17   The Curl-up. The curl-up involves only spinal flexion. With the chin on the chest and the arms straight (or crossed on the chest), simply sit up part way (about 30 degrees), and return slowly to the starting position. Do not anchor the feet. This exercise (*a*) involves the abdominals (the spinal flexors) and not the hip flexors. As you develop abdominal strength, increased resistance may be obtained by holding weights on the chest (*b*).

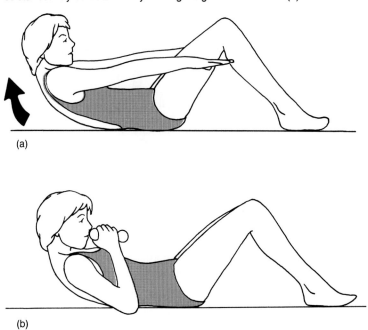

(a)

(b)

Figure 8.18   Bent-knee Sit-up. Lie on the back with knees bent and feet flat on the floor. Do the same movement as the curl-up in figure 8.17, but come all of the way up. Resistance in the sit-up may be increased as in figure 8.17*b* for the curl-up.

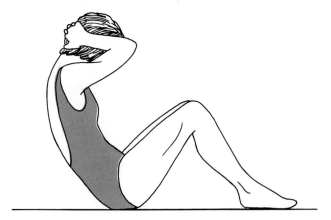

Figure 8.19 Slow Leg Lowering. Exercises such as this help to strengthen the abdominal muscles, but they may place a tremendous stress on the low back area. If you do exercises like this, keep the lower back flat against the floor throughout, i.e., always do the backward pelvic tilt.

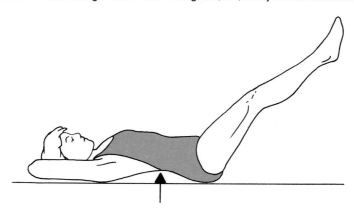

Individuals with lower levels of abdominal strength may need to progress gradually from the less strenuous to the more difficult abdominal exercises. For those with very low levels of abdominal strength, the pelvic tilt should be used as the primary exercise, with eventual progression through the various levels of the modified curl-up.

A. Backward Pelvic Tilt (fig. 8.5). Do 10 repetitions of 15 seconds each. This exercise may also be done periodically throughout the day, while sitting or standing.

B. Curl-Up with Modifications (fig. 8.17)
   For each level, work up to 50 repetitions before progressing to the next level.

   Level 1—Grasp back of both thighs with your hands and assist the curl-up by pulling yourself up. Go back slowly.
   Level 2—Place hands at sides of legs, arms straight as in figure 8.17a. Curl up with no pulling assistance. Go back down slowly.
   Level 3—Cross arms on stomach. Do curl-up. Go back down slowly.
   Level 4—Fold arms across chest. Do curl-up. Go back down slowly.
   Level 5—Place hands behind head. Do curl-up. Go back down slowly.
   Level 6—Place weights on chest. Do curl-up. Be sure lower back maintains contact with the floor. Go back down slowly. Only do this exercise after you are able to complete Level 5 comfortably. Start with light weights (e.g. 5 pounds) and follow the progression noted in chapter 7.

Many of the exercises in this chapter can be done anytime during the day. The flexibility exercises can be used during a stretch break at work, as can the backward pelvic tilt when you tuck in your hips. You are only limited by your imagination as to how these exercises may be worked into your daily schedule.

Assume a position as in figure 8.20. Bare feet should be flat against the surface. Knees should be kept flat on the floor, preferably by a partner who holds them down. Place one hand on top of the other and bend forward as far as you can with fingertips on the ruler. The ruler should extend 9 inches (23 centimeters) in front of the support. Measure the reach to the nearest centimeter or half inch. See the flexibility rating scale for interpretation of the results.

Figure 8.20   Position for the Sit-and-Reach Test of Flexibility in the Low Back and Hamstring Area

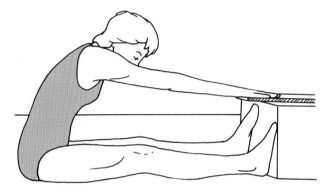

Flexibility Rating Scale

	Men		Women	
	Cm.	In.	Cm.	In.
Excellent	43	17	45	18
Good	35–42	14–16	38–44	15–17
Average	25–34	10–13	25–37	10–14
Poor	17–24	7–9	17–24	7–9
Very Poor	16 or less	6 or less	16 or less	6 or less

References

Beaulieu, J. "Developing a Stretching Program." *The Physician and Sportsmedicine* 9:59–69 (November 1981).

Blackburn, S. I., and Portney, L. "Electromyographic Activity of Basic Musculature during Williams' Flexion Exercises." *Physical Therapy* 61:878–85 (1981).

Block, I. *Low Back Pain—What It Is, What Can Be Done.* New York: Public Affairs Pamphlets, 1982.

Blush, K. "From the Clinic: Back School." *American Corrective Therapy Journal* 33:23–25 (1979).

Corbin, C.; Dowell, L.; Lindsey, R.; and Tolson, H. *Concepts in Physical Education.* Dubuque, IA: Wm. C. Brown Publishers, 1981.

Corbin, C., and Noble, L. "Flexibility." *Journal of Physical Education and Recreation* 51:23–24, 57–60 (June 1980).

Couch, J. "The Perfect Post-Run Stretching Routine." *Runners' World* 14:84–89 (April 1979).

Davies, J.; Gibson, T.; and Tester, L. "The Value of Exercises in the Treatment of Low Back Pain." *Rheumatology and Rehabilitation* 18:243–47 (1979).

Dukes-Dubos, F. "What Is the Best Way to Lift and Carry?" *Occupational and Health Safety* 46:16–18 (1977).

Fedo, M. "Understanding Lower-Back Pain." *Runner's World* 17:58–73 (February 1982).

Garg, A., and Saxena, U. "Effects of Lifting Frequency and Technique on Physical Fatigue with Special Reference to Psychophysical Methodology and Metabolic Rate." *American Industrial Hygiene Association* 40:894–903 (1979).

Goldberg, H.; Kohn, H.; Dehn, T.; and Seeds, R. "Diagnosis and Management of Low Back Pain." *Occupational and Health Safety* 49:14–31 (June 1980).

Grew, N. "Intraabdominal Pressure Response to Loads Applied to the Torso in Normal Subjects." *Spine* 5:149–54 (1980).

Grieve, D. "The Dynamics of Lifting." *Exercise and Sports Science Review* 5:157–79 (1977).

Halpern, A., and Bleck, E. "Sit-Up Exercises: An Electromyographic Study." *Clinical Orthopaedics* 145:172–78 (November-December 1979).

Hammond, J. *Understanding Human Engineering.* Vancouver: David and Charles, 1978.

Kraus, H.; Melleby, A.; and Gaston, S. "Basic Pain Correction and Prevention." *New York State Journal of Medicine* 77:1335–38 (1977).

Kroner, R. "Beware of Exercises that Do More Harm than Good." *Occupational and Health Safety* 49:32–35 (June 1980).

Poulsen, E. "Back Muscle Strength and Weight Limits in Lifting Burdens." *Spine* 6:73–75 (1981).

Pytel, J., and Kamon, E. "Dynamic Strength Test as a Predictor for Maximal and Acceptable Lifting." *Ergonomics* 24:663–72 (1981).

Ricci, B.; Marchetti, M.; and Figura, F. "Biomechanics of Sit-Up Exercises." *Medicine and Science in Sports and Exercise* 13:54–59 (1981).

Shultz, P. "Flexibility: Day of the Static Stretch." *The Physician and Sportsmedicine* 7:109 (November 1979).

Shyne, K. "Richard H. Dominguez, M.D.: To Stretch or Not To Stretch." *The Physician and Sportsmedicine* 10:137–40 (September 1982).

Stanitski, C. "Low Back Pain in Young Athletes." *The Physician and Sportsmedicine* 10:77–91 (October 1982).

Traywick, R. "Class Helps Many with Aching Backs." *Richmond Times-Dispatch* Cl (January 6 1983).

Verrill, D., and Pate, R. "Relationship between Duration of Static Stretch in the Sit and Reach Position and Biceps Femoris Electromyographic Activity." *Medicine and Science in Sports and Exercise* 14:124 (1982).

Witzig, K. "The Elevator—One Body Exercise against Backache." *Praxis* 67:1778–80 (1978).

Stress Reduction Techniques 9

Key Terms

assertiveness	negative addiction
autogenic relaxation	pituitary gland
Benson's relaxation response	progressive relaxation
caffeine	self-actualization
endorphins	state anxiety
homeostasis	stress
hypoglycemia	stress management
hypothalamus	stressor
imagery	stress response
inverted-U hypothesis	trait anxiety
mantra	Transcendental Meditation (TM)

Key Concepts

Although most of the stressors that our ancient ancestors faced are no longer with us (such as the threat of wild animals), our bodies still retain the physiological response to stress that can be evoked by other threats, such as threats to our esteem.

Both physical and mental stressors may evoke the stress response in which the body prepares for action by increasing muscular tension, increasing heart rate and blood pressure, and eliciting other physiological responses to help to counteract the stressor.

The stress response evolved as a normal reaction to stress and was vital in the survival of the fittest, but the constant physiological actions of the stress response, particularly in individuals with trait anxiety, may create a predisposition to certain health problems.

There are a variety of means to assess the tendency toward trait anxiety. One of the more practical is a self-assessment questionnaire.

There exists a wide variety of procedures to help manage stress, ranging from passive techniques, such as meditation, to active physical exercise. You should experiment with several to find those most appropriate for you.

Relaxation is a motor skill and needs to be learned, just like tennis. In order to be maximally effective, it must be practiced and perfected like any other motor skill.

One of the first steps in reducing stress is to try to remove the cause of the stress, which may be psychological, environmental or dietary.

Breathing exercises, concentrating upon a slow, deep inhalation followed by a slow, deep exhalation, is one of the simplest ways to induce a state of relaxation.

The major passive relaxation techniques involve meditation, imagery, and autogenic relaxation. Active techniques include progressive relaxation training and aerobic exercise.

In general, research has shown that both passive and active relaxation techniques may be helpful as stress management procedures.

Introduction

Abraham Maslow, a psychologist who has written extensively about motivation and personality development, has proposed a theory of motivation and behavior that is based upon a hierarchy of human needs. The hierarchy, in priority order from the lowest level to the level of **self-actualization,** is presented in table 9.1. According to Maslow, the ultimate goal for most individuals is to become self-actualized. In general, Maslow has characterized self-actualized individuals as being realistically-oriented, autonomous, independent, creative, democratic, spontaneous, not self-centered, having an air of detachment and a need for privacy, accepting themselves and the world for what they are, having a sincere appreciation of people, and experiencing deep, emotional, intimate relationships with a few specially loved people. In general, Maslow has noted that you must satisfy your needs at a lower level before you can concentrate on achieving satisfaction at the next highest level. Thus in order to become self-actualized, your needs at the lower four levels must be fulfilled first.

In prehistoric times, hunger, thirst, and danger were primary drives for human behavior. The quest for food, water, and safety was ever present. Man would often risk his life for food. In other words, basic physiological needs would take precedence over safety needs. In order to satisfy the needs at the first two levels, the human body had to be prepared for action, to fight for food or run to safety, whatever the case might have been. Through the process of evolution then, the human body developed a basic physiological response whenever some need, such as for safety, became great enough. This physiological response was designed to mobilize the body reserves for immediate activity. It was a beneficial response, because it could help to make the caveman run faster or fight more vigorously. Once the threat to safety was removed, so too was the basic physiological response.

In our modern society, hunger and thirst are no longer major needs driving our behavior, and although safety is still a concern, it is not as much a problem as it was in prehistoric times. However, the potential for the basic physiological response to these needs still remains with us. All of us can remember having been frightened by a sudden movement in the dark, and recall such obvious body reactions as a pounding heart, tightened musculature, and sweating palms. An anticipated danger activated this physiological response, but even later just walking by a dark alley or into a dark room may elicit the same response by simply thinking about the potential danger. In essence, a threat elicits a response similar to that elicited by the actual danger. More is said about this basic physiological response in the next section, but it is sufficient for now to realize that our thoughts, anticipating the threat of danger, may activate this response, even though an actual need for safety is not present.

Since most of our basic physiological and safety needs are satisfied by the benefits of modern society, the major drives for behavior originate in the next two levels—the needs for belongingness and love, and for esteem. Most of us want to belong to a loving family, to have friends, to share a special love with someone, and to achieve some degree of success and recognition in our vocations and avocations. If we perceive a threat in these areas, we may still experience the same basic physiological responses as we would if exposed to some actual danger. A classic example is the pounding heart, tight-

Table 9.1
Maslow's Hierarchy of Needs Involved in Human Motivation

Basic physiological needs
Safety needs
Belongingness and love needs
Esteem needs
Self-actualization needs

Figure 9.1 In the process of evolution, humans developed a physiological response to stress that prepared the body for action—to fight or take flight. This physiological response to stress helped in the survival of the fittest, but may be a cause of several major health problems if a prolonged response occurs in our modern stressful society.

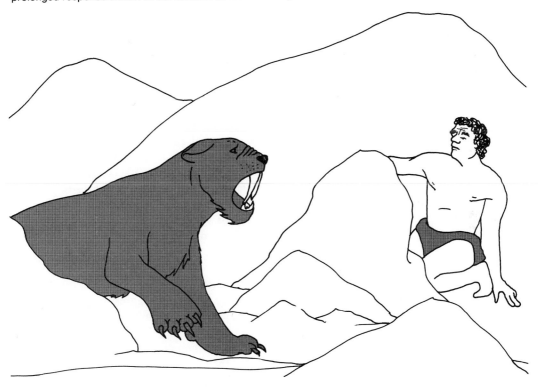

ened musculature, sweating palms, and dry mouth that often occurs before delivering a speech to a group of your peers. You may feel that your speech will be a failure, and this is a threat to your need for esteem.

Although there are some obvious threats to our personal safety in our external environment, it is important to realize that many of the threats we experience today are internally generated. They originate in our minds as perceived threats to our needs for fulfillment in love and esteem. Whatever the threat—external or internal—it imposes a stress upon our bodies that may eventually be harmful to our health. Current estimates suggest that 10 to 15 million Americans suffer from symptoms associated with such stress.

The purpose of this chapter is threefold: (1) to discuss the basic physiological response to stress, and relate it to possible medical problems; (2) to determine if you are prone to stress, and (3) to discuss various means that may be utilized to prevent or reduce stress levels.

Effects of Stress on the Body

Before we look at the actual effects that stress may cause in the body—the stress response—let us briefly discuss the general causes of stress. A **stressor** is anything that causes the stress response in any given individual. Stressors may be physical in nature (bodily pains or even exercise). Stressors may also be mental or emotional in nature, and affect the mind (worrying about an examination, a speech, or a first date). The key point is that both physical and mental stressors elicit a similar stress response in the body.

From a medical viewpoint, the stressor is the cause and **stress** is the physiological response (the stress response) the body makes to any stressor. Most of us associate other terms with the feeling of stress, such as strain, tension, and anxiety. These three terms are often used interchangeably to characterize the stress response.

The **stress response** is the mechanism whereby the body prepares for action to help counteract a stressor. The stressor may be external and be perceived by our senses, such as seeing a vicious dog coming at us while jogging; it may be internal, such as a change in our blood chemistry. Both external and internal stressors stimulate the **hypothalamus,** a key control area in the brain that helps regulate **homeostasis,** which is the normal functioning of our internal environment. The hypothalamus regulates homeostasis by two major pathways—the nervous system and the endocrine system.

The hypothalamus contains various clusters of nerve cells, called centers, which respond to specific stimuli. For example, there are centers for such basic physiological stimuli as hunger, thirst, and temperature. The hypothalamus also receives stimuli from the areas of the brain that control human emotions and, thus, contains centers that respond to such emotional feelings as pleasure, rage, and aggression. When any of these hypothalamic centers are activated by appropriate stimuli, a particular response is generated.

The hypothalamic centers stimulate the sympathetic nervous system. The primary function of the sympathetic nervous system is the maintenance of normal homeostasis; it affects almost all organs and glands in the body, including the heart and blood vessels. By activating the sympathetic nervous system, the hypothalamus is able to rapidly mobilize the body for action. The hypothalamus also exerts significant control over the **pituitary gland,** the so-called master gland of the endocrine system. The pituitary gland, in turn, exerts a significant effect upon many of the other endocrine glands in the body that are concerned with homeostasis, particularly the adrenal gland. Thus by regulating the activities of both the sympathetic nervous system and the pituitary gland, the hypothalamus can control the state of homeostasis in the body, and activate the stress response when stimulated by an appropriate stressor. An overview of the hypothalamic control mechanism is presented in figure 9.2.

Figure 9.2 The hypothalamus responds to physical or mental stress by stimulating the sympathetic nervous system and the pituitary gland, both of which may cause a number of physiological effects throughout the body.

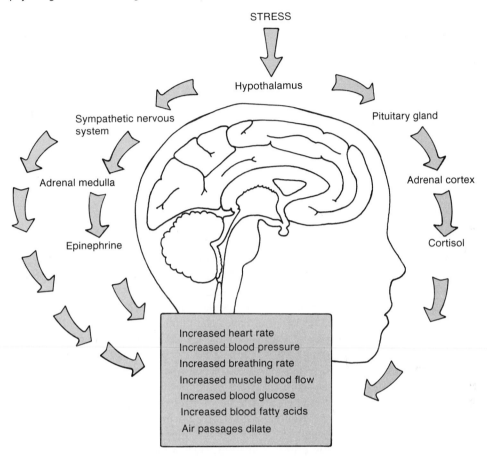

STRESS

Hypothalamus

Sympathetic nervous system

Pituitary gland

Adrenal medulla

Adrenal cortex

Epinephrine

Cortisol

Increased heart rate
Increased blood pressure
Increased breathing rate
Increased muscle blood flow
Increased blood glucose
Increased blood fatty acids
Air passages dilate

The major effect of the stress response is to mobilize the cardiovascular system to meet anticipated energy needs. In essence, the heart rate is increased and the heart pumps more forcefully with each beat. The blood flow to some parts of the body is increased, while decreased to others. Blood pressure is increased. Muscular tension is increased throughout the body, preparing the individual for rapid activation of muscle strength and power. This stress response is the body's way of preparing for activity, and has been instrumental in the preservation of the species through the process of evolution. Thus the stress response is natural, and it is good when an actual danger is encountered. When the danger is gone, the stress response fades away. However, the stress response may lead to certain health probelms if it persists for a prolonged period of time. Let us explore the stress response a little further by looking at the concepts of state and trait anxiety.

Figure 9.3 The inverted-U theory suggests that there is an optimal level of stress or anxiety that improves performance. Too little stress does not provide sufficient motivation for the task while too much stress may disrupt performance.
Source: Courtesy J. B. Oxendine.

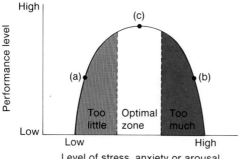

State and Trait Anxiety

Any situation may be a stressor for any one individual at any given time. **State anxiety** refers to any situational stressor that evokes the stress response. It is usually temporary and fades away when the stressor is removed. What may be a stressor for one individual may not be for another. For example, John may be very muscular and possess a great deal of upper body strength, but may not have good public speaking ability; Paul may possess excellent public speaking skills but have low levels of upper body strength. Climbing a 20 foot rope in gym class would be a major stressor for Paul; an oral book report in English class would evoke the stress response in John.

As mentioned earlier, the stress response is not considered to be an inappropriate body response. As a matter of fact, a little bit of stress may be necessary to obtain optimal levels of performance. Figure 9.3 illustrates the **inverted-U hypothesis** relative to stress, arousal, and performance. In certain activities, such as giving a speech or participating in some athletic events, too little stress may result in a lower level of arousal and, hence, the individual is not keyed up sufficiently to perform at an optimal level. On the other hand, too much stress may destroy performance, as forgetting your speech or being too nervous in a sport that requires precision. Thus there appears to be an optimal level of stress and arousal that results in optimal performance, and these appear to be dependent upon the individual and the type of task to be performed.

The key point is that an excessive stress response during a situation of state anxiety may be disruptive to performance. A schematic of excessive state anxiety is presented in figure 9.4. In essence, an excessive stress response can create both physical and mental alterations that will detract from optimal performance levels.

As is noted later in this chapter, many of the stress reduction techniques may be helpful in reducing the magnitude of the stress response during conditions of state anxiety.

Figure 9.4 Excessive state anxiety may elicit various bodily reactions so that physical and mental performance may be impaired.

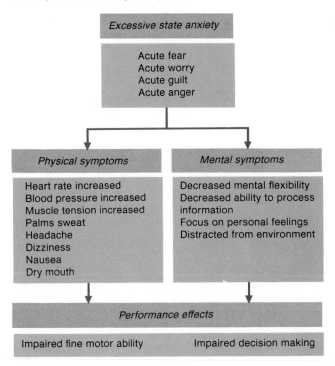

In contrast to state anxiety, which is considered to be a temporary condition, **trait anxiety** represents a general disposition of an individual to psychological stressors. Individuals who possess trait anxiety have a feeling of being threatened and are very prone to feelings of worry and guilt.

Hans Selye has conducted extensive research relative to the effects of excessive constant stress, or distress, on health. Selye developed a theory of stress that is based on three phases—the alarm phase, the adaptation phase, and the exhaustion phase. The alarm phase is the stress response discussed previously, which prepares the body for action. In state anxiety it is transitory. However, in trait anxiety it persists and the body necessarily has to adapt to this response in the second phase. Some of these adaptations, such as high blood pressure, are harmful to the health. If they persist they may lead to a third state, the exhaustion stage, possibly with severe health consequences.

Trait anxiety may cause physical and mental symptoms identical to those caused by excessive state anxiety. Many of these symptoms may persist and lead to other more severe health problems. Figure 9.5 presents a broad overview of some of the medical problems that may occur in certain individuals following prolonged trait anxiety. These medical problems may be caused directly by the effect of psychological stressors upon

Figure 9.5 Excessive trait anxiety over a period of time may be a contributing factor to a host of physical and mental health problems.

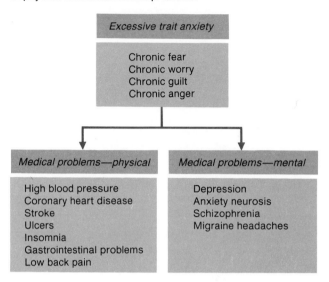

nervous and endocrine functions in the body, or indirectly through overeating and physical inactivity as responses to the imposed stress. Some of the major health problems are noted in figure 9.5. Selye's theory of stress suggests that almost any disease may be caused by the chronic excessive emotional stress that may be present in individuals with trait anxiety.

As with state anxiety, various relaxation techniques may be helpful in reducing, or possibly reversing, the adverse effects of chronic stress response in individuals with trait anxiety.

Your Stress Profile

There are a number of different ways that have been used to evaluate stress levels in an individual: measuring muscle tension by electromyographic techniques, voice analysis, certain blood tests for stress markers, and psychological interview techniques. However, several of the most practical techniques that have been developed involve self-assessment inventories in which the individual responds to some form of questionnaire designed to provide a general predisposition toward stress.

Laboratory Inventory 9.1 has four parts: measuring your vulnerability to stress from being frustrated; measuring your vulnerability to stress from being overloaded; testing for type A, or compulsive, time-urgent behavior; and evaluating how well you cope with stress in your life.

If the results of this Laboratory Inventory suggest that you are under stress, then the methods to help reduce stress (presented in the next section) should be of interest to you. Even if you do not appear to be prone to stress, passive relaxation techniques, such as breathing exercises and meditation, may be very useful in helping to reduce the stress response in cases of state anxiety.

Figure 9.6 A variety of relaxation techniques have been successful in reducing state anxiety. Exercise, meditation, and simple quiet reading have been equally effective in reducing state anxiety.
Source: From M. S. Bahrke and W. P. Morgan, "Anxiety Reduction Following Exercise and Medication," in *Cognitive Therapy and Research,* 2:323. Copyright © 1978 by Plenum Publishing Corporation. Reprinted by permission of the publisher and the author.

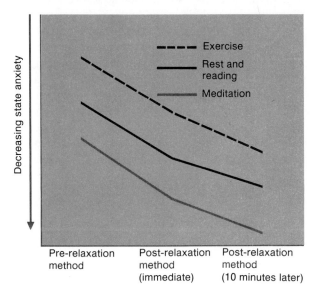

Methods to Reduce Stress

Now that you have a general idea of what stress is, how it may affect the body, and whether or not you have a general tendency toward trait anxiety, what can you do about its adverse effects? The general term for dealing with stress is known as **stress management.** In some cases, as discussed earlier in this chapter, the stress level may be increased in a given individual, such as an athlete prior to competition, in order to obtain an optimal performance level. A number of special motivational techniques have been developed for that purpose. However, for our purposes, we are interested in those stress management techniques that may reduce stress levels and their possible adverse effects on our mental and physical functioning.

A wide variety of techniques have been utilized to help reduce both state and trait anxiety, ranging on a continuum from active techniques such as strenuous exercise to very passive techniques such as meditation. In general, these two techniques, plus others on the continuum, have been shown to be equally effective in reducing stress. A number of theories have been advanced in attempts to explain how the stress reduction techniques work, but no major consensus of opinion appears to have been reached. For example, it has been suggested that exercise and meditation produce chemical changes in the brain, induce neuromuscular relaxation, train the parasympathetic nervous system, or provide a distraction—all of which may produce a relaxing effect on the mind and body. Some of these possible methods of stress reduction are integrated into the following discussion.

As noted above, there are many techniques for dealing with stress; some are desirable, some undesirable. Smoking, alcohol, tranquilizers, and other drugs may initially be helpful in stress reduction, but they may become a major health problem if they are abused. The techniques that are described in the following list have been utilized and found to be effective in many individuals. Not all techniques work with all people. You should become familiar with each technique and find which one works for you. An aerobic exercise program is advocated for other health benefits above and beyond the beneficial effects it may have as a means to reduce stress. If your aerobic exercise program helps to reduce your stress levels, that is all the better. However, one or more of the other techniques, such as meditation or breathing exercises, may be very useful additions to your stress reduction program.

Space does not permit a full detailed discussion of each stress reduction technique, but a basic explanation and/or example of each method is presented. For those desiring an expanded coverage, *Guide to Stress Reduction* by L. John Mason and *Controlling Stress and Tension* by D. Girdano and G. Everly are highly recommended. The common techniques are:

1. Removing the stressor
2. Rest and sleep
3. Breathing
4. Meditation
5. Imagery
6. Autogenic training
7. Progressive relaxation training
8. Active exercises

It is important to realize that relaxation is a motor skill that needs to be learned. In order to effectively use such techniques as breathing exercises, meditation, autogenic training, and progressive relaxation training, they must be practiced and perfected as must any other motor skill.

Removing the Stressor

Behind every stress response there is a cause, or stressor. The first step in any stress reduction program should be an attempt to remove this stressor, if possible. In order to be able to remove the stressor, however, you must first be able to identify it. In some cases you may not be able to identify the cause of your stress, since it may be the result of deep-seated and subconscious feelings of insecurity and distrust. In such cases, professional psychological help may be necessary to identify and remove these psychological causes.

Three general classes of stressors are psychological causes, environmental or situational causes, and dietary causes.

Psychological Stressors

Some identifiable psychological causes may be manifestations of the deep-seated causes noted previously, and may include such traits as excessive wants and desires, excessive drive and ambition, expectations of perfection from others, inability to make decisions, and negative thoughts about oneself. Volumes of books have been written about how to remove psychological stressors and become the person you want to be. The following general suggestions may help eliminate the most common psychological causes of stress.

1. Free yourself of worry and guilt. Both of these are useless emotions and may prevent you from being yourself. A good book to help you achieve this objective is *Your Erroneous Zones* by Dr. Wayne Dyer. Becoming more assertive helps remove feelings of guilt as you recognize the fact that you don't always have to conform to others' expectations. Worrying may be diminished by concentrating on the present, by enjoying the pleasures of where you are and who you are with now. Be content in the fact that the future will bring more pleasant experiences.

2. Become more assertive. **Assertiveness** is simply honest communication and should not be confused with aggressiveness. You are assertive when you express your feelings and desires in a straight-forward manner; you are aggressive when you demand your desires or express your feelings with undertones of threats and intimidation. You should recognize the fact that you have certain basic rights of assertiveness, such as the right to be treated with respect, to say no and not feel guilty, to act in ways to promote your self-respect, to express your feelings, to show your emotions, to change your mind, to ask for what you want, to make mistakes, and to feel good about yourself. You also have the responsibility not to violate the assertive rights of others. To become more assertive, you can take a basic class in assertiveness training or consult an appropriate book on the topic, such as *The Assertiveness Option: Your Rights and Responsibilities* by Patricia Jakubowski and Arthur Lange.

Environmental or Situational Stressors

Environmental or situational causes of stress may be many and varied. Too many un-solved problems and too many difficult responsibilities may be sources of worry and constant stress. Often this type of stress is a matter of disorganization and lack of priorities. Learn to take time during the week to establish priorities; decide what is worth your immediate attention and what is not. Set daily, weekly, or long-term goals that focus upon the most important issues and tasks. Five term papers or reports may seem mind-boggling when you think of doing them all at once, but will be much less stressful if you set daily and weekly goals to research and write them. A set routine, guided by realistic goals, will help to eliminate the stressful effects of disorganization.

Your workplace and home may also be situational stressors. Constant problems with your superiors at work, or with your parents or spouse at home may induce a stress response. A good approach to these types of problems is assertiveness. Honestly communicating your feelings and desires may help to resolve the problem. If not, then other solutions, such as finding a new job or moving out of the home should be tried, if feasible.

Noise and overcrowding may also be situational stressors. Finding a quiet place where you can be alone—which is necessary for some of the relaxation techniques discussed later in this chapter—will effectively reduce this stressor temporarily. If a noise bothers you, such as a stereo in the dorm room next door while you are attempting to study, be assertive and express your desires. Try to find ways to avoid the stress of overcrowding if it bothers you; drive to work or school a little earlier to avoid the morning traffic rush. The control of environmental stressors is dependent upon your individual situation, but if they are daily sources of stress for you, then you should take action to reduce or eliminate them.

The final situational stressor we shall mention is boredom. The basic cure for boredom is to have a life full of meaning and purpose. Develop a variety of interests, join clubs, become involved in community projects, or take up new recreational activities to safeguard against boredom. Also learn to entertain yourself, to feel content being alone once in a while with a good book. An active mind deters boredom.

Dietary Stressors

Certain substances in the diet may be stressors for some individuals. **Caffeine,** a natural stimulant, is found in coffee, tea, colas, and chocolate. Not everyone reacts the same way to caffeine, but it can cause nervousness and sleeplessness, particularly if consumed in large amounts. If caffeine appears to be an excessive stimulant in your diet, you can reduce your intake by switching to decaffeinated coffee, tea, and colas, which are the primary sources of caffeine in most diets. Caffeine is also found in certain over-the-counter drugs like aspirin, so be sure to check the labels.

Too much refined carbohydrate, such as table sugar, may create transient periods of **hypoglycemia,** or low blood sugar, in some persons. This may be accompanied by feelings of weakness and lethargy, which can be stressful to some individuals. Shifting to the type of diet suggested in chapter 5 will help to reduce the amount of refined carbohydrate you consume and thus reduce this potential dietary cause of stress.

Rest and Sleep

No extensive discussion of rest and sleep is offered here. However, you should recognize that adequate rest and sleep are necessary to avoid fatigue, which can be a stressor. You may take about 15 to 30 minutes each day and earmark it as a quiet time to rest. A short nap, closing your eyes and putting your feet on the desk, or quiet meditation may help to eliminate mental fatigue and restore vigor and enthusiasm for the task at hand.

A great deal has been written about the importance of sleep and the relative importance of various phases of sleep, such as deep sleep and dream sleep. There is no one general recommendation about how much sleep we need, but a ballpark figure is about 6 to 8 hours of restful sleep per night. Probably the best guideline as to whether or not you have had enough sleep is to decide if you feel rested when you awaken.

A well-rested body and mind is an important weapon against stress.

Breathing Exercises

One of the simplest ways to induce a state of relaxation is a breathing exercise. This technique may be particularly useful when you encounter a stressor, as in cases of state anxiety. However, you should learn to use it on a regular basis throughout the day.

Figure 9.7 In all passive relaxation exercises it is important to assume a relaxed position. For the sitting position, place your arms on your thighs, spread your fingers, let your head hang forward gently, and relax all of your muscles. For the lying position, use a bed or the floor and spread your legs, letting your feet roll to the outside, your arms should be away from the side of your body, palms down and fingers spread. You may wish to have a pillow or rolled towel placed under your neck, under the lower curve in your back, and under your knees and elbows for support.

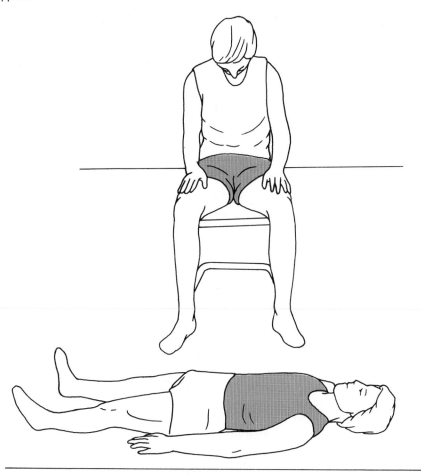

Breathing exercises for relaxation purposes should concentrate on a slow, deep inhalation followed by a slow, deep exhalation. The following steps illustrate a basic breathing exercise.

1. Assume a comfortable position, either sitting or lying on your back. Close your eyes throughout the exercise.
2. Inhale slowly and deeply through the nose. (You may inhale through the mouth also, if it is uncomfortable to inhale only through the nose.) As you inhale, slowly count mentally from one to five to insure that you do not rush your

breathing. Both your stomach and chest should expand considerably. You may place your hands on both to check their outward and upward motions. Focus your mind on the act of inhalation.

3. Once you have reached a full inhalation, hold that position for about 3 seconds and think to yourself, "My body is very calm and relaxed."

4. Exhale slowly through both the nose and mouth and again mentally count down from five to one. Concentrate upon expelling as much air as you possibly can. If you are alone, an alternate approach is to close your mouth and emit the sound OM. Make a long OOOOMMMMMM and vibrate the MMMMMM inside your skull.

Try it! Do you feel calmer and more relaxed? Do you feel less tension in your muscles? This technique may not reduce all of your stress, but it is a simple method to use and may be effective in many cases.

Meditation

Meditation is an Eastern religious technique of relaxation that was introduced to the United States as **Transcendental Meditation (TM)** in the 1960s by Maharishi Mahesh Yogi. In TM, each student is given a **mantra,** which is a particular word or sound to be used during the meditation session. For example, the OM sound in the breathing exercises could be a mantra. During the 20-minute meditation session, the student should concentrate solely on the mantra and eliminate all other distractions from his or her mind.

Dr. Herbert Benson studied TM and published his findings in a book entitled *The Relaxation Response.* The resultant meditation technique is known as **Benson's relaxation response.**

To practice meditation, the following guidelines may be helpful.

1. Find a quiet area. Sit quietly in a comfortable position with your eyes closed.

2. Do several repetitions of the breathing exercise discussed previously to start the relaxation process.

3. Think about your body and let all of your muscles relax. Let yourself go limp.

4. Choose a mantra that has little significance to you, such as the number "one." Concentrate on the mantra. You may associate the mantra with your breathing, mentally picturing the word "one" as you inhale and exhale. Do not think, feel, hear, or see anything but your mantra. Repeat it over and over again in your mind. Do not dwell on distracting thoughts; always return to your mantra.

5. After about 20 minutes, open your eyes, sit quietly for a minute or two as you phase out the mantra, make a fist with both hands and say to yourself, "I am totally awake, alert, and refreshed."

Imagery

Imagery for relaxation purposes involves the mental visualization of feelings that are relaxing to you. The basic principles of the meditation technique apply, but instead of a mantra, think of a relaxing scene, such as sinking into a soft cloud with the sun warming your whole body. Thoughts that convey feelings of floating, warmth, or heaviness of the body (such as sinking into a soft surface) are key points in imagery.

To practice imagery, simply follow the instructions for the meditation procedure noted above, substituting your mental image for the mantra.

Autogenic Relaxation Training

Autogenic means self-generating. In **autogenic relaxation,** you use a form of self-hypnosis to bring about specific body sensations that are associated with the state of relaxation. Autogenic training is closely associated with meditation and imagery. Quietness and feelings of warmth and heaviness are important components.

A basic autogenic relaxation technique follows. You may wish to tape-record the phrases so you can listen and possibly relax even more.

1. Assume a comfortable position seated or lying in a quiet area. Close your eyes.
2. Practice a few repetitions of the breathing exercises to induce the relaxation process.
3. Remove all distracting thoughts from your mind, repeating to yourself three times the phrase "I am totally relaxed and feel good about myself."
4. Progressively relax parts of your body by creating a feeling of warmth or heaviness. You may start at the top of your body and work down, or vice versa.

Slowly repeat in your mind each of the following phrases *three times* as you progressively move down the body. For example, think "My head and neck feel heavy. My head and neck feel heavy. My head and neck feel heavy."

My head and neck feel heavy.
My shoulders feel heavy.
My right arm feels heavy.
My left arm feels heavy.
My chest feels heavy.
My abdomen feels heavy.
My right leg feels heavy.
My left leg feels heavy.
My head and neck feel warm and calm.
My shoulders feel warm and calm.
My right arm feels warm and calm.
My left arm feels warm and calm.
My chest feels warm and calm.

My abdomen feels warm and calm.
My right leg feels warm and calm.
My left leg feels warm and calm.
My breathing is calm.
My heart rate is calm.
I am totally relaxed and feel good about myself.

As with meditation and imagery, you should end the session by saying to yourself, "I am totally awake, alert, and refreshed."

Progressive Relaxation Training

Dr. Edmund Jacobson, in his book *Progressive Relaxation,* describes a technique for reducing muscular tension through a series of exercises designed to teach muscle awareness and relaxation by tensing muscles in various parts of the body, and then consciously relaxing them. Jacobson theorizes that an anxious mind cannot exist in a relaxed body, so relaxing the muscles will reduce stress. The technique can be practiced in a fashion similar to those already mentioned, for about 20 minutes per day. Once you have mastered this technique, it may be utilized when you feel excessive muscular tension during moments of mental or emotional stress. For example, if you are sitting in a meeting and feel tension beginning to develop in the back of your neck, you can isolate those muscles, tense them, and then consciously relax them.

Jacobson utilized over two hundred exercises in his full program, and the following technique is one of the most often used adaptations. In essence, you contract and relax various muscle groups, moving progressively from the lower part to the upper part of the body. There are also three levels of muscle contraction—maximal, half-strength, and very light.

1. The first step is to assume a relaxed position lying on your back. Put a small pillow or some support under your neck or knees if needed. Your legs should be straight, arms at your side, and eyes closed. Let your body go limp.
2. Practice a few repetitions of the breathing exercises to induce the relaxation response.
3. Remove any distracting thoughts from your mind. Say to yourself "I am completely relaxed."
4. For each of the following muscle actions, you should use this procedure:
   A. Take a deep breath. Contract the muscles as hard as possible and hold for 5 seconds. Concentrate on the muscular tension you have developed. After 5 seconds, slowly release the contraction and relax the muscles as you exhale slowly. After you have exhaled, concentrate on the full state of relaxation in that muscular area of the body.
   B. Repeat A, but only utilize about one-half of your maximal strength.
   C. Repeat A, but only utilize a very light amount of muscular force.
   As you perform A, B, and C, be aware of the different sensations during tension and relaxation. Learn the feeling of muscular relaxation and reduced muscular tension.

5. Do the following muscular contractions and movements in sequence, developing the force slowly. Try to isolate the contraction to only that body part. Try not to contract other muscle groups.
   A. Curl just your toes in your right foot.
   B. Curl just your toes in your left foot.
   C. Bend your right foot upward toward your face as far as possible.
   D. Bend your left foot upward toward your face as far as possible.
   E. Extend the right foot downward as far as possible.
   F. Extend the left foot downward as far as possible.
   G. Tense your upper right leg.
   H. Tense your upper left leg.
   I. Tense your buttocks, squeezing in.
   J. Tense your stomach muscles by flattening your lower back against the floor.
   K. Bring your shoulders as far forward as possible, keeping your head and elbows in place.
   L. Push your shoulders back as far as possible, trying to pull your shoulder blades together.
   M. Spread the fingers on your right hand.
   N. Spread the fingers on your left hand.
   O. Make a fist with your right hand.
   P. Make a fist with your left hand.
   Q. Bring your head forward, chin to chest, as far as possible.
   R. Push your head back against the mat.
   S. Open your mouth as wide as possible.
   T. Pucker your lips.
   U. Clench your teeth.
   V. Wrinkle your forehead.
   W. Press your eyes tightly closed.

This relaxation technique is a motor skill to be learned, but with practice you should be able to isolate most of these muscular movements. You may even develop your own exercises and incorporate them into your routine. For a more detailed discussion of this procedure, consult Jacobson's book, *Progressive Relaxation*.

If you find, however, that this procedure creates tension in you due to its active nature, then you may wish to stay with some of the more passive procedures described earlier.

Active Exercise

As we mentioned previously, exercise in itself can be a stressor. However, exercise may also be a very effective means to reduce stress. According to Dr. William P. Morgan, a sports psychologist at the University of Wisconsin, the present clinical and experimental evidence overwhelmingly supports the view that a bout of vigorous exercise can reduce the levels of state anxiety in both normal and clinically anxious individuals. Moreover, a chronic training program may also decrease trait anxiety. A number of

Figure 9.8 Running in a quiet peaceful environment may be helpful as a means to reduce stress.

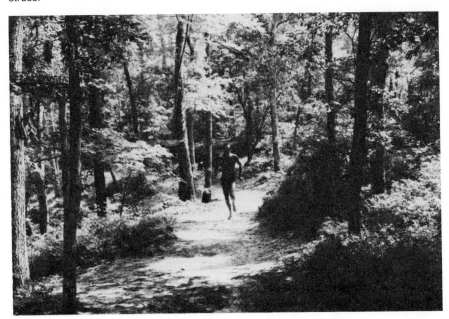

studies have shown that aerobic exercise programs, particularly running, decrease trait anxiety characteristics such as depression, tension, and obsessive-compulsive behavior. Subjects become more relaxed, self-confident, and assertive.

The recommended type of exercise program is one that is aerobic in nature. The guidelines presented in chapter 4 are appropriate for determining the intensity, duration, and frequency of such an exercise program. You may also attempt to learn to meditate while exercising. An isolated area, away from noise and traffic, is preferred (a park or nature trail). If you are running, start slowly and build up to a comfortable pace. Think about your breathing and your body movements: they should blend together in a relaxed, comfortable synchrony. Look around you as you run, and take in the beauty of your surroundings. As you continue to run, think about the muscles in various parts of the body, such as your neck, shoulders, and arms, and relax them. As you relax your body, turn your thoughts inward and think peaceful thoughts about your environment or something that is pleasing to you. Do not create stress by reviewing arguments in your mind, or thinking about how much work you have to do later. Learning to relax and meditate while you exercise may help to reduce some of the stress-producing effects of the exercise itself.

You may ask the question, "If exercise is a stressor, how can it possibly reduce stress?" We can look at the answer from two viewpoints—reducing state anxiety and reducing trait anxiety.

A single bout of exercise has been shown to decrease state anxiety. One theory is that the exercise may simply be a diversion, freeing your mind from the stressors contributing to state anxiety. Another theory suggests that the feeling of accomplishment—taking the time and effort to do something for your body—is a key factor. Still another theory suggests that exercise reduces muscular tension and induces a state of muscular relaxation. Finally, there may be some chemical changes in the brain that occur during exercise that may reduce stress levels. Some earlier research suggested that naturally-produced tranquilizers in the brain called **endorphins** may be involved. However recent findings question the role of the endorphins in this regard, and suggest that other chemicals in the brain, which act as stimulants, may be involved. Possibly all of these causes are involved in one way or another, but whatever the cause, aerobic exercise does appear to reduce state anxiety. Try it the next time you feel stressed.

The major theory underlying the reduction of trait anxiety by chronic exercise training centers around the effects such training may have on the body. The physical development that occurs (decreased body weight and better appearance), and the physiological changes that make you feel better, enhance the way you feel about yourself. The feelings brought by personal accomplishment of long-range exercise goals (such as completing a 10 kilometer race or a marathon), also improve your self-concept. The improvements in self-assurance and self-confidence are critical to the reduction of trait anxiety. Moreoever, the beneficial physiological adaptations in the body to chronic exercise training, such as increased efficiency of the heart, provide increased resistance to the stress of exercise, as well as to other stressors, such as emotional stressors.

It is important to note, however, that exercise may become a major source of stress, particularly if you overexercise. Adherence to the principles and guidelines in chapter 4 will help you to develop an optimal exercise program, so exercise will be a positive factor in your Positive Health Life-style. However, for some individuals exercise may become a negative factor, a **negative addiction.** They may begin to need more and more exercise, need to run more miles, in order to continue to achieve a feeling of accomplishment or well-being. This addiction to exercise is not necessarily harmful or undesirable in itself, providing it does not become so obsessive or compulsive that you begin to sacrifice your job, family, and friends. Moreover, if you become injured and cannot run, for example, you may go through withdrawal symptoms that may lead to anxiety and depression.

A properly designed aerobic exercise program can produce many beneficial physiological, as well as psychological, effects. In order to do so, however, the program must be within your capacity so that you are not overstressed. It must not lead to staleness and chronic fatigue or injuries, and it must not become obsessive.

In summary, there are a number of different ways to reduce stress levels. A good aerobic exercise program may be all that you need, but even though it may not reduce your stress levels, it is still an important component of your Positive Health Life-style as it relates to other factors, such as coronary heart disease and body weight control. If aerobic exercise is not enough, then incorporate one or more of the other techniques, such as meditation or progressive relaxation training, into your Positive Health Life-style.

This is a four-part test. The first three parts are designed to measure your vulnerability to certain types of stress, and to increase your awareness of stress and how it affects you. The fourth part gives you some idea of how well you cope with stressful situations.

These tests were developed by Dr. Daniel Girdano and Dr. George Everly at The University of Maryland, and may be found in their text *Controlling Stress and Tension.*

If you have any concerns or questions about your answers to this assessment you may want to discuss them with a qualified counselor, your family physician, or other medical professionals. For additional information on stress, you may wish to write to the National Institute of Mental Health, Public Inquiries Section, 5600 Fishers Lane, Rockville, MD 20857.

Stress Test Part One
Read and choose the most appropriate answer for each of the ten questions as it actually pertains to you.

1. When I can't do something "my way," I simply adjust to do it the easiest way.
   a) Almost always true, b) Usually true, c) Usually false, d) Almost always false.

2. I get "upset" when someone in front of me drives slowly.
   a) Almost always true, b) Usually true, c) Usually false, d) Almost always false.

3. It bothers me when my plans are dependent upon others.
   a) Almost always true, b) Usually true, c) Usually false, d) Almost always false.

4. Whenever possible, I tend to avoid large crowds.
   a) Almost always true, b) Usually true, c) Usually false, d) Almost always false.

5. I am uncomfortable when I have to stand in long lines.
   a) Almost always true, b) Usually true, c) Usually false, d) Almost always false.

6. Arguments upset me.
   a) Almost always true, b) Usually true, c) Usually false, d) Almost always false.

7. When my plans don't "flow smoothly," I become anxious.
   a) Almost always true, b) Usually true, c) Usually false, d) Almost always false.

8. I require a lot of room (space) to live and work in.
   a) Almost always true, b) Usually true, c) Usually false, d) Almost always false.

9. When I am busy at some task, I hate to be disturbed.
   a) Almost always true, b) Usually true, c) Usually false, d) Almost always false.

10. I believe that "All good things are worth waiting for."
    a) Almost always true, b) Usually true, c) Usually false, d) Almost always false.

Scoring Part One
To score: 1 and 10: a=1 pt, b=2 pts, c=3 pts, d=4 pts
            2 through 9: a=4 pts, b=3 pts, c=2 pts, d=1 pt.
This test measures your vulnerability to the stress of being "frustrated," i.e., inhibited. Scores in excess of 25 seem to suggest some vulnerability to this source of stress.

Stress Test Part Two

Circle the letter of the response option that best answers the following ten questions.
How often do you

1. Find yourself with insufficient time to complete your work?
   a) Almost always, b) Very often, c) Seldom, d) Never
2. Find yourself becoming confused and unable to think clearly because too many things are happening at once?
   a) Almost always, b) Very often, c) Seldom, d) Never
3. Wish you had help to get everything done?
   a) Almost always, b) Very often, c) Seldom, d) Never
4. Feel your boss/professor simply expects too much from you?
   a) Almost always, b) Very often, c) Seldom, d) Never
5. Feel your family/friends expect too much from you?
   a) Almost always, b) Very often, c) Seldom, d) Never
6. Find your work infringing upon your leisure hours?
   a) Almost always, b) Very often, c) Seldom, d) Never
7. Find yourself doing extra work to set an example for those around you?
   a) Almost always, b) Very often, c) Seldom, d) Never
8. Find yourself doing extra work to impress your superiors?
   a) Almost always, b) Very often, c) Seldom, d) Never
9. Have to skip a meal so that you can get work completed?
   a) Almost always, b) Very often, c) Seldom, d) Never
10. Feel that you have too much responsibility?
    a) Almost always, b) Very often, c) Seldom, d) Never

Scoring Part Two

To score: a=4 pts, b=3 pts, c=2 pts, d=1 pt.
　　　　　Total up your score for this exercise.
This test measures your vulnerability to "overload" (having too much to do.) Scores in excess of 25 seem to indicate vulnerability to this source of stress.

Stress Test Part Three

Answer all questions as is generally true for you.

1. I hate to wait in lines.
   a) Almost always true, b) Usually true, c) Seldom true, d) Never true
2. I often find myself "racing" against the clock to save time.
   a) Almost always true, b) Usually true, c) Seldom true, d) Never true
3. I become upset if I think something is taking too long.
   a) Almost always true, b) Usually true, c) Seldom true, d) Never true

4. When under pressure, I tend to lose my temper.
   a) Almost always true, b) Usually true, c) Seldom true, d) Never true

5. My friends tell me that I tend to get irritated easily.
   a) Almost always true, b) Usually true, c) Seldom true, d) Never true

6. I seldom like to do anything unless I can make it competitive.
   a) Almost always true, b) Usually true, c) Seldom true, d) Never true

7. When something needs to be done, I'm the first to begin even though the details may still need to be worked out.
   a) Almost always true, b) Usually true, c) Seldom true, d) Never true

8. When I make a mistake, it is usually because I've rushed into something without giving it enough thought and planning.
   a) Almost always true, b) Usually true, c) Seldom true, d) Never true

9. Whenever possible, I try to do two things at once, like eating while working, or planning while driving or bathing.
   a) Almost always true, b) Usually true, c) Seldom true, d) Never true

10. When I go on a vacation, I usually take some work along just in case I get a chance.
    a) Almost always true, b) Usually true, c) Seldom true, d) Never true

Scoring Part Three
To score: a = 4 pts, b = 3 pts, c = 2 pts, d = 1 pt.
This test measures the presence of compulsive, time-urgent, and excessively aggressive behavioral traits. Scores in excess of 25 suggest the presence of one or more of these traits.

Stress Test Part Four

How do you cope with the stress in your life? There are numerous ways, some more effective than others. Some coping strategies may actually be as harmful as the stress they are used to alleviate. This scale was created largely on the basis of results compiled by clinicians and researchers who sought to identify how individuals effectively cope with stress. This scale is an educational tool, not a clinical instrument. Therefore, its purpose is to inform you, the reader, of ways by which you can effectively and healthfully cope with the stress in your life. At the same time, a point system gives you some indication of the relative desirability of the coping strategies you are currently using. Simply follow the instructions given for each of the fourteen items listed on the following page. When you have completed all of the items, total your points and consult the scoring procedure.

_____ 1. Give yourself 10 points if you feel that you have a supportive family around you. .

_____ 2. Give yourself 10 points if you actively pursue a hobby.

_____ 3. Give yourself 10 points if you belong to some social or activity group (other than your family) that meets at least once a month.

_____ 4. Give yourself 15 points if you are within 5 pounds of your "ideal" body weight, considering your height and bone structure.

_____ 5. Give yourself 15 points if you practice some form of "deep relaxation" at least 3 times a week. Deep relaxation exercises include meditation, imagery, yoga, etc.

_____ 6. Give yourself 5 points for each time you exercise for 30 minutes or longer during the course of an average week.

_____ 7. Give yourself 5 points for each nutritionally balanced and wholesome meal you consume during the course of an average day.

_____ 8. Give yourself 5 points if you do something that you really enjoy, and that is "just for you" during the course of an average week.

_____ 9. Give yourself 10 points if you have some place in your home that you can go in order to relax and/or be by yourself.

_____ 10. Give yourself 10 points if you practice time management techniques in your daily life.

_____ 11. Subtract 10 points for each pack of cigarettes you smoke during the course of an average day.

_____ 12. Subtract 5 points for each evening during the course of an average week that you take any form of medication or chemical substance (including alcohol) to help you sleep.

_____ 13. Subtract 10 points for each day during the course of an average week that you consume any form of medication or chemical substance (including alcohol) to reduce your anxiety or just calm you down.

_____ 14. Subtract 5 points for each evening during the course of an average week that you bring work home—work that was meant to be done at your place of employment.

Scoring Part Four
Calculate your total score. A "perfect" score is 115 points. If you scored in the 50–60 range, you probably have an adequate collection of coping strategies for most common sources of stress. However, you should keep in mind that the higher your score the greater your ability to cope with stress in an effective and healthful manner.

References

Bahrke, M. "Exercise, Meditation and Anxiety Reduction: A Review." *American Corrective Therapy Journal* 33:41–44 (1979).

Bahrke, M., and Morgan, W. P. "Anxiety Reduction following Exercise and Meditation." *Cognitive Therapy and Research* 2:323–33 (1978).

Benson, H. *The Relaxation Response.* New York: William Morrow and Co., 1975.

Berger, B. "Facts and Fancy: Mood Alteration through Exercise." *Journal of Physical Education, Recreation and Dance* 53:47–48 (November-December, 1982).

Clark, M. (ed). "Coping with Stress through Leisure." *Journal of Physical Education, Recreation and Dance* 53:31–61 (October 1982).

Coben, J., and Robertson, R. "Effect of Maximal Voluntary Exercise upon Physiological Response to Stress." *Medicine and Science in Sports and Exercise* 14:166 (1982).

deVries, H. "A Review of the Tranquilizer Effect of Exercise." *Journal of Physical Education and Recreation* 46:53–54 (September 1975).

deVries, H.; Wiswell, R.; Bulbulian, R.; and Moritani, T. "Tranquilizer Effect of Exercise. Acute Effects of Moderate Aerobic Exercise on Spinal Reflex Activation Level." *American Journal of Physical Medicine* 50:57–66 (1981).

Dishman, R. "Biologic Influences of Exercise Adherence." *Research Quarterly for Exercise and Sport* 52:143–59 (1981).

Dyer, W. *Your Erroneous Zones.* New York: Funk and Wagnalls, 1976.

Eliot, R.; Forker, A.; and Robertson, R. "Aerobic Exercise as a Therapeutic Modality in the Relief of Stress." *Advances in Cardiology* 18:231–42 (1976).

Folkins, C., and Amsterdam, E. "Control and Modification of Stress Emotions through Chronic Exercise." In *Exercise in Cardiovascular Health and Disease,* edited by E. Amsterdam, J. Wilmore, A. DeMaria. New York: Yorke Medical Books, 1977.

Folkins, C. H., and Sime, W. "Physical Fitness Training and Mental Health." *American Psychologist* 36:373–89 (1981).

Friedman, M., and Rosenman, R. *Type A Behavior and Your Heart.* New York: Alfred A. Knopf, 1974.

Girdano, D., and Everly, G. *Controlling Stress and Tension.* Englewood Cliffs, NJ: Prentice Hall, 1979.

Goldstein, A. "Opioid Peptides (Endorphins) in Pituitary and Brain." *Science* 193:1081–86 (1976).

Greist, J.; Klein, M.; Eischens, R.; Faris, J.; Gurman, A.; and Morgan, W. "Running as Treatment for Depression." *Comprehensive Psychiatry* 20:41–54 (1979).

Holmes, T., and Rahe, R. "The Social Readjustment Rating Scale." *Journal of Psychosomatic Research* 11:213–18 (1967).

———. *Psychiatry and Behavioral Science.* Seattle, WA: University of Washington Medical School, 1979.

Jacobson, E. *Progressive Relaxation.* Chicago: University of Chicago Press, 1956.

Jakubowski, P., and Lange, A. *The Assertiveness Option: Your Rights and Responsibilities.* Champaign, IL: Research Press, 1978.

Jarrett, P. "Some Mental Aspects of Physical Fitness." *Journal of the Florida Medical Association* 67:378–81 (1980).

Jones, R., and Weinhouse, S. "Running as Self Therapy." *Journal of Sports Medicine and Physical Fitness* 19:397–404 (1979).

Layman, E. "Psychological Effects of Physical Activity." *Exercise and Sport Science Review* 2:33–70 (1974).

Levin, S., and Gimino, F. "Psychological Effects of Aerobic Exercise on Schizophrenic Patients." *Medicine and Science in Sports and Exercise* 14:116 (1982).

Levine, S. "Stress and Behavior." *Scientific American* 224:26–31 (January 1971).

Lion, L. "Psychological Effects of Jogging: A Preliminary Study." *Perceptual and Motor Skills* 47:1215–18 (1978).

Markoff, R.; Ryan, P.; and Young, T. "Endorphins and Mood Changes in Long-distance Running." *Medicine and Science in Sports and Exercise* 14:11–15 (1982).

Maslow, A. *Motivation and Personality*. New York: Harper and Row, 1954.

Merzbacher, C. "A Diet and Exercise Regimen: Its Effects upon Mental Acuity and Personality, A Pilot Study." *Perceptual and Motor Skills* 48:367–71 (1979).

Morgan, W. "Psychophysiology of Self-Awareness during Vigorous Physical Activity." *Research Quarterly for Exercise and Sport* 52:385–427 (1981).

Morgan, W.; Horstman, D.; Cymerman, A.; and Stokes, J. "Use of Exercise as a Relaxation Technique." *Journal of the South Carolina Medical Association* 75:596–601 (1979).

Morgan, W.; Roberts, J.; and Feinerman, A. "Psychologic Effect of Acute Physical Activity." *Archives for Physical and Mental Rehabilitation* 52:422–25 (1971).

Pitts, F. "The Biochemistry of Anxiety." *Scientific American* 220:69–75 (February 1969).

Ransford, C. "A Role for Amines in the Antidepressant Effect of Exercise: A Review." *Medicine and Science in Sports and Exercise* 14:1–10 (1982).

Schwartz, G.; Davidson, R.; and Goleman, J. "Patterning of Cognitive and Somatic Processes in the Self-Regulation of Anxiety: Effects of Meditation Versus Exercise." *Psychosomatic Medicine* 40:321–28 (1978).

Selye, H. *The Stress of Life*. New York: McGraw-Hill, 1956.

Singer, R. "Thought Processes and Emotions in Sport. *The Physician and Sportsmedicine* 10:75–88 (July 1982).

Smith, A., and Brandt, S. "Physical Activity: A Tool in Promoting Mental Health." *Journal of Psychiatric Nursing* 17:24–25 (November 1979).

Tucker, L. "Exercise—One Way to Cope with Stress. *American Pharmacy* 19:17 (August 1979).

Vitale, F. *Individualized Fitness Programs*. Englewood Cliffs, NJ: Prentice Hall, 1973.

Weltman, A., and Stamford, B. "Psychological Effects of Exercise." *The Physician and Sportsmedicine* 11:175 (January 1983).

Wiese, J.; Singh, M.; and Yendall, L. "Occipital and Parietal Alpha Power before, during and after Exercise." *Medicine and Science in Sports and Exercise* 15:117 (1983).

10 The Physically Active Female

Key Terms

anorexia nervosa
dysmenorrhea
estrogen
nulliparity

oligomenorrhea
secondary amenorrhea
testosterone

Key Concepts

The design of an exercise program for cardiovascular endurance, flexibility or strength, and a dietary-exercise program for weight control is the same for both males and females.

The major physical differences between males and females that influence physical performance, such as strength, body fat, and aerobic capacity, develop after the onset of puberty.

Women will respond to and benefit from most types of exercise programs in a fashion very similar to men, with the major exception that weight training programs will not produce the type of muscular hypertrophy seen in males.

Exercise need not be stopped during different phases of the menstrual cycle, although some women may feel the need to decrease the intensity of training during the pre-flow and flow phases.

Although the cause of secondary amenorrhea in physically active females has not been determined, several associated factors are prior menstrual problems, increased stress, weight loss, low body fat, inadequate dietary fat and protein, high intensity and/or increased duration of exercise.

Proper exercise may lead to a healthier pregnancy, but the key is to develop a high level of fitness before conception and to consult your physician about the intensity and duration of exercise during the pregnancy period.

All females need to consume foods rich in iron and those above age thirty should consume foods rich in calcium as well.

Introduction

Differences between males and females have been studied from a variety of viewpoints, including psychological, emotional, social, intellectual, and physiological. With the exception of the obvious sex differences and several other genetic factors, most reviews have reported that males and females are more alike than they are dissimilar. Many of the conceptual differences between males and females may be attributed to cultural factors. For example, in the United States strenuous physical activity was at one time considered unfeminine and women were generally discouraged from participation in sports or heavy physical training. However, the recent physical fitness boom has no sex barriers, and millions of women are involved in a variety of exercise programs, including long-distance running. As a result of their successful involvement in running, the previously held concept that women could not withstand the rigors of long-distance running has been conclusively discredited, and the women's marathon race became an Olympic event for the first time in 1984. Similar misconceptions are being disproven as more and more women become physically active.

In general, the principles and guidelines advanced in this book are applicable to both males and females. The design of an exercise program for cardiovascular endurance, flexibility or strength, and a dietary program for weight control are identical for both sexes. Nevertheless, several aspects of exercise and nutrition are of special concern to women. This chapter briefly addresses these concerns.

Basic Sexual Differences and Physical Performance

In relation to physical performance, the physical and physiological differences between boys and girls are minimal, at least until the age of puberty. Height, weight, strength, blood hemoglobin levels, oxygen uptake, and other measures related to athletic potential are fairly similar, but these characteristics begin to change markedly during adolescence. Girls reach puberty earlier than boys, usually by age twelve compared to age fourteen for boys, and for a brief time may possess greater physical characteristics, such as height and weight. However, the boys eventually become taller, heavier, and stronger.

The sex differences after puberty are due to the differential effects of the major hormones secreted in the body. Both females and males produce **estrogen,** the major female sex hormone, and **testosterone,** the major male sex hormone. However, the quantities of estrogen and testosterone are greater in the female and male, respectively. Estrogen secretion is responsible for the development of the female secondary sex characteristics, one of which is an increase in the amount of body fat and another is the onset of menstruation; both of these changes have implications for physical performance. Testosterone is a major anabolic hormone. Its effect in the male is to rapidly increase the growth rate and formation of muscular tissue, physical changes that are accompanied by a great increase in strength. In addition, testosterone increases the production of red blood cells so that the oxygen-carrying capacity of the blood increases.

Figure 10.1 In relation to physical performance, the physical and physiological differences between young boys and girls are relatively insignificant. However, at puberty, physical and physiological changes that are associated with improvement in athletic performance increase more markedly in boys than in girls. For example, increases in muscle mass and hemoglobin levels are important factors in the increased differences in maximal oxygen uptake.

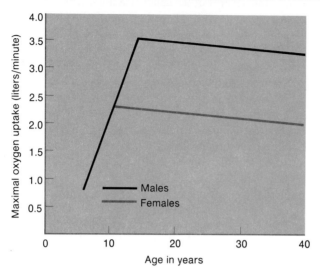

Throughout adolescence, the male becomes taller and heavier, primarily through increased muscle mass, and although the female also becomes taller and heavier, a proportionately greater amount of her weight is body fat. Moreover, the hemoglobin level becomes significantly greater in males. Translated into practical terms, boys possess the capacity for more strength, speed, power, and endurance. These characteristics also persist through adulthood. However, women generally possess a greater degree of flexibility than men.

Note that these characteristics are general differences between the sexes and that many individual differences do exist. For example, men generally have a greater endurance capacity than women, but some women possess a greater capacity than 99 percent of the male population. Good examples would be some of the excellent female long-distance runners performing today. Everyone, both male and female, has a certain capacity or potential for the different physical and physiological characteristics that we inherit from our parents. However, it is up to us to maximize that potential by exercise training and diet. In regard to the ability to maximize our own personal potential, there appears to be no difference between the sexes.

In the past decade, we have witnessed a tremendous increase in the participation of females in sports and fitness activities. The old cultural concepts have changed markedly, and now it is not only acceptable, but highly desirable for girls and women to be physically active. Ten years ago there were very few research studies available about women and physical performance. However, as a result of the increased emphasis on fitness and sports for women and an increase in the number of women involved in sports medicine, more research has been generated. The results of such research have dispelled many myths concerning women and participation in exercise.

Figure 10.2 Many women who start running for health and weight control become involved in the competitive aspects of the sport.

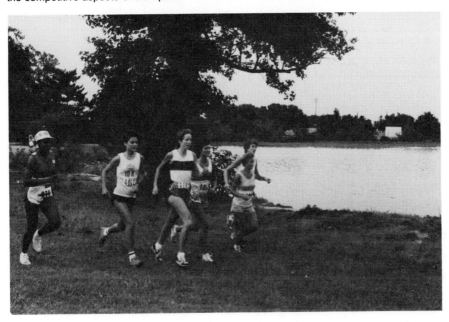

In general, women will realize the same physiological benefits from exercise training as men. An aerobic exercise program will increase their $\dot{V}O_2$ max, hemoglobin levels, cardiovascular efficiency, and other associated factors. Weight training will increase women's strength proportionately comparable to the increases experienced by males. However, women will not experience a comparable muscular hypertrophy, or muscle bulk, as males do. Thus both types of training may be recommended for women; aerobic exercises for cardiovascular health and weight control, and weight training for toning the muscles that are not developed by running.

The Menstrual Cycle and Exercise

The interaction of the menstrual cycle and exercise can be viewed from two points. First, what is the effect of the menstrual cycle on physical performance? Second, what effect does exercise have upon the menstrual cycle?

A number of research studies have been conducted about the first question, and probably the best conclusion is that the effects of the different phases of the menstrual cycle on physical performance depend on the individual. Some evidence suggests that performance in aerobic endurance events may be impaired in the phase just before menstrual flow, which may be related to the increased water retention and body weight at that time. Although performance during menstrual flow is worse in some women, others have achieved record-breaking performances during the active-flow period. For some women, performance seems to be best during the phase immediately following menstrual flow, particularly in high-intensity exercise.

There appear to be no physical or physiological reasons that a woman cannot exercise during any phase of the menstrual cycle. Each woman should monitor her physical condition during each phase, particularly as it relates to her feelings toward exercise and her ability to exercise. In particular, she should evaluate differences between the pre-menstrual flow and post-menstrual flow period, where the most marked differences are likely to occur.

Can exercise influence the menstrual cycle? **Secondary amenorrhea,** a clinical condition in female athletes and exercisers, has received considerable attention in the past ten years. Secondary amenorrhea refers to the condition in those women who have menstruated but stop for at least three regular cycles. Secondary amenorrhea has been observed primarily in runners and ballet dancers, but has been noted in other female athletes as well. **Oligomenorrhea** refers to infrequent bleeding, missing about two months, and also appears to occur more frequently among physically active females. However, only a small percentage of athletes, about 3–4 percent, experience these clinical symptoms. At the present time, the cause of amenorrhea and oligomenorrhea is not known, although it may have many predisposing factors. Among the potential factors are:

1. Prior menstrual problems. Individuals with irregular periods before initiating an exercise training program may be more susceptible.
2. Stress. As noted in chapter 9, stress can create a number of hormonal changes in the body by affecting the hypothalamus. These hormonal changes may disrupt the normal menstrual cycle.
3. Weight loss and low body weight or low body fat. Women who lose body weight rapidly or have low levels of body fat appear to be more prone to amenorrhea. Fat cells produce estrogen, so a decreased amount of fat may influence the levels of this hormone.
4. Distance and intensity of exercise. Runners who log over 30 miles per week or do high-intensity exercises are more likely to be amenorrheic. The distance and intensity of exercise may increase stress in some individuals.
5. Inadequate fat and protein in the diet. The low fat levels may decrease cholesterol production that is necessary for the formation of estrogen. Low dietary protein may signal the body that there are insufficient stores to support pregnancy, so the menstrual cycle may cease.
6. Increased body temperature during exercise. The increased temperature may disrupt optimal functioning of the hypothalamus and hence create a hormonal imbalance.
7. Young age and nulliparity. The condition appears to be more prevalent in the young, and in those who never have had children (**nulliparity**). Young girls who undertake strenuous physical training before puberty are also more susceptible.

In general, the amenorrhea experienced by runners and other athletes appears to be reversible once training has stopped. However, as a point of caution, there may be a number of other reasons why a woman becomes amenorrheic, which may have serious medical implications. If you do develop amenorrhea, it is highly recommended

Figure 10.3 Aerobic exercise may be performed into the latter stages of pregnancy, if approved by your physician.

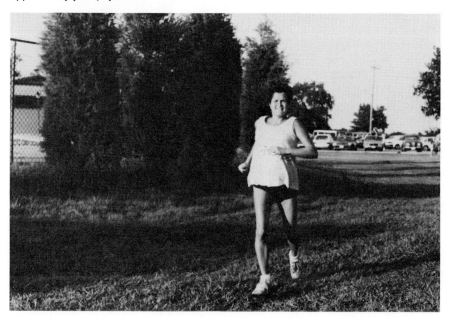

that you consult a gynecologist, preferably one who is sports oriented, for a full medical checkup to determine if there is a medical problem not associated with your exercise program.

Some women periodically experience **dysmenorrhea,** or painful cramps associated with menstruation. Exercise does not appear to aggravate the condition, but the individual may wish to exercise less strenuously if it exists. Flexibility exercises for the lower back and pelvic area may help to alleviate the symptoms. Women who are more physically fit seem to experience this problem less frequently.

Exercise and Pregnancy

Exercise and pregnancy are not mutually exclusive. Most women who are exercising can continue to exercise through the eighth or ninth month, although their exercise intensity will need to be curtailed. Mona Shangold, a gynecologist and marathon runner, has noted that the key to fitness during pregnancy is to become fit before pregnancy. By being physically fit, your body has already adapted to the stress of exercise. One of the benefits will be less decrease of blood flow to your body organs during exercise, so your body will not be deprived of oxygen when you exercise. Shangold also indicates that fitness will increase the safety of giving birth. Giving birth is hard work, and a high level of fitness will help you tolerate it better.

Check with your physician about beginning or continuing an exercise program during pregnancy. Exercise is advisable only if your pregnancy is normal and uncomplicated. Shangold suggests you listen to your body at all times, and stop exercising immediately if you develop pain, begin to bleed, or rupture membranes and release water. If any of these happen, check with your physician immediately.

Brief mention should be made that jogging or running may suppress ovulation in some women. A recent case report revealed that two women were able to resume ovulation when they stopped jogging, and that this point should be considered by physicians who are treating women who want to become pregnant.

Dietary Concerns

The major concern of the average female is to obtain a sufficient amount of iron in the diet. Iron is the major nutrient deficiency in the American diet, primarily for women who need almost twice the dietary intake than men. The increased need is due to the iron loss through menstrual bleeding. Thus women should include foods in their diet that are high in iron content, as highlighted on pages 131 and 143.

Women who are pregnant or lactating (breast feeding) need additional amounts of Calories, protein, iron, and calcium in their diets. Recommended amounts may be found in appendix A. These nutrients are essential for the growth and development of the child and for the production of milk. Weight gain should not be excessive during pregnancy. The guidance of a physician is crucial during this very important time in a woman's life.

As a woman enters her late thirties, an adequate supply of calcium is essential in the diet to help prevent osteoporosis, a condition discussed on pages 44–45. Foods high in calcium include dairy products, such as milk and cheese, and dark green leafy vegetables. Exercise, as noted in chapter 2, may also be an effective means to counteract the development of osteoporosis.

A potential nutritional concern that primarily afflicts young females is **anorexia nervosa,** a loss of appetite not explainable by any specific disease process. Most victims have a psychological obsession, classified as a neurosis, with extreme thinness. The cause of the obsession is not known, but may be related to family or societal pressures to be thin. Anorexia nervosa is an extreme form of malnutrition in which the individual intentionally starves herself or uses regurgitation to achieve low body weight, often as little as 70 pounds or less. The condition may lead to irreversible brain damage or death. Expert treatment by a physician is necessary and may involve forced feeding. Psychotherapy is used with the individual and the family in order to find and eliminate the underlying cause; this is often difficult because the patient is usually self-assured and claims to be in excellent health. Anorexia nervosa has a tendency to recur. Although reduction of excess body fat is one of the goals of a Positive Health Life-style, an excessive loss of body weight, as in anorexia nervosa, is not compatible with such a life-style, since it may lead to some serious health problems.

Summary

Both men and women develop coronary heart disease. However, compared to males, females have a greater degree of protection against its development, which may be attributed to hormonal influences. Estrogen is associated with higher concentrations of HDL cholesterol that helps to delay the onset of CHD to a later age. However, this advantage may be suppressed in individuals whose health behaviors are not in accord with a Positive Health Life-style. In particular, recent evidence has suggested that the increased incidence of cigarette smoking by women is a major factor leading to an earlier onset of CHD. Not smoking is a major health behavior that will help women retain their natural protective effect. The adoption of other health behaviors in a Positive Health Life-style, such as a sound exercise-nutrition program, will also help in the prevention of CHD and other diseases.

Of more contemporary importance to many women, a Positive Health Life-style stressing an aerobic exercise program, flexibility and strength training, and a nutritional diet will help them to maintain an optimal body weight and to participate fully in today's physically active life-style.

References

American College of Sports Medicine. "The Female Athlete in Long Distance Running." *The Physician and Sportsmedicine* 8:135–36 (January 1980).

Andersen, A. "Anorexia Nervosa and Bulimia." *Journal of Adolescent Health Care* 4:15–21 (1983).

Baker, E. R. "Menstrual Dysfunction and Hormonal Status in Athletic Women: A Review." *Fertility and Sterility* 36:691–96 (1981).

Bruch, H. "Anorexia Nervosa: A Review." *Dietetic Currents, Ross Timesaver* 4:7–11 (March–April 1977).

Calabrese, L.; Kirkendall, D.; Floyd, M.; Rapoport, S.; Weiker, G.; and Bergfield, J. "Menstrual Abnormalities and Body Composition in Professional Ballet Dancers." *Medicine and Science in Sports and Exercise* 14:145 (1982).

Clarke, H. "Physical Activity during Menstruation and Pregnancy." *Physical Fitness Research Digest* 8:1–25 (July 1978).

———. "Physical and Motor Sex Differences." *Physical Fitness Research Digest* 9:1–27 (1979).

Drinkwater, B. "Menstrual Changes in Athletes." *The Physician and Sportsmedicine* 9:99–112 (November 1981).

Fraccaroli, G. "Sport Performance in Women during Menstrual Cycle." *Minerva Medica* 71:3557–66 (1980).

Gelman, D. "Just How the Sexes Differ." *Newsweek* 97:72–83 (May 1981).

Jurkowski, J.; Jones, N.; Toews, C.; and Sutton, J. "Effects of Menstrual Cycle on Blood Lactate, O_2 Delivery, and Performance during Exercise." *Journal of Applied Physiology* 51:1493–99 (1981).

Korcok, M. "Add Exercise to Calcium in Osteoporosis Prevention." *Journal of the American Medical Association* 247:1106 (1982).

Luter, J., and Cushman, S. "Menstrual Patterns in Female Runners." *The Physician and Sportsmedicine* 10:60–72 (September 1982).

Morgan, W. "Research Studies on the Female Athlete." *Journal of Physical Education and Recreation* 46:32–46 (January 1975).

O'Herlihy, C. "Jogging and Suppression of Ovulation." *New England Journal of Medicine* 306:50–51 (1982).

Pate, R.; Barnes, C.; and Miller, W. "A Physiological Comparison of Performance-matched Male and Female Distance Runners." *Medicine and Science in Sports and Exercise* 14:139 (1982).

Russell, C. "Doctors Warn of Pregnancy Hazards, from Foods to Nonfoods." *Washington Post* (November 4, 1982) A3.

Ryan, A. "Research Studies on the Female Athlete. Gynecological Considerations." *Journal of Physical Education and Recreation* 46:40–44 (January 1975).

———. "Sports during Pregnancy, Other Questions Explored." *The Physician and Sportsmedicine* 4:82 (March 1976).

Schuwater, B.; Cumming, D.; Riordan, E.; Selye, M.; Yen, S.; and Rebar, R. "Exercise-associated Amenorrhea: A Distinct Entity?" *American Journal of Obstetrics and Gynecology* 141:662–70 (1981).

Shangold, M. "Menstrual Irregularity in Athletics: Basic Principles, Evaluation and Treatment." *Canadian Journal of Applied Sports Sciences* 7:68–73 (1982).

———. "Women's Running." *Runner's World* 17:20 (August 1982).

———. "Women's Running." *Runner's World* 17:18 (November 1982).

Shephard, R., and Sidney, K. "Exercise and Aging." *Exercise and Sport Science Review* 6:1–57 (1978).

Smith, E.; Reddan, W.; and Smith, P. "Physical Activity and Calcium Modalities for Bone Mineral Increase in Aged Women." *Medicine and Science in Sports and Exercise* 13:60–64 (1981).

Stillman, R.; Lohman, T.; Slaughter, M.; and Massey, B. "The Relationship of Bone Mineral Content and Physical Activity in Women over the Age of Thirty." *Medicine and Science in Sports and Exercise* 15:149 (1983).

Wells, C., and Plowman, S. "Sexual Differences in Athletic Performance: Biological or Behavioral?" *The Physician and Sportsmedicine* 11:52–63 (August 1983).

Wilmore, J. "Inferiority of the Female Athlete: Myth or Reality." *Sports Medicine Bulletin* 10:7–8 (April 1975).

Wynne, T. "Effect of a Controlled Exercise Program on Serum Lipoprotein Levels in Women on Oral Contraceptives." *Metabolism* 29:1267–71 (1980).

A Lifetime Positive Health Life-style

11

Key Concepts

Knowledge of the why and how of a Positive Health Life-style is important, but in order for this knowledge to be of any benefit to you, you must do it.

Aerobic exercise is the key to a Positive Health Life-style, for it will increase cardiovascular fitness, decrease body fat, and help to reduce stress and muscular tension.

If exercise has personal value to you, if you have established realistic goals, if it is fun, and if it is practical to you in terms of location, time and money, then you are more likely to make it a lifetime habit.

With adequate knowledge, you should be able to design your own exercise or diet program, but if you feel the need to join a commercial exercise or weight loss facility, be sure to investigate the qualifications of the personnel involved and look over the facilities and equipment available.

The principles underlying a sound aerobic exercise program and a healthy diet are the same for males and females—children, adolescents, young adults, and older adults.

Many young children, as young as six or seven, and adolescents already have coronary heart disease risk factors such as hypertension, obesity, and elevated blood lipid levels.

Although the principles underlying the development and initiation of an aerobic exercise program for older adults are the same as for younger adults, the basic recommendation is to start at a lower intensity level and progress slowly; initially an aerobic walking program is highly recommended.

Health benefits will be provided no matter what stage of life the Positive Health Life-style is initiated, but for optimal results, the earlier in life it is started, the better, preferably with young children.

Introduction

By now you have been exposed to a considerable amount of information and techniques about the development of your personal Positive Health Life-style. You have learned that a sound nutrition program and a properly designed exercise program may be an effective means to help prevent some of the chronic debilitating diseases in the United States and subsequently improve your chances for an increased life expectancy. You have also learned that a Positive Health Life-style may confer some immediate benefits, such as an improvement in fitness, a change in physical appearance, a reduction of stress, and an improved psychological well-being. Since exercise and nutrition are such important components of the Positive Health Life-style, most of this chapter will deal with the topics of adherence to an exercise and nutrition program and the importance of lifetime fitness.

Adherence

Of all the people who start some type of health improvement program, such as a supervised diet, a smoking-cessation plan, or an aerobic exercise program, nearly 50 percent or more usually drop out within the first 3 to 6 months. If you have been involved in a Positive Health Life-style program involving aerobic exercise for the past 3 months, your body is beginning to reap some of the benefits. However, if you stop your exercise program after the semester is over, those benefits will be lost within a month or so. Aerobic exercise, to be truly effective as a positive health factor, must be a lifetime commitment. How can you prevent yourself from being a dropout?

Exercise Programs

There are a number of personal and situational factors that may influence an individual's decision to adhere to an exercise program. Recent research has revealed two of these factors: your degree of self-motivation and your degree of leanness, the latter measured by your body weight and percent body fat. Individuals who are highly self-motivated and lean are more likely to adhere to an exercise program on a long-range basis. Laboratory Inventory 11.1 will give you a general idea of your degree of self-motivation, while Laboratory Inventories 6.1 and 6.2 will help you assess your degree of leanness.

What if the results of the laboratory inventories reveal that you have a low self-motivation level and/or you are carrying more weight and body fat than is desirable? If this is the case, you should use the results to motivate you to stay with your program, not as a sign of predestined failure. Having a score of low self-motivation and/or an excessive amount of body weight or body fat should be viewed as a motivating factor to continue exercising. Overcome this predisposition to quit. If you stay with the program long enough, body fat and body weight should be reduced or eliminated as you attain your desirable body weight.

Figure 11.1   To become a lifelong habit, exercise should be enjoyable.

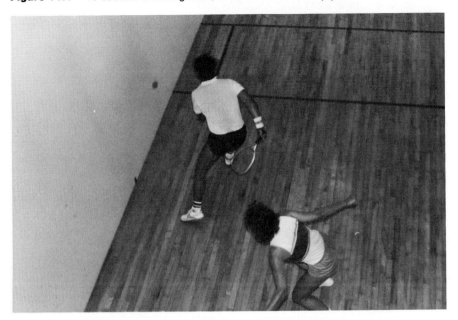

Here are some strategies to help you avoid being a drop-out.

1. Personal Value—One of the most important considerations is that you must believe the exercise program will be of personal value to you, such as improving your physical appearance.

2. Realistic Goals—Establish some realistic goals for yourself. The guidelines of the American College of Sports Medicine are realistic: Intensity of 60–90 percent of your heart rate reserve, duration of 15–60 minutes, and a frequency of 3–4 times per week. Be patient in attaining these goals. Don't expect too much too soon. Remember, fitness takes time. Think in terms of months, not days or weeks. Faithfulness to your goals is a key: it takes time and effort, so you must value the outcome.

3. Practicality—Location, time, and money may be important factors. Select a place to exercise that is convenient so that you do not have to spend much time just getting there. The closer you are to the exercise facility, the more likely you will use it. The value of a running program is that you can do it anywhere.

   Money may also be a concern, particularly if you need expensive equipment or want to join a commercial exercise facility. Again, running is one of the more practical activities in this regard. Although the cost of running shoes has increased rather rapidly in the last several years, they are the only major investment needed by those who run for health reasons.

4. People—Do you like to exercise alone, in a social atmosphere with another person, or with a group of people? Decide which is best for you and plan your program accordingly.

5. Fun—An important factor is enjoyment of the exercise. To be effective in the long run, select an activity that you enjoy and that will meet the ACSM standards mentioned under point two above. For example, you may not enjoy jogging or running, but fast walking (with vigorous arm action), swimming, bicycling, tennis, handball, or racquetball may be more fun for you. Enjoy your exercise, make it a lifelong habit, and do a variety of fitness activities if possible.

6. Contract—You may make an exercise contract with yourself, for example, running 2 miles per day/4 days per week; or you may have an exercise contract designed for you by a specialist (a physical educator or an exercise instructor). An example of such a contract may be found on page 112.

7. Knowledge—Review previous chapters about the design and implementation of your personal exercise program. The more you know about exercise and what to expect, the better prepared you will be to respond to setbacks or problems.

Dieting

If a new diet is part of your Positive Health Life-style, the general principles about adherence to an exercise program are also applicable to a diet program to attain a desirable weight. A review of chapters 5 and 6 will reinforce the principles and guidelines underlying the development and implementation of a healthy diet.

Commercial Fitness and Weight Loss Organizations

With the soaring popularity of physical fitness in the past decade, it was not long before fitness studios, health spas, weight-control centers, and other similar businesses appeared in large numbers to meet public demand and to reap some of the financial rewards. Is it worthwhile to join one of these organizations to develop physical fitness or control your body weight, and if so, how do you select a reputable one?

Most individuals who are interested in improved physical fitness and nutrition can develop their own programs; the principles and guidelines in this book demonstrate how, so for many individuals there is no need to join a health club. On the other hand, some individuals may benefit from such a move. If you enjoy the comfort of a well-equipped, temperature-controlled facility, the sociability and support of other people while exercising or dieting, or the guidance of an exercise specialist or weight-control counselor, then these organizations may be beneficial to you. However, keep in mind that not all of these commercial operations are reputable; there are a large number of incompetent operators, and consumer fraud is not uncommon. The Federal Trade Commission has over 8,000 pages of written complaints from consumers throughout the country. The major problems involve deceptive advertising, sales tactics, cancellations of contracts, and many facility closures leaving the customers with no place to go. One of the major underlying causes of these problems is that there are no legal guidelines as to who can open a fitness or weight-control center.

Figure 11.2 A commercial exercise facility may offer a sound program, but you should use some guidelines to select one.

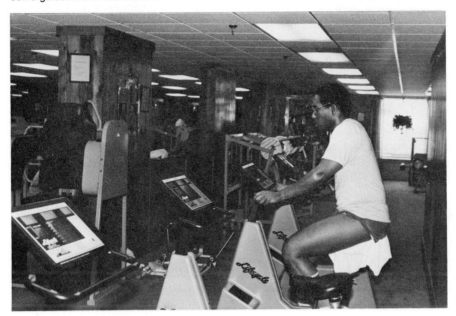

If you want to join one, here are some guidelines:

1. First, keep in mind that joining such an organization is a long-term commitment. To reap the benefits of an exercise program, you must use the facility on a regular basis, so be sure it is in a convenient location.

2. Check your telephone directory under Health Clubs and Spas, or Exercise and Physical Fitness for a listing of local operations. Also contact your local YMCA or YWCA, as well as your local parks-and-recreation department for their programs. Some colleges and universities also have ongoing fitness programs.

3. Once you have made a list, call or visit the operation and obtain information about the following:
   a. Equipment and facilities—Does the club have what is necessary for your fitness or weight-control program? Ask to use it on a trial basis if possible, for example, on a one-month membership.
   b. Personnel—What are the qualifications of the instructors? Do they have degrees in exercise-related fields or nutrition? Are weight-control programs supervised by medical doctors or registered dieticians?
   c. Availability—When is the facility available—what hours, how many days per week? Visit the club at the time when you would most likely use it to see if it is overcrowded.
   d. Rates—How much does it cost? Are there additional use fees for some facilities like racketball courts or Nautilus equipment? You may get similar facilities for a lower fee by comparing rates.

e. Contracts—Can you void the contract and get a return of some of your money if dissatisfied with the program? Check the contract for ambiguous terms; get a copy and have your lawyer review it if possible before you sign.

f. Precautions—Be suspicious of those operations that make extravagant claims such as rapid body weight loss, or physical fitness the easy way. Be wary of hard-sell organizations. If you can, get a financial statement to determine if it is a stable operation and will be in business for a while. Do they have a reciprocal agreement with other operations in the area so you will have a place to go if they do go out of business?

Thinking through these guidelines should enable you to determine whether or not a particular organization meets your needs. Well-run operations can be very helpful in guiding you through a physical fitness and/or weight-control program, but a shaky operation can take your money and give you nothing in return.

Exercise for a Lifetime

Although this material has been written with the young adult in mind, there are some special concerns for other age groups that may be of interest to you. For example, you may want to involve your children, younger brothers and sisters, parents or grand-parents in an exercise program and you may wonder if vigorous aerobic exercise is suitable for them. In general, the principles and guidelines that have been presented in this book are applicable to all age groups because everyone can benefit from proper exercise and balanced nutrition.

Childhood

Let's start with the kids. Children need several hours of vigorous physical activity per day in order to achieve optimal growth and physical development. In the first five to six years of life, this is the responsibility of the parents or others who care for the children. But all too often in our busy society, the television set or other inactive modes of entertainment are used to occupy the child's time. In such cases, the adverse effects of physical inactivity, such as childhood obesity, may begin at a very early age. Dr. Thomas Gilliam, director of a long-term research program about exercise for children, has noted that many young children, even six- and seven-year-olds, have coronary heart disease risk factors such as hypertension, obesity, and elevated blood lipids.

Thus as a parent or as an older brother or sister, you should see that young children get some vigorous play daily. It does not have to be a structured exercise program, but children should be exposed to a physically stimulating environment with other children to run, jump, climb, and perform other such physical activities. Moreover, sound nutritional practices can be initiated early: fresh fruits and vegetables and other nutritious foods or snacks should be available. The principles of sound nutrition apply to young children as well as adults. Of special dietary concern for young children are foods rich in protein, calcium, and iron, all very important during periods of growth.

Figure 11.3 Children may reap the benefits of aerobic exercise through strenuous games such as soccer.

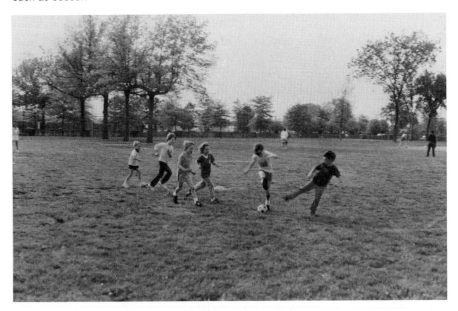

When young children enter school for the first time, we may think that their exercise needs will be satisfied by a physical education program. However, this is often not the case because the physical education program may be weak or nonexistent. And even if a physical education program does exist with a qualified physical educator, there may not be much emphasis upon physical fitness per se. Elementary school physical education over the past decade has been characterized by the concept of movement education, a program that is designed to give the children meaningful and varied movement experiences so that they learn to control their bodies. The theory was that the better control children have over their bodies, the more likely they are to be successful in sports later (for example, tennis, baseball, basketball, gymnastics). The idea is to teach the basic skills, and as the student practices the skills, physical fitness will follow naturally.

Although movement education is a sound approach to physical education and should be continued, it might not incorporate the type of sustained aerobic exercise that is the key to health-related fitness. Thus many physical educators are now incorporating aerobic programs, such as endurance running, in their elementary school programs as early as the first grade.

In his research with children, Dr. Gilliam noted that most children are not spontaneously active. He used a heart-rate monitor on over 300 children for a 12-hour period and found that their heart rates rarely achieved the level needed to get a training effect for the heart. However, in an experimental exercise training and diet project with children in the second, fifth, and seventh grades, Dr. Gilliam noted that the second grade students made significant increases in physical activity and also reduced the amount of sodium and cholesterol in their diets. (The changes were not as noticeable in the fifth and seventh grade students.) Thus Dr. Gilliam suggests that we should attempt to teach the principles of a Positive Health Life-style to children as early as possible.

Are the elementary schools in your area teaching sound exercise and nutrition practices? Your school system needs to promote vigorous physical activity in their physical education programs as well as during recess periods. Dr. Gilliam offered the following suggestions to encourage this activity.

1. Set up an exercise trail on the school grounds.
2. Set up a large clock so children can check their pulse rates.
3. Have the children jog around the playground before beginning recess.

If you have any influence on children, help them start on their Positive Health Life-style at the earliest possible age. In its Statement on Exercise, the American Heart Association recommended that parents be aware of the health benefits of regular aerobic exercise and incorporate such a program in their own lives. This commitment to exercise by parents will provide an incentive, set an example, and help develop a positive attitude in children toward exercise.

Adolescence

As children get older they usually become less physically active. Dr. Gilliam noted that patterns of physical inactivity begin as early as fourth and fifth grade. In a recent survey, Dr. Wynn Updyke found that physical fitness levels for children begin to plateau or decline when children enter puberty. The reasons for this plateau or decline in fitness may be similar to those in younger children; that is, these young adolescents acquire new interests that may not involve strenuous exercise. Moreover, Dr. Updyke believes that high school physical education programs may be partially to blame, because the emphasis appears to be on teaching a skill, such as tennis. This type of learning is desirable, since the student will have a lifelong sport that will confer fitness benefits later in life. However in the meantime, physical fitness levels are stagnant. Dr. Updyke believes that this situation can be improved if we educate adolescents about the benefits of exercise, the experience of being physically fit, and how to control their body weight. Fitness should not be just a unit in a physical education class but should become a part of the student's life-style.

Nutritional needs for adolescents are similar to those for adults. They still need significant amounts of protein, iron, and calcium, so foods rich in these nutrients should be included in the diet. Teenagers are notorious for raiding the refrigerator or cupboards, so plan to have nutritious snacks available. Growing teenagers also need more Calories, particularly if they are physically active, and sweets have a place in their diet, but should be limited. Other high-Calorie nutritious foods that are sweet, such as orange juice and bran muffins, may be good substitutes. Moreover, fast foods such as pizza, hamburgers, and milk shakes may be good sources of nutrients that teenagers need; although they are high in Calories, many teenagers need the additional energy. In essence, the principles of sound nutrition discussed in chapters 5 and 6 are pertinent to the teenager and will serve as a useful guide.

Adolescents are generally very self-conscious, particularly concerning their physical appearance. Exercise and nutrition can play an important role in improving the teenager's appearance, whether it is to lose weight or to gain weight. The concern for their appearance can serve as a good basis for learning the major principles of a Positive Health Life-style.

The Younger Adult

Young is a relative term, but for the purpose of this discussion the age range of eighteen to forty will be construed to be the younger adult. As mentioned before, this book was written for college classes in lifetime fitness, so the principles are directly relevant to their age group, particularly the early twenties. As you approach the forties, be particularly aware of the need for a medical examination before initiating a vigorous exercise program.

Some of the major concerns of the young adult are beginning a career, becoming successful in it, and starting a family. Thus a physically active individual often becomes less active as exercise takes a lower priority in comparison to work and family. He or she becomes too busy to exercise. Dietary practices may also change: more processed foods, high-Calorie meals on the run, and greater quantities of alcohol. Years of physical inactivity and poor nutrition may eventually contribute to obesity and other health problems as noted in chapter 2.

A relevant phrase that has been around for years is that nothing is as important as your health. This is a broad statement, of course, but your health status will impact on your job and your family life. The health benefits of a Positive Health Life-style should make you more effective in the other important aspects of your life.

Take the time to learn the techniques of a Positive Health Life-style. The gains you achieve will be well worth the investment. If you can, also teach the life-style to others.

The Older Adult

As with the word young, old is a relative term. We have all known young seventy-year-olds and old forty-year-olds. Chronologically, we shall define the older adult as being in the range forty and over, although it is recognized that there may be vast differences in physical capacity between a forty-year-old and an eighty-year-old.

Unfortunately, many older Americans have relatively poor knowledge and poor attitudes about exercise. According to C. Carson Conrad, executive director of the President's Council on Fitness and Sports, most older Americans believe that they need little or no exercise as they get older; they vastly exaggerate the risks involved in vigorous exercise; they overrate the value of light exercise such as bowling; and they underrate their own ability and capacity.

The major point for this age group is that you are never too old to exercise, and the benefits, both physiological and psychological, that you attain by a proper exercise program are similar for all age groups. Moreover, the older you are, the more significant these benefits are to your overall health. An individual may be chronologically old but physiologically and psychologically young. You may review some of the beneficial effects of exercise for older adults on page 98, but in general, physically active older individuals are more independent: they get out and do more, have a greater sense of well-being, have fewer illnesses, and have greater levels of strength, flexibility and endurance.

The older you are, the more precautions you should take before initiating a vigorous exercise program. In general, a medical examination is recommended. (See pages 80–81 for guidelines.) The recommended exercise program is identical to that recommended for younger adults, including both aerobic activities and exercises to increase strength and flexibility in the low-back area. The guidelines presented in chapters 3 and 4 are pertinent to the older adult, but the intensity level may be reduced and the progression may be slower.

Dr. Herbert deVries is an expert on exercise for older adults. His basic recommendation for those just beginning to exercise is a walk-jog program that has four phases.

1. A slow warm-up period. Start the walk at a slow pace.
2. A stimulus period. Dr. deVries suggests that the minimum heart rate should be only 40 percent of the target heart rate range, while the maximum should be only 75 percent. The average target heart rate should be 60 percent. (See pages 85–87 to use this method.)
3. A warm-down period. Warm down by doing light exercises or slower walking.
4. A static-stretching period. Slowly stretch the muscles in the lower back area and the back of the thigh and calf. (See chapter 8 for recommended exercises.)
5. Progression should be slow. The walking program in table 4.6 or the walk-jog program in table 4.7 are highly recommended, but possibly each level could be two weeks in duration.

The basic principles of sound nutrition still apply. The older adult may need less Calories, particularly if physically inactive, but the nutrient requirements remain similar, so foods with high nutrient value should be selected for the diet. A good source of calcium is also important, particularly for women, so dairy foods are an important item. The physically active individual will be able to consume more Calories due to the increased energy expenditure during exercise, and thus will be better able to secure the necessary amounts of required nutrients.

The later years in life, particularly those in the post-retirement senior years, should be happy ones. If you are in good, vigorous health, you will be more likely to enjoy those years. Initiating a Postive Health Life-style early in life, including a sound exercise and nutrition program, will pay dividends in your senior years.

Figure 11.4 The older adult may reap the same type of benefits from aerobic exercise as the younger individual.

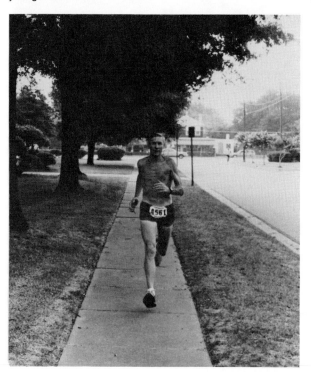

Summary

Chronologically we get older every day; it is unavoidable. If we live a sedentary life-style and do not eat properly, we will also age physiologically every day, becoming not only old, but fat, weak, and ill as well. However, we can minimize physiological aging by adopting a Positive Health Life-style.

The two keys to a Positive Health Life-style are exercise and nutrition. The preceding chapters have presented the essential information about the design and implementation of sound exercise and nutrition programs, and the health benefits that result from such programs. However, in order for these programs to be effective and to serve as personal preventive medicine, they must be lifelong. An old Chinese proverb notes that a journey of 1000 miles begins with a single step. So too, a Positive Health Life-style may begin with that first jogging or aerobic walking step. Make such a personal commitment now. Your body and mind will thank you for years to come.

Read the following statements and circle the *number beneath the letter* that corresponds to how characteristic that behavior is to you. Answer every item and be as honest as possible, keeping your responses to yourself.

A. extremely uncharacteristic of me
B. somewhat uncharacteristic of me
C. neither characteristic nor uncharacteristic of me
D. somewhat characteristic of me
E. extremely characteristic of me

Self-Motivation Assessment Scale

A	B	C	D	E	
5	4	3	2	1	1. I get discouraged easily.
5	4	3	2	1	2. I don't work any harder than I have to.
1	2	3	4	5	3. I seldom, if ever, let myself down.
5	4	3	2	1	4. I'm just not the goal-setting type.
1	2	3	4	5	5. I'm good at keeping promises, especially the ones I make to myself.
5	4	3	2	1	6. I don't impose much structure on my activities.
1	2	3	4	5	7. I have a very hard-driving, aggressive personality.

Scoring: Simply add the total of your seven scores. If the total is 24 or less, you are more subject to dropping out. The lower the score, the greater the possibility you will drop out.

Source: Rod K. Dishman, Ph.D., University of Georgia; William Ickes, Ph.D., University of Texas.

References

Berg, K.; Sady, S.; Beal, D. et al. "Developing an Elementary School CHD Prevention Program." *The Physician and Sportsmedicine* 11:99–105 (October 1983).

Bortz, W. "Effect of Exercise on Aging—Effect of Aging on Exercise." *Journal of the American Geriatric Society* 28:49–51 (1980).

Carter, R. "Exercise and Happiness." *Journal of Sports Medicine and Physical Fitness* 17:307–13 (1977).

Clarke, H. "Exercise and Aging." *Physical Fitness Research Digest* 7:1–27 (April 1977).

deVries, H. "Physiological Effects of an Exercise Training Regimen upon Men Aged 52–88." *Journal of Gerontology* 25:325–36 (1970).

———. "Tips on Prescribing Exercise Regimens for Your Older Patient." *Geriatrics* 34:75–81 (1979).

Dishman, R., and Gettman, L. "Psychobiologic Influences on Exercise Adherence." *Journal of Sports Psychology* 2:295–310 (1980).

Falls, H.; Baylor, A.; and Dishman, R. *Essential of Fitness*. Philadelphia: Saunders College Publishing, 1980.

Fries, J., and Crapo, L. *Vitality and Aging*. San Francisco: W. H. Freeman, 1981.

Gettman, L.; Pollock, M.; and Ward, A. "Adherence to Unsupervised Exercise." *The Physician and Sportsmedicine* 11:56–66 (October 1983).

Gilliam, T.; MacConnie, S.; Geenen, D.; Pels, A.; and Freedson, P. "Exercise Programs for Children: A Way to Prevent Heart Disease?" *The Physician and Sportsmedicine* 10:96–108 (September 1982).

Legwold, G. "Little Bodies and Healthy Hearts: Counseling in the Schools." *The Physician and Sportsmedicine* 10:128–32 (May 1982).

———. "New Verse, Same Chorus: Children Aren't Fit." *The Physician and Sportsmedicine* 11:153–55 (May 1983).

Montgomery, D.; Ismail, A.; and Corrigan, D. "Physical Fitness over a 10-Year Period—A Longitudinal Comparison of Exercises and Drop-outs." *Medicine and Science in Sports and Exercise* 15:109 (1983).

Morris, A.; Vaccaro, P.; and Harris, R. "Life Quality Changes of Older Adults during Various Physical Activity Programs." *Medicine and Science in Sports and Exercise* 15:117 (1983).

President's Council on Physical Fitness. *Adult Physical Fitness—A Program for Men and Women*. Washington, D.C.: U.S. Government Printing Office.

President's Council on Physical Fitness and Sports. *The Fitness Challenge in the Later Years. An Exercise Program for Older Americans*. Washington, D.C.: U.S. Government Printing Office, 1968.

Shephard, R., and Sidney, K. "Exercise and Aging." *Exercise and Sport Science Review* 6:1–57 (1978).

"The Skinning You Can Get at a Health Club." *Changing Times* 35:64–66 (September 1981).

Tu, J., and Rothstein, A. "Improvement of Jogging Performance through Application of Personality Specific Motivational Techniques." *Research Quarterly* 50:97–103 (1979).

Weltman, A., and Stamford, B. "Exercise and the Cigarette Smoker." *The Physician and Sportsmedicine* 10:153 (December 1982).

Wood, P. "Adding Years to Life and Life to Years through Running and Physical Fitness." *Runner's World* 18:45 (December 1983).

Appendix A
The 1980 Recommended Dietary Allowances

Recommended Daily Dietary Allowance[a] Revised 1980

	Age (years)	Weight (kg)	Weight (lbs)	Height (cm)	Height (in)	Fat-soluble Vitamins — Protein (g)	Vitamin A (μg R.E.)[b]	Vitamin D (μg)[c]	Vitamin E (mg α T.E.)[d]	Water-soluble Vitamins — Vitamin C (mg)	Thiamin (mg)
Infants	0.0–0.5	6	13	60	24	kg×2.2	420	10	3	35	0.3
	0.5–1.0	9	20	71	28	kg×2.0	400	10	4	35	0.5
Children	1–3	13	29	90	35	23	400	10	5	45	0.7
	4–6	20	44	112	44	30	500	10	6	45	0.9
	7–10	28	62	132	52	34	700	10	7	45	1.2
Males	11–14	45	99	157	62	45	1,000	10	8	50	1.4
	15–18	66	145	176	69	56	1,000	10	10	60	1.4
	19–22	70	154	177	70	56	1,000	7.5	10	60	1.5
	23–50	70	154	178	70	56	1,000	5	10	60	1.4
	51+	70	154	178	70	56	1,000	5	10	60	1.2
Females	11–14	46	101	157	62	46	800	10	8	50	1.1
	15–18	55	120	163	64	46	800	10	8	60	1.1
	19–22	55	120	163	64	44	800	7.5	8	60	1.1
	23–50	55	120	163	64	44	800	5	8	60	1.0
	51+	55	120	163	64	44	800	5	8	60	1.0
Pregnant						+30	+200	+5	+2	+20	+0.4
Lactating						+20	+400	+5	+3	+40	+0.5

[a]The allowances are intended to provide for individual variations among most normal persons as they live in the United States under usual environmental stresses. Diets should be based on a variety of common foods in order to provide other nutrients for which human requirements have been less well defined.

[b]Retinol equivalents. 1 Retinol equivalent = 1 μg retinol or 6 μg carotene.

[c]As cholecalciferol. 10 μg cholecalciferol = 400 I.U. vitamin D.

[d]α tocopherol equivalents. 1 mg d-α-tocopherol = 1αT.E.

[e]1 NE (niacin equivalent) is equal to 1 mg of niacin or 60 mg of dietary tryptophan.

[f]The folacin allowances refer to dietary sources as determined by *Lactobacillus casei* assay after treatment with enzymes ("conjugases") to make polyglutamyl forms of the vitamin available to the test organism.

[g]The RDA for vitamin B_{12} in infants is based on average concentration of the vitamin in human milk. The allowances after weaning are based on energy intake (as recommended by the American Academy of Pediatrics) and consideration of other factors such as intestinal absorption.

[h]The increased requirement during pregnancy cannot be met by the iron content of habitual American diets nor by the existing iron stores of many women; therefore the use of 30–60 mg of supplement iron is recommended. Iron needs during lactation are not substantially different from those of non-pregnant women, but continued supplementation of the mother for 2–3 months after parturition is advisable in order to replenish stores depleted by pregnancy.

Source: From Food and Nutrition Board, National Academy of Sciences, National Research Council, Washington, D.C.

Water-soluble Vitamins / Minerals

Riboflavin (mg)	Niacin (mg N.E.)e	Vitamin B$_6$ (mg)	Folacinf (µg)	Vitamin B$_{12}$(µg)	Calcium (mg)	Phosphorus (mg)	Magnesium (mg)	Iron (mg)	Zinc (mg)	Iodine (µg)
0.4	6	0.3	30	0.5g	360	240	50	10	3	40
0.6	8	0.6	45	1.5	540	360	70	15	5	50
0.8	9	0.9	100	2.0	800	800	150	15	10	70
1.0	11	1.3	200	2.5	800	800	200	10	10	90
1.4	16	1.6	300	3.0	800	800	250	10	10	120
1.6	18	1.8	400	3.0	1,200	1,200	350	18	15	150
1.7	18	2.0	400	3.0	1,200	1,200	400	18	15	150
1.7	19	2.2	400	3.0	800	800	350	10	15	150
1.6	18	2.2	400	3.0	800	800	350	10	15	150
1.4	16	2.2	400	3.0	800	800	350	10	15	150
1.3	15	1.8	400	3.0	1,200	1,200	300	18	15	150
1.3	14	2.0	400	3.0	1,200	1,200	300	18	15	150
1.3	14	2.0	400	3.0	800	800	300	18	15	150
1.2	13	2.0	400	3.0	800	800	300	18	15	150
1.2	13	2.0	400	3.0	800	800	300	10	15	150
+0.3	+2	+0.6	+400	+1.0	+400	+400	+150	h	+5	+25
+0.5	+5	+0.5	+100	+1.0	+400	+400	+150	h	+10	+50

1980 RDAs—Mean Heights and Weights and Recommended Energy Intake

Category	Age (years)	Weight (kg)	Weight (lb)	Height (cm)	Height (in)	Energy Needs (with range) (Calories)	(MG)
Infants	0.0–0.5	6	13	60	24	kg × 115 (95–145)	kg × .48
	0.5–1.0	9	20	71	28	kg × 105 (80–135)	kg × .44
Children	1–3	13	29	90	35	1,300 (900–1,800)	5.5
	4–6	20	44	112	44	1,700 (1,300–2,300)	7.1
	7–10	28	62	132	52	2,400 (1,650–3,300)	10.1
Males	11–14	45	99	157	62	2,700 (2,000–3,700)	11.3
	15–18	66	145	176	69	2,800 (2,100–3,900)	11.8
	19–22	70	154	177	70	2,900 (2,500–3,300)	12.2
	23–50	70	154	178	70	2,700 (2,300–3,100)	11.3
	51–75	70	154	178	70	2,400 (2,000–2,800)	10.1
	76 +	70	154	178	70	2,050 (1,650–2,450)	8.6
Females	11–14	46	101	157	62	2,200 (1,500–3,000)	9.2
	15–18	55	120	163	64	2,100 (1,200–3,000)	8.8
	19–22	55	120	163	64	2,100 (1,700–2,500)	8.8
	23–50	55	120	163	64	2,000 (1,600–2,400)	8.4
	51–75	55	120	163	64	1,800 (1,400–2,200)	7.6
	76 +	55	120	163	64	1,600 (1,200–2,000)	6.7
Pregnant						+300	
Lactating						+500	

1980 RDAs—Estimated Safe and Adequate Daily Dietary Intakes of Additional Selected Vitamins and Minerals[a]

Subjects		Vitamins				Trace Elements[b]			
	Age (years)	Vitamin K (µg)	Biotin (µg)	Panto-thenic Acid (mg)		Copper (mg)	Manganese (mg)	Fluoride (mg)	Chromium (mg)
Infants	0–0.5	12	35	2		0.5–0.7	0.5–0.7	0.1–0.5	0.01–0.04
	0.5–1	10–20	50	3		0.7–1.0	0.7–1.0	0.2–1.0	0.02–0.06
Children and Adolescents	1–3	15–30	65	3		1.0–1.5	1.0–1.5	0.5–1.5	0.02–0.08
	4–6	20–40	85	3–4		1.5–2.0	1.5–2.0	1.0–2.5	0.03–0.12
	7–10	30–60	120	4–5		2.0–2.5	2.0–3.0	1.5–2.5	0.05–0.2
	11	50–100	100–200	4–7		2.0–3.0	2.5–5.0	1.5–2.5	0.05–0.2
Adults		70–140	100–200	4–7		2.0–3.0	2.5–5.0	1.5–4.0	0.05–0.2

[a]Because there is less information on which to base allowances, these figures are not given in the main table of the RDA and are provided here in the form of ranges of recommended intakes.

[b]Since the toxic levels for many trace elements may be only several times usual intakes, the upper levels for the trace elements given in this table should not be habitually exceeded.

From: Recommended Dietary Allowances, Revised 1980. Food and Nutrition Board, National Academy of Sciences-National Research Council, Washington, D.C.

Trace Elements[b]		Electrolytes		
Selenium (mg)	Molybdenum (mg)	Sodium (mg)	Potassium (mg)	Chloride (mg)
0.01–0.04	0.03–0.06	115–350	350–925	275–700
0.02–0.06	0.04–0.08	250–750	425–1275	400–1200
0.02–0.08	0.05–0.1	325–975	550–1,650	500–1,500
0.03–0.12	0.06–0.15	450–1,350	775–2,325	700–2,100
0.05–0.2	0.10–0.3	600–1,800	1,000–3,000	925–2,775
0.05–0.2	0.15–0.5	900–2,700	1,525–4,575	1,400–4,200
0.05–0.2	0.15–0.5	1,100–3,300	1,875–5,625	1,700–5,100

The data in this table (page 297, bottom) has been assembled from the observed median heights and weights of children, together with desirable weights for adults for the mean heights of men (70 inches) and women (64 inches), between the ages of 18 to 34 years as surveyed in the U.S. population (HEW/NCHS data).

The energy allowances for the young adults are for men and women doing light work. The allowances for the two older age groups represent mean energy needs over these age spans, allowing for a 2 percent decrease in basal (resting) metabolic rate per decade and a reduction in activity of 200 Calories/years and 400 Calories for women over 75. The customary range of daily energy output is shown for adults in parentheses, and is based on a variation in energy needs of ±400 Calories at any one age, emphasizing the wide range of energy intakes appropriate for any group of people.

Energy allowances for children through age 18 are based on median energy intakes of children these ages followed in longitudinal growth studies. The values in parentheses are 10th and 90th percentiles of energy intake, to indicate the range of energy consumption among children of these ages.

Appendix B
The Food Exchange Lists

Exchange lists represent groups of foods, in specific measured amounts, that contain approximately the same amount of energy, carbohydrate, fat, and protein. Thus foods within a particular exchange list may be substituted for one another.

Meals should be planned so they contain a selection from each of the exchange groups. A balanced selection should be used to total your daily caloric intake. The exchange list is patterned after the Basic Four Food Groups, and the principles discussed in chapters 5 and 6 are relevant for sound nutritional practices and dieting. The Exchange Lists for Meal Planning were prepared by a number of organizations, primarily the American Dietetic Association and the American Diabetes Association in cooperation with the National Institute of Arthritis, Metabolism, and Digestive Diseases and the National Heart and Lung Institute; National Institutes of Health, Public Health Service; and the United States Department of Health, Education, and Welfare.

---

(1) The Milk List
A MILK EXCHANGE is a serving of food that is equivalent to one cup of skim milk in its energy nutrient content. One milk exchange contains substantial amounts of carbohydrate and protein and about 80 Calories. (12 grams carbohydrate, 8 grams protein)

Nonfat Fortified Milk
1 cup	skim or nonfat milk
1 cup	buttermilk made from skim milk
1 cup	yogurt made from skim milk (plain, unflavored)
1/3 cup	powdered, nonfat dry milk, before adding liquid
1/2 cup	canned evaporated skim milk, before adding liquid

Low-fat Fortified Milk
1 cup	1% fat fortified milk (add 1/2 fat exchange)*
1 cup	2% fat fortified milk (add 1 fat exchange)*
1 cup	yogurt made from 2% fortified milk (plain, unflavored) (add 1 fat exchange*)

Whole Milk (add 2 fat exchanges*)
1 cup	whole milk
1 cup	buttermilk made from whole milk
1 cup	yogurt made from whole milk (plain, unflavored)
1/2 cup	canned, evaporated whole milk, before adding liquid

---

*These foods contain more fat than skim milk. When calculating fat values, add fat exchanges as indicated. (1 fat exchange = 5 grams fat.)

(2) The Vegetable List

A VEGETABLE EXCHANGE is a serving of any vegetable that contains a moderate amount of carbohydrate, a small but significant amount of protein, and about 25 Calories. (5 grams carbohydrate, 2 grams protein)

1/2 cup asparagus	1/2 cup okra	**Greens**
1/2 cup bean sprouts	1/2 cup onions	1/2 cup beet greens
1/2 cup beets	1/2 cup rhubarb	1/2 cup chards
1/2 cup broccoli	1/2 cup rutabaga	1/2 cup collard greens
1/2 cup Brussels sprouts	1/2 cup sauerkraut	1/2 cup dandelion greens
1/2 cup cabbage	1/2 cup string beans, green or yellow	1/2 cup kale
1/2 cup carrots	1/2 cup summer squash	1/2 cup mustard greens
1/2 cup cauliflower	1/2 cup tomatoes	1/2 cup spinach
1/2 cup celery	1/2 cup tomato juice	1/2 cup turnip greens
1/2 cup cucumbers	1/2 cup turnips	
1/2 cup eggplant	1/2 cup vegetable juice cocktail	
1/2 cup green pepper	1/2 cup zucchini	
1/2 cup mushrooms		

The following vegetables may be assumed to have negligible carbohydrate, protein, and Calories:

chicory	lettuce
Chinese cabbage	parsley
endive	radishes
escarole	watercress

Starchy vegetables are found in the Bread Exchange List.

(3) The Fruit List

A FRUIT EXCHANGE is a serving of fruit that contains about 10 grams of carbohydrate and 40 Calories. The protein and fat content of fruit is negligible. (10 grams carbohydrate)

1 small	apple	1/8 medium	honeydew melon
1/3 cup	apple juice	1/2 small	mango
1/2 cup	applesauce (unsweetened)	1 small	nectarine
2 medium	apricots, fresh	1 small	orange
4 halves	apricots, dried	1/2 cup	orange juice
1/2 small	banana	3/4 cup	papaya
1/2 cup	blackberries	1 medium	peach
1/2 cup	blueberries	1 small	pear
1/4 small	cantaloupe melon	1 medium	persimmon
10 large	cherries	1/2 cup	pineapple
1/3 cup	cider	1/3 cup	pineapple juice
2	dates	2 medium	plums
1	fig, fresh	2 medium	prunes
1	fig, dried	1/4 cup	prune juice
1 half	grapefruit	2 tbsp	raisins
1/2 cup	grapefruit juice	1/2 cup	raspberries
12	grapes	3/4 cup	strawberries
1/4 cup	grape juice	1 medium	tangerine
		1 cup	watermelon

Cranberries may be assumed to have negligible carbohydrate and Calories if used without sugar.

(4) The Bread List (Includes Bread, Cereals, and Starchy Vegetables)

A BREAD EXCHANGE is a serving of bread, cereal, or starchy vegetable that contains appreciable carbohydrate and a small but significant amount of protein, totaling about 70 Calories. (15 grams carbohydrate, 2 grams protein)

Bread

1 slice	white (including French and Italian)
1 slice	whole wheat
1 slice	rye or pumpernickel
1 slice	raisin
1 half	small bagel
1 half	small English muffin
1	plain roll, bread
1 half	frankfurter roll
1 half	hamburger bun
3 tbsp	dried bread crumbs
1 6-inch	tortilla

Cereal

1/2 cup	bran flakes
3/4 cup	other ready-to-eat cereal, unsweetened
1 cup	puffed cereal (unfrosted)
1/2 cup	cereal (cooked)
1/2 cup	grits (cooked)
1/2 cup	rice or barley (cooked)
1/2 cup	pasta (cooked): spaghetti, noodles, or macaroni
3 cups	popcorn (popped, no fat added)
2 tbsp	cornmeal (dry)
2 1/2 tbsp	flour
1/4 cup	wheat germ

Crackers

3	arrowroot
2	graham, 2 1/2" square
1 half	matzoh, 4" × 6"
20	oyster
25	pretzels, 3 1/8" long × 1/8" diameter
3	rye wafers, 2" × 3 1/2"
6	saltines
4	soda, 2 1/2" square

Dried Beans, Peas, and Lentils

1/2 cup	beans, peas, lentils (dried and cooked)
1/4 cup	baked beans, no pork (canned)

Starchy Vegetables

1/3 cup	corn
1 small	corn on cob
1/2 cup	lima beans
2/3 cup	parsnips
1/2 cup	peas, green (canned or frozen)
1 small	potato, white
1/2 cup	potato (mashed)
3/4 cup	pumpkin
1/2 cup	squash winter, acorn, or butternut
1/4 cup	yam or sweet potato

Prepared Foods*

1 biscuit, 2" diameter (add 1 fat exchange)
1 corn bread, 2" × 2" × 1" (add 1 fat exchange)
1 corn muffin, 2" diameter (add 1 fat exchange)
5 crackers, round butter type (add 1 fat exchange)
1 muffin, plain, small (add 1 fat exchange)
8 potatoes, French fried, length 2" by 3 1/2" (add 1 fat exchange)
15 potato chips or corn chips (add 2 fat exchanges)
1 pancake, 5" × 1/2" (add 1 fat exchange)
1 waffle, 5" × 1/2" (add 1 fat exchange)

---

*These foods contain more fat than bread. When calculating fat values, add fat exchanges as indicated.
(1 fat exchange = 5 grams fat.)

(5) The Meat List

A MEAT EXCHANGE is a serving of protein-rich food that contains negligible carbohydrate, but a significant amount of protein and fat, roughly equivalent to the amounts in one ounce of lean meat: contains about 55 Calories.
(7 grams protein, 3 grams fat)

Low-fat Meat

1 ounce beef	baby beef (very lean), chipped beef, chuck, flank steak, tenderloin, plate ribs, plate skirt steak, round (bottom, top), all cuts rump, spare ribs, tripe
1 ounce lamb	leg, rib, sirloin, loin (roast and chops), shank, shoulder
1 ounce pork	leg (whole rump, center shank), ham, smoked (center slices)
1 ounce veal	leg, loin, rib, shank, shoulder, cutlets
1 ounce poultry	meat (without skin) of chicken, turkey, cornish hen, guinea hen, pheasant
1 ounce fish	any fresh or frozen
1/4 cup fish	canned salmon, tuna, mackerel, crab, and lobster
5 (or 1 ounce)	clams, oysters, scallops, shrimp
3	sardines, drained
1 ounce cheese	containing less than 5% butterfat
1/4 cup	cottage cheese, dry and 2% butterfat
1/2 cup	dried beans and peas (add 1 bread exchange*)

Medium-fat Meat (Add 1/2 Fat Exchange*)

1 ounce beef	ground (15% fat), corned beef (canned), rib eye, round (ground commercial)
1 ounce pork	loin (all cuts tenderloin), shoulder arm (picnic), shoulder blade, Boston butt, Canadian bacon, boiled ham
1 ounce	liver, heart, kidney, and sweetbreads (these are high in cholesterol)
1/4 cup	cottage cheese, creamed
1 ounce cheese	mozzarella, ricotta, farmer's cheese, Neufchatel
3 tbsp	Parmesan cheese
1	egg (high in cholesterol)

High-fat Meat (Add 1 Fat Exchange*)

1 ounce beef	brisket, corned beef (brisket), ground beef (more than 20% fat), hamburger (commercial), chuck (ground commercial), roasts (rib), steaks (club and rib)
1 ounce lamb	breast
1 ounce pork	spare ribs, loin (back ribs), pork (ground), country style ham, deviled ham
1 ounce veal	breast
1 ounce poultry	capon, duck (domestic), goose
1 ounce cheese	cheddar types
1 slice	cold cuts, 4 1/2″ × 1/8″ slice
1 small	frankfurter

Peanut Butter

2 tbsp	peanut butter (add 2 1/2 fat exchanges*)

*These foods contain more carbohydrate or fat than lean meat. When calculating carbohydrate or fat values, add bread or fat exchanges as indicated.

(6) The Fat List

A FAT EXCHANGE is a serving of any food that contains negligible carbohydrate and protein, but appreciable fat, totaling about 45 Calories. (5 grams fat)

Polyunsaturated Fat

1 tsp margarine, soft, tub, or stick*
1 eighth avocado (4″ in diameter)†
1 tsp oil, corn, cottonseed, safflower, soy, sunflower
1 tsp oil, olive†
1 tsp oil, peanut†
5 small olives†

10 whole almonds†
2 large whole pecans†
20 whole peanuts, Spanish†
10 whole peanuts, Virginia†
6 small walnuts
6 small nuts, other†

Saturated Fat

1 tsp margarine, regular stick
1 tsp butter
1 tsp bacon fat
1 strip bacon, crisp
2 tbsp cream, light
2 tbsp cream, sour
1 tbsp cream, heavy

1 tbsp cream cheese
1 tbsp French dressing‡
1 tbsp Italian dressing‡
1 tsp lard
1 tsp mayonnaise‡
2 tsp salad dressing, mayonnaise type‡
3/4 inch salt pork cube

*Made with corn, cottonseed, safflower, soy, or sunflower oil only.

†Fat content is primarily monounsaturated.

‡If made with corn, cottonseed, safflower, soy, or sunflower oil, can be assumed to contain polyunsaturated fat.

Unlimited Foods

These are *free foods* that contain negligible carbohydrate, protein, and fat, and therefore negligible Calories.

diet Calorie-free beverage
coffee
tea
bouillon without fat
unsweetened gelatin
unsweetened pickles
salt and pepper
red pepper

paprika
garlic
celery salt
parsley
nutmeg
lemon
mustard

chili powder
onion salt or powder
horseradish
vinegar
mint
cinnamon
lime

Appendix C
American College of Sports Medicine "Position Stand on Proper and Improper Weight Loss Programs"[1]

Millions of individuals are involved in weight reduction programs. With the number of undesirable weight loss programs available and a general misconception by many about weight loss, the need for guidelines for proper weight loss programs is apparent.

Based on the existing evidence concerning the effects of weight loss on health status, physiologic processes and body composition parameters, the American College of Sports Medicine makes the following statements and recommendations for weight loss programs.

For the purposes of this position stand, body weight will be represented by two components, fat and fat-free (water, electrolytes, minerals, glycogen stores, muscular tissue, bone, etc.):

1. Prolonged fasting and diet programs that severely restrict caloric intake are scientifically undesirable and can be medically dangerous.
2. Fasting and diet programs that severely restrict caloric intake result in the loss of large amounts of water, electrolytes, minerals, glycogen stores, and other fat-free tissue (including proteins within fat-free tissues), with minimal amounts of fat loss.
3. Mild calorie restriction (500–1000 kcal less than the usual daily intake) results in a smaller loss of water, electrolytes, minerals, and other fat-free tissue, and is less likely to cause malnutrition.
4. Dynamic exercise of large muscles helps to maintain fat-free tissue, including muscle mass and bone density, and results in losses of body weight. Weight loss resulting from an increase in energy expenditure is primarily in the form of fat weight.
5. A nutritionally sound diet resulting in mild calorie restriction coupled with an endurance exercise program along with behavioral modification of existing eating habits is recommended for weight reduction. The rate of sustained weight loss should not exceed 1 kg (2 lb) per week.
6. To maintain proper weight control and optimal body fat levels, a lifetime commitment to proper eating habits and regular physical activity is required.

[1]**Source:** American College of Sports Medicine. "Position Stand on Proper and Improper Weight Loss Programs." *Medicine and Science in Sports and Exercise* 15, no. 1:ix-x (1983).

Research Background for the Position Stand

Each year millions of individuals undertake weight loss programs for a variety of reasons. It is well known that obesity is associated with a number of health-related problems. These problems include impairment of cardiac function due to an increase in the work of the heart and to left ventricular dysfunction; hypertension; diabetes; renal disease; gall bladder disease; respiratory dysfunction; joint diseases and gout; endometrial cancer; abnormal plasma lipid and lipoprotein concentrations; problems in the administration of anesthetics during surgery; and impairment of physical working capacity. As a result, weight reduction is frequently advised by physicians for medical reasons. In addition, there are a vast number of individuals who are on weight reduction programs for aesthetic reasons.

It is estimated that 60–70 million American adults and at least 10 million American teenagers are overfat. Because millions of Americans have adopted unsupervised weight loss programs, it is the opinion of the American College of Sports Medicine that guidelines are needed for safe and effective weight loss programs. This position stand deals with desirable and undesirable weight loss programs. Desirable weight loss programs are defined as those that are nutritionally sound and result in maximal losses in fat weight and minimal losses of fat-free tissue. Undesirable weight loss programs are defined as those that are not nutritionally sound, that result in large losses of fat-free tissue, that pose potential serious medical complications, and that cannot be followed for long-term weight maintenance.

Therefore, a desirable weight loss program is one that:

1. Provides a caloric intake not lower than 1200 kcal·d^{-1} for normal adults in order to get a proper blend of foods to meet nutritional requirements. (Note: this requirement may change for children, older individuals, athletes, etc.).
2. Includes foods acceptable to the dieter from the viewpoints of socio-cultural background, usual habits, taste, cost, and ease in acquisition and preparation.
3. Provides a negative caloric balance (not to exceed 500–1000 kcal·d^{-1} lower than recommended), resulting in gradual weight loss without metabolic derangements. Maximal weight loss should be 1 kg·wk^{-1}.
4. Includes the use of behavior modification techniques to identify and eliminate dieting habits that contribute to improper nutrition.
5. Includes an endurance exercise program of at least 3 d/wk, 20–30 min in duration, at a minimum intensity of 60% of maximum heart rate (refer to ACSM Position Stand on the Recommended Quantity and Quality of Exercise for Developing and Maintaining Fitness in Healthy Adults, *Med. Sci. Sports* 10:vii, 1978).
6. Provides that the new eating and physical activity habits can be continued for life in order to maintain the achieved lower body weight.

1. Since the early work of Keys et al. and Bloom, which indicated that marked reduction in caloric intake or fasting (starvation or semistarvation) rapidly reduced body weight, numerous fasting, modified fasting, and fad diet and weight loss programs have emerged. While these programs promise and generally cause rapid weight loss, they are associated with significant medical risks.

    The medical risks associated with these types of diet and weight loss programs are numerous. Blood glucose concentrations have been shown to be markedly reduced in obese subjects who undergo fasting. Further, in obese non-diabetic subjects, fasting may result in impairment of glucose tolerance. Ketonuria begins within a few hours after fasting or low-carbohydrate diets are begun and hyperuricemia is common among subjects who fast to reduce body weight. Fasting also results in high serum uric acid levels with decreased urinary output. Fasting and low-calorie diets also result in urinary nitrogen loss and a significant decrease in fat-free tissue (see section 2). In comparison to ingestion of a normal diet, fasting substantially elevates urinary excretion of potassium. This, coupled with the aforementioned nitrogen loss, suggests that the potassium loss is due to a loss of lean tissue. Other electrolytes, including sodium, calcium, magnesium, and phosphate have been shown to be elevated in urine during prolonged fasting. Reductions in blood volume and body fluids are also common with fasting and fad diets. This can be associated with weakness and fainting. Congestive heart failure and sudden death have been reported in subjects who fasted or markedly restricted their caloric intake. Myocardial atrophy appears to contribute to sudden death. Sudden death may also occur during refeeding. Untreated fasting has also been reported to reduce serum iron binding capacity, resulting in anemia. Liver glycogen levels are depleted with fasting and liver function and gastrointestinal tract abnormalities are associated with fasting. While fasting and calorically restricted diets have been shown to lower serum cholesterol levels, a large portion of the cholesterol reduction is a result of lowered HDL-cholesterol levels. Other risks associated with fasting and low-calorie diets include lactic acidosis, alopecia, hypoalaninemia, edema, anuria, hypotension, elevated serum bilirubin, nausea and vomiting, alterations in thyroxine metabolism, impaired serum triglyceride removal and production, and death.

2. The major objective of any weight reduction program is to lose body fat while maintaining fat-free tissue. The vast majority of research reveals that starvation and low-calorie diets result in large losses of water, electrolytes, and other fat-free tissue. One of the best controlled experiments was conducted from 1944 to 1946 at the Laboratory of Physiological Hygiene at the University of Minnesota. In this study subjects had their base-line caloric intake cut by 45% and body weight and body composition changes were followed for 24 wk. During the first 12 wk of semistarvation, body weight declined by 25.4 lb (11.5 kg) with only an 11.6-lb (5.3 kg) decline in body fat. During the second 12-wk period, body weight declined an additional 9.1 lb (4.1 kg) with only a 6.1-lb (2.8 kg) decrease in body fat. These data clearly demonstrate that fat-free tissue significantly contributes to weight loss from semistarvation. Similar

results have been reported by several other investigators. Buskirk et al. reported that the 13.5-kg weight loss in six subjects on a low-calorie mixed diet averaged 76% fat and 24% fat-free tissue. Similarly, Passmore et al. reported results of 78% of weight loss (15.3 kg) as fat and 22% as fat-free tissue in seven women who consumed a 400-kcal·d^{-1} diet for 45 d. Yang and Van Itallie followed weight loss and body composition changes for the first 5 d of a weight loss program involving subjects consuming either an 800-kcal mixed diet, an 800-kcal ketogenic diet, or undergoing starvation. Subjects on the mixed diet lost 1.3 kg of weight (59% fat loss, 3.4% protein loss, 37.6% water loss), subjects on the ketogenic diet lost 2.3 kg of weight (33.2% fat, 3.8% protein, 63.0% water), and subjects on starvation regimens lost 3.8 kg of weight (32.3% fat, 6.5% protein, 61.2% water). Grande and Grande et al. reported similar findings with a 1000-kcal carbohydrate diet. It was further reported that water restriction combined with 1000-kcal·d^{-1} of carbohydrate resulted in greater water loss and less fat loss.

Recently, there has been some renewed speculation about the efficacy of the very-low-calorie diet (VLCD). Krotkiewski and associates studied the effects on body weight and body composition after 3 wk on the so-called Cambridge diet. Two groups of obese middle-aged women were studied. One group had a VLCD only, while the second group had a VLCD combined with a 55-min/d, 3-d/wk exercise program. The VLCD-only group lost 6.2 kg in 3 wk, of which only 2.6 kg was fat loss, while the VLCD-plus-exercise group lost 6.8 kg in 3 wk with only a 1.9-kg body fat loss. Thus it can be seen that VLCD results in undesirable losses of body fat, and the addition of the normally protective effect of chronic exercise to VLCD does not reduce the catabolism of fat-free tissue. Further, with VLCD, a large reduction (29%) in HDL-cholesterol is seen.

3. Even mild calorie restriction (reduction of 500–1000 kcal·d^{-1} from base-line caloric intake), when used alone as a tool for weight loss, results in the loss of moderate amounts of water and other fat-free tissue. In a study by Goldman et al., 15 female subjects consumed a low-calorie mixed diet for 7–8 wk. Weight loss during this period averaged 6.43 kg (0.85 kg·wk^{-1}), 88.6% of which was fat. The remaining 11.4% represented water and other fat-free tissue. Zuti and Golding examined the effect of 500 kcal·d^{-1} calorie restriction on body composition changes in adult females. Over a 16-wk period the women lost approximately 5.2 kg; however, 1.1 kg of the weight loss (21%) was due to a loss of water and other fat-free tissue. More recently, Weltman et al. examined the effects of 500 kcal·d^{-1} calorie restriction (from base-line levels) on body composition changes in sedentary middle-aged males. Over a 10-wk period subjects lost 5.95 kg, 4.03 kg (68%) of which was fat loss and 1.92 kg (32%) was loss of water and other fat-free tissue. Further, with calorie restriction only, these subjects exhibited a decrease in HDL-cholesterol. In the same study, the two other groups who exercised and/or dieted and exercised were able to maintain their HDL-cholesterol levels. Similar results for females have been presented by Thompson et al. It should be noted that the decrease seen in HDL-cholesterol with weight loss may be an acute effect. There are data that indicate that stable weight loss has a beneficial effect on HDL-cholesterol.

Further, an additional problem associated with calorie restriction alone for effective weight loss is the fact that it is associated with a reduction in basal metabolic rate. Apparently exercise combined with calorie restriction can counter this response.

4. There are several studies that indicate that exercise helps maintain fat-free tissue while promoting fat loss. Total body weight and fat weight are generally reduced with endurance training programs while fat-free weight remains constant or increases slightly. Programs conducted at least 3 d/wk, of at least 20-min duration and of sufficient intensity and duration to expend at least 300 kcal per exercise session have been suggested as a threshold level for total body weight and fat weight reduction. Increasing caloric expenditure above 300 kcal per exercise session and increasing the frequency of exercise sessions will enhance fat weight loss while sparing fat-free tissue. Leon et al. had six obese male subjects walk vigorously for 90 min, 5 d/wk for 16 wk. Work output progressed weekly to an energy expenditure of 1000–1200 kcal/session. At the end of 16 wk, subjects averaged 5.7 kg of weight loss with a 5.9-kg loss of fat weight and a 0.2-kg gain in fat-free tissue. Similarly, Zuti and Golding followed the progress of adult women who expended 500 kcal/exercise session 5 d/wk for 16 wk of exercise. At the end of 16 wk the women lost 5.8 kg of fat and gained 0.9 of fat-free tissue.

5. Review of the literature cited above strongly indicates that optimal body composition changes occur with a combination of calorie restriction (while on a well-balanced diet) plus exercise. This combination promotes loss of fat weight while sparing fat-free tissue. Data of Zuti and Golding and Weltman et al. support this contention. Calorie restriction of 500 $kcal \cdot d^{-1}$ combined with 3–5 d of exercise requiring 300–500 kcal per exercise session results in favorable changes in body composition. Therefore, the optimal rate of weight loss should be between 0.45–1 kg (1–2 lb) per wk. This seems especially relevant in light of the data which indicates that rapid weight loss due to low caloric intake can be associated with sudden death. In order to institute a desirable pattern of calorie restriction plus exercise, behavior modification techniques should be incorporated to identify and eliminate habits contributing to obesity and/or overfatness.

6. The problem with losing weight is that, although many individuals succeed in doing so, they invariably put the weight on again. The goal of an effective weight loss regimen is not merely to lose weight. Weight control requires a lifelong commitment, an understanding of our eating habits and a willingness to change them. Frequent exercise is necessary, and accomplishment must be reinforced to sustain motivation. Crash dieting and other promised weight loss cures are ineffective.

Appendix D
Scoring Tables for Cooper's Distance
Tests of Aerobic Capacity

Table D.1
1.5 Mile Run Test
Time (Minutes)

Fitness Category		Age (Years)					
		13–19	20–29	30–39	40–49	50–59	60+
Very poor	(men)	>15:31*	>16:01	>16:31	>17:31	>19:01	>20:01
	(women)	>18:31	>19:01	>19:31	>20:01	>20:31	>21:01
Poor	(men)	12:11–15:30	14:01–16:00	14:44–16:30	15:36–17:30	17:01–19:00	19:01–20:00
	(women)	18:30–16:55	19:00–18:31	19:30–19:01	20:00–19:31	20:30–20:01	21:00–21:30
Fair	(men)	10:49–12:10	12:01–14:00	12:31–14:45	13:01–15:35	14:31–17:00	16:16–19:00
	(women)	16:54–14:31	18:30–15:55	19:00–16:31	19:30–17:31	20:00–19:01	20:30–19:30
Good	(men)	9:41–10:48	10:46–12:00	11:01–12:30	11:31–13:00	12:31–14:30	14:00–16:10
	(women)	14:30–12:30	15:54–13:31	16:30–14:31	17:30–15:56	19:00–16:31	19:30–17:30
Excellent	(men)	8:37– 9:40	9:45–10:45	10:00–11:00	10:30–11:30	11:00–12:30	11:15–13:50
	(women)	12:29–11:50	13:30–12:30	14:30–13:00	15:55–13:45	16:30–14:30	17:30–16:30
Superior	(men)	< 8:37	< 9:45	<10:00	<10:30	<11:00	<11:15
	(women)	<11:50	<12:30	<13:00	<13:45	<14:30	<16:30

*< Means "less than"; > means "more than."

Source: From *The Aerobics Program for Total Well-Being* by Dr. Kenneth H. Cooper. Reprinted by permission of the publisher, M. Evans and Co., Inc., New York, N.Y. 10017

Table D.2
3 Mile Walking Test (No Running)
Time (Minutes)

Fitness Category		Age (Years)					
		13–19	20–29	30–39	40–49	50–59	60+
Very poor	(men)	>45:00*	>46:00	>49:00	>52:00	>55:00	>60:00
	(women)	>47:00	>48:00	>51:00	>54:00	>57:00	>63:00
Poor	(men)	41:01–45:00	42:01–46:00	44:31–49:00	47:01–52:00	50:01–55:00	54:01–60:00
	(women)	43:01–47:00	44:01–48:00	46:31–51:00	49:01–54:00	52:01–57:00	57:01–63:00
Fair	(men)	37:31–41:00	38:31–42:00	40:01–44:30	42:01–47:00	45:01–50:00	48:01–54:00
	(women)	39:31–43:00	40:31–44:00	42:01–46:30	44:01–49:00	47:01–52:00	51:01–57:00
Good	(men)	33:00–37:30	34:00–38:30	35:00–40:00	36:30–42:00	39:00–45:00	41:00–48:00
	(women)	35:00–39:30	36:00–40:30	37:30–42:00	39:00–44:00	42:00–47:00	45:00–51:00
Excellent	(men)	<33:00	<34:00	<35:00	<36:30	<39:00	<41:00
	(women)	<35:00	<36:00	<37:30	<39:00	<42:00	<45:00

*< Means "less than"; > means "more than."

The Walking test, covering 3 miles in the fastest time possible without running, can be done on a track or anywhere with an accurately measured distance.

Source: From *The Aerobics Program for Total Well-Being* by Dr. Kenneth H. Cooper. Reprinted by permission of the publisher, M. Evans and Co., Inc., New York, N.Y. 10017

Table D.3
Predicted VO$_2$ max (ml O$_2$/kg) on Basis of Cooper's Fitness Categories

Fitness Category		Age (Years)					
		13–19	20–29	30–39	40–49	50–59	60+
Very poor	(men)	<35.0	<33.0	<31.5	<30.2	<26.1	<20.5
	(women)	<25.0	<23.6	<22.8	<21.0	<20.2	<17.5
Poor	(men)	35.0–38.3	33.0–36.4	31.5–35.4	30.2–33.5	26.1–30.9	20.5–26.0
	(women)	25.0–30.9	23.6–28.9	22.8–26.9	21.0–24.4	20.2–22.7	17.5–20.1
Fair	(men)	38.4–45.1	36.5–42.4	35.5–40.9	33.6–38.9	31.0–35.7	26.1–32.2
	(women)	31.0–34.9	29.0–32.9	27.0–31.4	24.5–28.9	22.8–26.9	20.2–24.4
Good	(men)	45.2–50.9	42.5–46.4	41.0–44.9	39.0–43.7	35.8–40.9	32.2–36.4
	(women)	35.0–38.9	33.0–36.9	31.5–35.6	29.0–32.8	27.0–31.4	24.5–30.2
Excellent	(men)	51.0–55.9	46.5–52.4	45.0–49.4	43.8–48.0	41.0–45.3	36.5–44.2
	(women)	39.0–41.9	37.0–40.9	35.7–40.0	32.9–36.9	31.5–35.7	30.3–31.4
Superior	(men)	>56.0	>52.5	>49.5	>48.1	>45.4	>44.3
	(women)	>42.0	>41.0	>40.1	>37.0	>35.8	>31.5

Source: From *The Aerobics Way* by Dr. Kenneth H. Cooper. Copyright © 1982 by Kenneth H. Cooper. Reprinted by permission of the publisher, M. Evans and Company, Inc., New York, N.Y. 10017

Appendix E
Approximate Metabolic Cost
of Various Occupational
and Recreational Activities in METS

METS	Occupation	Exercise or Recreational Activity
1–2	Desk work Light housework Sewing, knitting Light office work	Strolling, 1 mile/hour Standing Playing cards
2–3	Light janitorial work Auto repair Bartending Woodworking, light Bakery work, general	Walking, 2 miles/hour Golf, motor cart Horseback riding (walk) Easy canoeing
3–4	Moderate housework, cleaning windows Yard work, power mower Electrical work Machine tooling	Walking, 3 miles/hour Cycling, 6 miles/hour Golf, pull cart Horseback riding (trot) Badminton (doubles)
4–5	Light carpentry Painting, masonry work Raking leaves Hoeing garden	Walking, 3.5 miles/hour Cycling, 8 miles/hour Golf, carrying clubs Tennis, doubles Dancing
5–6	Moderate gardening, shoveling Farming, general	Walking, 4 miles/hour Cycling, 10 miles/hour
6–7	Heavy shoveling Splitting wood Snow shoveling Lawn mowing, hand mower Forestry, general	Walking, 5 miles/hour Cycling, 11 miles/hour Tennis, singles Folk dancing
7–8	Digging ditches Sawing wood, lumber work	Jogging, 5 miles/hour Cycling, 12 miles/hour Horseback riding, gallop Basketball Climbing hills
8–9		Running, 5.5 miles/hour Cycling, 13 miles/hour Cross-country skiing, 4 miles/hour Squash, handball
10+		Running, over 6 miles/hour Cycling, over 14 miles/hour Cross-country skiing, over 5 miles/hour Competitive squash and handball

Source: Modified from Fox, S.; Naughton, J.; and Gorman, P. "Physical Activity and Cardiovascular Health. III. The Exercise Prescription; Frequency and Type of Activity." *Modern Concepts of Cardiovascular Disease* 41:25 (1972). Reprinted by permission of the American Heart Association.

Appendix F
Caloric Expenditure per Minute for Various Physical Activities

Body Weight

Kg		45	48	50	52	55	57	59	61	64	66	68	70
Pounds		100	105	110	115	120	125	130	135	140	145	150	155
Sedentary Activities													
lying quietly		.99	1.0	1.1	1.1	1.2	1.3	1.3	1.4	1.4	1.5	1.5	1.5
sitting and writing, card playing, etc.		1.2	1.3	1.4	1.5	1.5	1.6	1.7	1.7	1.8	1.8	1.9	2.0
standing with light work, cleaning, etc.		2.7	2.9	3.0	3.1	3.3	3.4	3.5	3.7	3.8	3.9	4.1	4.2
Physical Activities													
archery		3.1	3.3	3.5	3.6	3.8	4.0	4.1	4.3	4.5	4.6	4.8	4.9
badminton													
recreational singles		3.6	3.8	4.0	4.2	4.4	4.6	4.7	4.9	5.1	5.3	5.4	5.6
social doubles		2.7	2.9	3.0	3.1	3.3	3.4	3.5	3.7	3.8	3.9	4.1	4.2
competitive		5.9	6.1	6.4	6.7	7.0	7.3	7.6	7.9	8.2	8.5	8.8	9.1
baseball													
player		3.1	3.3	3.4	3.6	3.8	4.0	4.1	4.3	4.4	4.5	4.7	4.8
pitcher		3.9	4.1	4.3	4.5	4.7	4.9	5.1	5.3	5.5	5.7	5.9	6.0
basketball													
half court		3.0	3.1	3.3	3.5	3.6	3.8	3.9	4.1	4.2	4.4	4.5	4.7
recreational		4.9	5.2	5.5	5.7	6.0	6.2	6.5	6.7	7.0	7.2	7.5	7.7
vigorous competition		6.5	6.8	7.2	7.5	7.8	8.2	8.5	8.8	9.2	9.5	9.9	10.2
bicycling, level													
(MPH)	(Min/mile)												
5	12:00	1.9	2.0	2.1	2.2	2.3	2.4	2.5	2.6	2.7	2.8	2.9	3.0
6	10:00	2.7	2.8	3.0	3.1	3.2	3.4	3.5	3.6	3.8	3.9	4.0	4.2
8	7:30	3.4	3.6	3.8	4.0	4.1	4.3	4.5	4.7	4.8	5.0	5.2	5.4
10	6:00	4.2	4.4	4.6	4.8	5.1	5.3	5.5	5.7	5.9	6.1	6.4	6.6
11	5:28	5.0	5.2	5.5	5.7	6.0	6.2	6.5	6.7	7.0	7.2	7.5	7.8
12	5:00	5.7	6.0	6.3	6.6	6.9	7.2	7.5	7.8	8.1	8.4	8.7	9.0
13	4:37	6.8	7.1	7.5	7.8	8.2	8.5	8.8	9.2	9.5	9.9	10.2	10.6
bowling		2.7	2.8	3.0	3.1	3.3	3.4	3.5	3.7	3.8	3.9	4.1	4.2
calisthenics													
light type		3.4	3.6	3.8	4.0	4.1	4.3	4.5	4.7	4.8	5.0	5.2	5.4
timed, vigorous		9.7	10.1	10.6	11.1	11.6	12.1	12.6	13.1	13.6	14.1	14.6	15.1
canoeing													
(MPH)	(Min/mile)												
2.5	24	1.9	2.0	2.1	2.2	2.3	2.4	2.5	2.6	2.7	2.8	2.9	3.0
4.0	15	4.4	4.6	4.9	5.1	5.3	5.5	5.8	6.0	6.2	6.4	6.7	6.9
5.0	12	5.7	6.0	6.3	6.6	6.9	7.2	7.5	7.8	8.1	8.4	8.7	9.0
dancing													
moderately (waltz)		3.1	3.3	3.5	3.6	3.8	4.0	4.1	4.3	4.5	4.6	4.8	4.9
active (square, disco)		4.5	4.7	5.0	5.2	5.4	5.6	5.9	6.1	6.3	6.6	6.8	7.0
aerobic (vigorously)		6.0	6.3	6.7	7.0	7.3	7.6	7.9	8.2	8.5	8.8	9.1	9.4

Source: From Williams, Melvin H., *Nutrition for Fitness and Sport*. © 1983 Wm. C. Brown Publishers, Dubuque, Iowa. All Rights Rese Reprinted by permission.

| 73 | 75 | 77 | 80 | 82 | 84 | 86 | 89 | 91 | 93 | 95 | 98 | 100 |
160	165	170	175	180	185	190	195	200	205	210	215	220
1.6	1.6	1.7	1.7	1.8	1.8	1.9	1.9	2.0	2.0	2.1	2.1	2.2
2.0	2.1	2.2	2.2	2.3	2.4	2.4	2.5	2.5	2.6	2.7	2.7	2.8
4.4	4.5	4.6	4.8	4.9	5.0	5.2	5.3	5.4	5.6	5.7	5.9	6.0
5.1	5.3	5.4	5.6	5.7	5.9	6.0	6.2	6.4	6.5	6.7	6.9	7.0
5.8	6.0	6.2	6.4	6.6	6.7	6.9	7.1	7.3	7.4	7.6	7.8	8.0
4.4	4.5	4.6	4.8	4.9	5.0	5.2	5.3	5.4	5.6	5.7	5.9	6.0
9.4	9.7	10.0	10.3	10.6	10.9	11.2	11.5	11.8	12.1	12.4	12.7	13.0
5.0	5.2	5.3	5.5	5.6	5.8	5.9	6.1	6.3	6.4	6.6	6.8	6.9
6.3	6.5	6.7	6.9	7.1	7.3	7.4	7.7	7.9	8.0	8.2	8.5	8.6
4.8	5.0	5.1	5.3	5.4	5.6	5.7	5.9	6.0	6.2	6.4	6.5	6.7
8.0	8.2	8.5	8.7	9.0	9.2	9.5	9.7	10.0	10.2	10.5	10.7	11.0
10.5	10.9	11.2	11.5	11.9	12.2	12.5	12.9	13.2	13.5	13.8	14.2	14.5
3.1	3.2	3.3	3.4	3.5	3.6	3.7	3.8	3.9	4.0	4.1	4.2	4.3
4.3	4.4	4.6	4.7	4.9	5.0	5.1	5.3	5.4	5.5	5.7	5.8	6.0
5.5	5.7	5.9	6.1	6.3	6.4	6.6	6.8	6.9	7.1	7.3	7.5	7.7
6.8	7.0	7.2	7.4	7.6	7.9	8.1	8.3	8.5	8.7	8.9	9.1	9.4
8.0	8.3	8.5	8.8	9.0	9.3	9.5	9.8	10.0	10.3	10.6	10.8	11.1
9.3	9.5	9.8	10.1	10.4	10.7	11.0	11.3	11.6	11.9	12.2	12.5	12.8
10.9	11.3	11.6	12.0	12.3	12.6	13.0	13.3	13.7	14.0	14.4	14.7	15.0
4.4	4.5	4.6	4.8	4.9	5.0	5.2	5.3	5.5	5.6	5.7	5.9	6.0
5.5	5.7	5.9	6.1	6.3	6.4	6.6	6.8	7.0	7.1	7.3	7.5	7.7
15.6	16.1	16.6	17.1	17.6	18.1	18.6	19.1	19.6	20.0	20.5	21.0	21.5
3.1	3.2	3.3	3.4	3.5	3.6	3.7	3.8	3.9	4.0	4.1	4.2	4.3
7.1	7.4	7.6	7.8	8.0	8.2	8.5	8.7	8.9	9.1	9.4	9.6	9.8
9.3	9.5	9.8	10.1	10.4	10.7	11.0	11.3	11.6	11.9	12.2	12.5	12.8
5.1	5.3	5.4	5.6	5.7	5.9	6.0	6.2	6.4	6.5	6.7	6.9	7.0
7.3	7.5	7.7	7.9	8.2	8.4	8.6	8.9	9.1	9.3	9.5	9.8	10.0
9.7	10.0	10.3	10.6	10.9	11.2	11.5	11.8	12.1	12.4	12.7	13.0	13.3

Body Weight

		Kg	45	48	50	52	55	57	59	61	64	66	68	70
		Pounds	100	105	110	115	120	125	130	135	140	145	150	155
fencing														
	moderately		3.3	3.5	3.6	3.8	4.0	4.1	4.3	4.5	4.6	4.8	5.0	5.2
	vigorously		6.6	7.0	7.3	7.7	8.0	8.3	8.7	9.0	9.4	9.7	10.0	10.4
field hockey			5.0	6.3	6.7	7.0	7.3	7.6	7.9	8.2	8.5	8.8	9.1	9.4
football														
	moderate		3.3	3.5	3.6	3.8	4.0	4.1	4.3	4.5	4.6	4.8	5.0	5.2
	touch, vigorous		5.5	5.8	6.1	6.4	6.6	6.9	7.2	7.5	7.8	8.0	8.3	8.6
golf														
	2-some (carry clubs)		3.6	3.8	4.0	4.2	4.4	4.6	4.7	4.9	5.1	5.3	5.4	5.6
	4-some (carry clubs)		2.7	2.9	3.0	3.1	3.3	3.4	3.5	3.7	3.8	3.9	4.1	4.2
	power cart		1.9	2.0	2.1	2.2	2.3	2.4	2.5	2.6	2.7	2.8	2.9	3.0
handball														
	moderate		6.5	6.8	7.2	7.5	7.8	8.2	8.5	8.8	9.2	9.5	9.9	10.2
	competitive		7.7	8.0	8.4	8.8	9.2	9.6	10.0	10.4	10.8	11.1	11.5	11.9
hiking, pack (3 MPH)			4.5	4.7	5.0	5.2	5.4	5.6	5.9	6.1	6.3	6.6	6.8	7.0
hockey, ice			6.6	7.0	7.3	7.7	8.0	8.3	8.7	9.0	9.4	9.7	10.0	10.4
horseback riding														
	walk		1.9	2.0	2.1	2.2	2.3	2.4	2.5	2.6	2.7	2.8	2.9	3.0
	sitting to trot		2.7	2.9	3.0	3.1	3.3	3.4	3.5	3.7	3.8	3.9	4.1	4.2
	posting to trot		4.2	4.4	4.6	4.8	5.1	5.3	5.5	5.7	5.9	6.1	6.4	6.6
	gallop		5.7	6.0	6.3	6.6	6.9	7.2	7.5	7.8	8.1	8.4	8.7	9.0
horseshoes			2.5	2.6	2.8	2.9	3.0	3.1	3.3	3.4	3.5	3.7	3.8	3.9
jogging (see running)														
judo			8.5	8.9	9.3	9.8	10.2	10.6	11.0	11.5	11.9	12.3	12.8	13.2
karate			8.5	8.9	9.3	9.8	10.2	10.6	11.0	11.5	11.9	12.3	12.8	13.2
mountain climbing			6.5	6.8	7.2	7.5	7.8	8.2	8.5	8.8	9.2	9.5	9.8	10.2
paddle ball			5.7	6.0	6.3	6.6	6.9	7.2	7.5	7.8	8.1	8.4	8.7	9.0
pool (billiards)			1.5	1.6	1.6	1.7	1.8	1.9	1.9	2.0	2.1	2.2	2.2	2.3
racketball			6.5	6.8	7.1	7.5	7.8	8.1	8.4	8.8	9.1	9.4	9.8	10.1
roller skating (9 MPH)			4.2	4.4	4.6	4.8	5.1	5.3	5.5	5.7	5.9	6.1	6.4	6.6
running (steady state)														
(MPH)	(Min/mile)													
5.0	12:00		6.0	6.3	6.6	7.0	7.3	7.6	7.9	8.2	8.5	8.8	9.1	9.4
5.5	10:55		6.7	7.0	7.3	7.7	8.0	8.4	8.7	9.0	9.4	9.7	10.0	10.4
6.0	10:00		7.2	7.6	8.0	8.4	8.7	9.1	9.5	9.8	10.2	10.6	10.9	11.3
7.0	8:35		8.5	8.9	9.3	9.0	10.2	10.6	11.0	11.5	11.9	12.3	12.8	13.2
8.0	7:30		9.7	10.2	10.7	11.2	11.6	12.1	12.6	13.1	13.6	14.1	14.6	15.1
9.0	6:40		10.8	11.3	11.9	12.4	12.9	13.5	14.0	14.6	15.1	15.7	16.2	16.8
10.0	6:00		12.1	12.7	13.3	13.9	14.5	15.1	15.7	16.4	17.0	17.6	18.2	18.8
11.0	5:28		13.3	14.0	14.6	15.3	16.0	16.7	17.3	18.0	18.7	19.4	20.0	20.7
12.0	5:00		14.5	15.2	16.0	16.7	17.4	18.2	18.9	19.7	20.4	21.1	21.9	22.6
sailing, small boat			2.7	2.9	3.0	3.1	3.3	3.4	3.5	3.7	3.8	3.9	4.1	4.2
skating, ice (9 MPH)			4.2	4.4	4.6	4.8	5.1	5.2	5.5	5.7	5.9	6.1	6.4	6.6

73 160	75 165	77 170	80 175	82 180	84 185	86 190	89 195	91 200	93 205	95 210	98 215	100 220
5.3	5.5	5.7	5.8	6.0	6.2	6.3	6.5	6.7	6.8	7.0	7.1	7.3
10.7	11.0	11.4	11.7	12.1	12.4	12.7	13.1	13.4	13.8	14.1	14.4	14.8
9.7	10.0	10.3	10.6	10.9	11.2	11.5	11.8	12.1	12.4	12.7	13.0	13.3
5.3	5.5	5.7	5.8	6.0	6.2	6.3	6.5	6.7	6.8	7.0	7.1	7.3
8.9	9.2	9.4	9.7	10.0	10.3	10.6	10.8	11.1	11.4	11.7	12.0	12.2
5.8	6.0	6.2	6.4	6.6	6.7	6.9	7.1	7.3	7.4	7.6	7.8	8.0
4.4	4.5	4.6	4.8	4.9	5.0	5.2	5.3	5.4	5.6	5.7	5.9	6.0
3.1	3.2	3.3	3.4	3.5	3.6	3.7	3.8	3.9	4.0	4.1	4.2	4.3
10.5	10.9	11.2	11.5	11.9	12.2	12.5	12.9	13.2	13.5	13.8	14.2	14.5
12.3	12.7	13.1	13.5	13.9	14.3	14.7	15.0	15.4	15.8	16.2	16.6	17.0
7.3	7.5	7.7	7.9	8.2	8.4	8.6	8.9	9.1	9.3	9.5	9.8	10.0
10.7	11.0	11.4	11.7	12.1	12.4	12.7	13.1	13.4	13.8	14.1	14.4	14.8
3.1	3.2	3.3	3.4	3.5	3.6	3.7	3.8	3.9	4.0	4.1	4.2	4.3
4.4	4.5	4.6	4.8	4.9	5.0	5.2	5.3	5.4	5.6	5.7	5.9	6.0
6.8	7.0	7.2	7.4	7.6	7.9	8.1	8.3	8.5	8.7	8.9	9.1	9.4
9.3	9.5	9.8	10.1	10.4	10.7	11.0	11.3	11.6	11.9	12.2	12.5	12.8
4.0	4.2	4.3	4.4	4.5	4.7	4.8	4.9	5.2	5.2	5.3	5.4	5.6
13.6	14.1	14.5	14.9	15.4	15.8	16.2	16.6	17.1	17.5	17.9	18.4	18.8
13.6	14.1	14.5	14.9	15.4	15.8	16.2	16.6	17.1	17.5	17.9	18.4	18.8
10.5	10.8	11.2	11.5	11.8	12.1	12.5	12.8	13.1	13.5	13.8	14.1	14.5
9.3	9.5	9.8	10.1	10.4	10.7	11.0	11.2	11.6	11.9	12.2	12.5	12.8
2.4	2.5	2.6	2.6	2.7	2.8	2.9	2.9	3.0	3.1	3.2	3.2	3.3
10.4	10.7	11.1	11.4	11.7	12.0	12.4	12.7	13.0	13.4	13.7	14.0	14.4
6.8	7.0	7.2	7.4	7.6	7.9	8.1	8.3	8.5	8.7	8.9	9.1	9.4
9.7	10.0	10.3	10.6	10.9	11.2	11.6	11.9	12.2	12.5	12.8	13.1	13.4
10.7	11.1	11.4	11.7	12.1	12.4	12.8	13.1	13.4	13.8	14.1	14.5	14.8
11.7	12.0	12.4	12.8	13.1	13.5	13.8	14.3	14.6	15.0	15.4	15.7	16.1
13.6	14.1	14.5	14.9	15.4	15.8	16.2	16.6	17.1	17.5	17.9	18.4	18.8
15.6	16.1	16.6	17.1	17.6	18.1	18.5	19.0	18.5	20.0	20.5	21.0	21.5
17.3	17.9	18.4	19.0	19.5	20.1	20.6	21.2	21.7	22.2	22.8	23.3	23.9
19.4	20.0	20.7	21.3	21.9	22.5	23.1	23.7	24.2	24.8	25.4	26.0	26.7
21.4	22.1	22.7	23.4	24.1	24.8	25.4	26.1	26.8	27.5	28.1	28.8	29.5
23.3	24.1	24.8	25.6	26.3	27.0	27.8	28.5	29.2	30.0	30.7	31.5	32.2
4.4	4.5	4.6	4.8	4.9	5.0	5.2	5.3	5.4	5.6	5.7	5.9	6.0
6.8	7.0	7.2	7.4	7.6	7.9	8.1	8.3	8.5	8.7	8.9	9.1	9.4

Body Weight

Kg		45	48	50	52	55	57	59	61	64	66	68	70
Pounds		100	105	110	115	120	125	130	135	140	145	150	155
skiing, cross-country													
(MPH)	(Min/mile)												
2.5	24:00	5.0	5.2	5.5	5.7	6.0	6.2	6.5	6.7	7.0	7.2	7.5	7.8
4.0	15:00	6.5	6.8	7.2	7.5	7.8	8.2	8.5	8.8	9.2	9.5	9.9	10.2
5.0	12:00	7.7	8.0	8.4	8.8	9.2	9.6	10.0	10.4	10.8	11.1	11.5	11.9
skiing, downhill		6.5	6.8	7.2	7.5	7.8	8.2	8.5	8.8	9.2	9.5	9.9	10.2
soccer		5.9	6.2	6.6	6.9	7.2	7.5	7.8	8.1	8.4	8.7	9.0	9.3
squash													
normal		6.7	7.0	7.3	7.7	8.0	8.4	8.7	9.1	9.5	9.8	10.1	10.5
competition		7.7	8.0	8.4	8.8	9.2	9.6	10.0	10.4	10.8	11.1	11.5	11.9
swimming (Yards/min)													
backstroke													
25		2.5	2.6	2.8	2.9	3.0	3.1	3.3	3.4	3.5	3.7	3.8	3.9
30		3.5	3.7	3.9	4.1	4.2	4.4	4.6	4.8	4.9	5.1	5.3	5.5
35		4.5	4.7	5.0	5.2	5.4	5.6	5.9	6.1	6.3	6.6	6.8	7.0
40		5.5	5.8	6.1	6.4	6.6	6.9	7.2	7.5	7.8	8.0	8.3	8.6
breaststroke													
20		3.1	3.3	3.5	3.6	3.8	4.0	4.1	4.3	4.5	4.6	4.8	4.9
30		4.7	5.0	5.2	5.4	5.7	5.9	6.2	6.4	6.7	6.9	7.1	7.4
40		6.3	6.7	7.0	7.3	7.6	8.0	8.3	8.6	8.9	9.3	9.6	9.9
front crawl													
20		3.1	3.3	3.5	3.6	3.8	4.0	4.1	4.3	4.5	4.6	4.8	4.9
25		4.0	4.2	4.4	4.6	4.8	5.0	5.2	5.4	5.6	5.8	6.0	6.2
35		4.8	5.1	5.4	5.6	5.9	6.1	6.4	6.6	6.8	7.0	7.3	7.5
45		5.7	6.0	6.3	6.6	6.9	7.2	7.5	7.8	8.1	8.4	8.7	9.0
50		7.0	7.4	7.7	8.1	8.5	8.8	9.2	9.5	9.9	10.3	10.6	11.0
table tennis		3.4	3.6	3.8	4.0	4.1	4.3	4.5	4.7	4.8	5.0	5.2	5.4
tennis													
singles, recreational		5.0	5.2	5.5	5.7	6.0	6.2	6.5	6.7	7.0	7.2	7.5	7.8
doubles, recreational		3.4	3.6	3.8	4.0	4.1	4.3	4.5	4.7	4.8	5.0	5.2	5.4
competition		6.4	6.7	7.1	7.4	7.7	8.1	8.4	8.7	9.1	9.4	9.8	10.1
volleyball													
moderate, recreational		2.9	3.0	3.2	3.3	3.5	3.6	3.8	3.9	4.1	4.2	4.4	4.5
vigorous, competition		6.5	6.8	7.1	7.5	7.8	8.1	8.4	8.8	9.1	9.4	9.8	10.1

| 73 | 75 | 77 | 80 | 82 | 84 | 86 | 89 | 91 | 93 | 95 | 98 | 100 |
160	165	170	175	180	185	190	195	200	205	210	215	220
8.0	8.3	8.5	8.8	9.0	9.3	9.5	9.8	10.0	10.3	10.6	10.8	11.1
10.5	10.9	11.2	11.5	11.9	12.2	12.5	12.9	13.2	13.5	13.8	14.2	14.5
12.3	12.7	13.1	13.5	13.9	14.3	13.7	15.0	15.4	15.8	16.2	16.6	17.0
10.5	10.9	11.2	11.5	11.9	12.2	12.5	12.9	13.2	13.5	13.8	14.2	14.5
9.6	9.9	10.2	10.5	10.8	11.1	11.4	11.7	12.0	12.3	12.6	12.9	13.2
10.8	11.2	11.5	11.8	12.2	12.5	12.9	13.2	13.5	13.9	14.2	14.6	14.9
12.3	12.7	13.1	13.5	13.9	14.3	14.7	15.0	15.4	15.8	16.2	16.6	17.0
4.0	4.2	4.3	4.4	4.5	4.7	4.8	4.9	5.1	5.2	5.3	5.4	5.6
5.6	5.8	6.0	6.2	6.4	6.5	6.7	6.9	7.1	7.2	7.4	7.6	7.8
7.3	7.5	7.7	7.9	8.2	8.4	8.6	8.9	9.1	9.3	9.5	9.8	10.0
8.9	9.2	9.4	9.7	10.0	10.3	10.6	10.8	11.1	11.4	11.7	12.0	12.2
5.1	5.3	5.4	5.6	5.7	5.9	6.0	6.2	6.4	6.5	6.7	6.9	7.0
7.6	7.9	8.1	8.3	8.6	8.8	9.1	9.3	9.5	9.8	10.0	10.3	10.5
10.2	10.5	10.9	11.2	11.5	11.9	12.2	12.5	12.8	13.1	13.5	13.8	14.1
5.1	5.3	5.4	5.6	5.7	5.9	6.0	6.2	6.4	6.5	6.7	6.9	7.0
6.4	6.6	6.8	7.0	7.2	7.4	7.6	7.8	8.0	8.2	8.4	8.6	8.8
7.8	8.0	8.3	8.5	8.8	9.0	9.2	9.4	9.7	9.9	10.2	10.4	10.7
9.3	9.5	9.8	10.1	10.4	10.7	11.0	11.3	11.6	11.9	12.2	12.5	12.8
11.3	11.7	12.0	12.4	12.8	13.1	13.5	13.8	14.2	14.5	14.9	15.2	15.6
5.5	5.7	5.9	6.1	6.3	6.4	6.6	6.8	7.0	7.1	7.3	7.5	7.7
8.0	8.3	8.5	8.8	9.0	9.3	9.5	9.8	10.0	10.3	10.6	10.8	11.1
5.5	5.7	5.9	6.1	6.3	6.4	6.6	6.8	7.0	7.1	7.3	7.5	7.7
10.4	10.8	11.1	11.4	11.8	12.1	12.4	12.8	13.1	13.4	13.7	14.1	14.4
4.7	4.8	5.0	5.1	5.3	5.4	5.6	5.7	5.9	6.0	6.1	6.3	6.4
10.4	10.7	11.1	11.4	11.7	12.0	12.4	12.7	13.0	13.4	13.7	14.0	14.4

Glossary

abdominal and low back-hamstring musculoskeletal function The concept that optimal strength and flexibility of the abdominal muscles, the muscles in the low back area, and the hamstring muscles will help to prevent the low back pain syndrome.

acclimatization The ability of the body to undergo physiological adaptations so that the stress of a given environment, such as high environmental temperature, is less severe.

acetaldehyde An intermediate breakdown product of alcohol.

acetyl CoA The major fuel for the oxidative processes in the body. It is derived from the breakdown of glucose and fatty acids.

Achilles tendinitis An inflammation in the Achilles tendon in the lower back portion of the leg.

acute muscular soreness The muscle soreness, or pain, that may occur during a very strenuous exercise bout. It is usually temporary. Compare to delayed muscle soreness.

additives Substances added to food to improve color, texture, stability, or for similar purposes.

adenosinetriphosphate *See* ATP.

ADH The antidiuretic hormone secreted by the pituitary gland; its major action is to conserve body water by decreasing urine formation.

adrenalin A hormone secreted by the adrenal medulla gland; it is a stimulant and prepares the body for "fight or flight."

adult-onset obesity Obesity that occurs during adulthood, usually the hypertrophy-type obesity. *See also* creeping obesity.

aerobic Relating to energy processes that occur in the presence of oxygen.

aerobic capacity The capacity of the individual to utilize oxygen to produce energy. *See also* VO_2 max.

aerobic exercise The term coined by Dr. Kenneth Cooper to mean those exercise activities that use the oxygen system in order to improve the health of the cardio-vascular-respiratory system.

aerobic walking Rapid walking designed to elevate the HR so that a training effect would occur; more strenuous than ordinary leisure walking.

alanine A nonessential amino acid.

alcohol A colorless liquid with depressant effects; ethyl alcohol (or ethanol) is the alcohol designed for human consumption.

aldosterone The main electrolyte-regulating hormone secreted by the adrenal cortex; primarily controls sodium and potassium balance.

alpha-tocopherol The most biologically active alcohol in vitamin E.

alveoli The tiny air sacs in the lungs where the exchange of gases between the blood and the lungs takes place.

amenorrhea Cessation or abnormal stoppage of normal menstrual blood flow.

amino acids The chief structural material of protein, consisting of an amino group (NH_2) and an acid group (COOH) plus other components.

amino group The nitrogen-containing component of amino acids (NH_2).

aminostatic theory A theory suggesting that hunger is controlled by the presence or absence of amino acids in the blood acting upon a receptor in the hypothalamus.

anabolic steroids Drugs designed to mimic the actions of testosterone to build muscle tissue (anabolism) while minimizing the androgenic effects (masculinization).

anabolism Constructive metabolism, the process whereby simple body compounds are formed into more complex ones.

anaerobic Relating to energy processes that occur in the absence of oxygen.

anemia In general, below normal levels of circulating RBCs and hemoglobin; there are many different types of anemia.

anorexia nervosa A serious eating disorder, particularly among teenage girls, marked by a loss of appetite and leading to various degrees of emaciation.

antidiuretic hormone *See* ADH.

apoplexy *See* stroke.

appetite A pleasant desire for food for the purpose of enjoyment that is developed through previous experience; controlled in humans by an appetite center, or appestat, in the hypothalamus.

arteriosclerosis Hardening of the arteries. *See also* atherosclerosis.

artery The major blood vessels that transport blood away from the heart to various parts of the body.

arthritis An inflammation in the joints between bones.

ascorbic acid Vitamin C.

assertiveness The quality of being assertive and positive, or expressing your feelings honestly and openly to others.

atherosclerosis A specific form of arteriosclerosis characterized by the formation of plaque on the inner layers of the arterial wall.

ATP Adenosinetriphosphate, a high-energy phosphate compound found in the body; one of the major forms of energy available for immediate use in the body.

ATP-PC system The energy system for fast, powerful muscle contractions; uses ATP as the immediate energy source, the spent ATP being quickly regenerated by breakdown of the PC. ATP and PC are high energy phosphates in the muscle cell.

autogenic relaxation A technique to induce relaxation in which you attempt to relax specific body parts in a set sequence, such as starting with the muscles in the head and progressing to the feet.

BAL Blood alcohol level; the concentration of alcohol in the blood.

ballistic A rapid motion, often used in conjunction with flexibility exercises, in which the muscle is stretched rapidly.

basal metabolic rate *See* BMR.

Basic Four Food Groups Grouping of foods into four categories that can be used as a means to educate individuals how to obtain essential nutrients. The four groups are meat, milk, bread-cereals, and fruit-vegetable.

behavior modification Relative to weight-control methods, personal behavioral patterns may be modified to help achieve weight loss.

Benson's relaxation response A meditation technique used for relaxation purposes; similar to Transcendental Meditation.

bile A fluid secreted into the intestine by the liver that aids in the breakdown process of fats.

biotin A component of the B complex.

blood alcohol level *See* BAL.

blood glucose Blood sugar; the means by which carbohydrate is carried in the blood; normal range is 70–120 mg/ml.

blood pressure The pressure of the blood in the various blood vessels; usually means arterial blood pressure. *See also* systolic blood pressure and diastolic blood pressure.

BMR The basal metabolic rate; measurement of energy expenditure in the body under resting, post-absorptive conditions; indicative of the energy needed to maintain life under these basal conditions.

body building A sport designed to increase muscle size and definition for aesthetic competition; weight training is the primary mode of training.

body composition The analysis of the body into two primary components,— body fat and lean body mass. Body mass is primarily muscle and bone tissue.

body image The image or impression the individual has of his or her body. A poor body image may lead to personality problems.

caffeine A stimulant drug found in many food products such as coffee, tea, and colas; stimulates the central nervous system.

calciferol A synthetic form of vitamin D, vitamin D_2.

calcium A silver-white metallic element essential to human nutrition.

caloric concept of weight control The concept that Calories are the basis of weight control. Excess Calories will add body weight while caloric deficiencies will contribute to weight loss.

Calorie A Calorie is a measure of heat energy. A small calorie represents the amount of heat needed to raise one gram of water one degree Celsius. A large Calorie (kilocalorie, KC, or C) is 1,000 small calories.

calorimeter A device used to measure the caloric value of a given food or to measure heat production of animals or man.

capillary The smallest blood vessels in the body where nutrients, gases, and waste products are exchanged between the blood and the tissues.

carbohydrate A group of compounds containing carbon, hydrogen, and oxygen. Glucose, glycogen, sugar, starches, fiber, cellulose, and the various saccharides are all carbohydrates.

carbohydrate loading A dietary method utilized by endurance-oriented athletes to help increase the carbohydrate (glycogen) levels in their muscles and liver.

cardiac output The amount of blood pumped by the heart per minute.

cardiovascular endurance The ability of the cardiovascular system to provide sufficient energy to sustain aerobic exercise for prolonged periods of time. *See also* aerobic exercise.

catabolism Destructive metabolism whereby complex chemical compounds in the body are degraded to simpler compounds.

cellulose The fibrous carbohydrate that provides the structural backbone for plants; plant fiber.

central circulation The role of the heart, or center, in pumping blood to the periphery. *See also* peripheral circulation.

cerebral thrombosis A blood clot in a cerebral artery. *See also* stroke.

cerebral vascular accident A stroke caused by a thrombus in a cerebral artery.

CHD Coronary heart disease; a degenerative disease of the heart caused primarily by arteriosclerosis or atherosclerosis of the coronary vessels of the heart.

chloride A compound of chlorine present in a salt form carrying a negative charge; Cl^-.

cholesterol A fatlike pearly substance, an alcohol, found in all animal fats and oils; a main constituent of some body tissues and body compounds.

chromium A whitish metal essential to human nutrition; it is involved in carbohydrate metabolism via its role with insulin.

chronic diseases Diseases that develop over prolonged periods of time, such as coronary heart disease and lung cancer. (A Positive Health Life-style may help to retard their development.)

chronic training effect Repeated bouts of exercise will elicit physiological changes in the body that will help make the body more efficient during exercise.

cirrhosis A degenerative disease of the liver; one cause is excessive consumption of alcohol.

cobalamin The cobalt-containing complex common to all members of the vitamin B_{12} group; often used to designate cyanocobalamin.

cobalt A gray, hard metal that is a component of vitamin B_{12}.

coenzyme An activator of an enzyme; many vitamins are coenzymes.

collateral circulation A secondary or accessory blood vessel, such as a small side branch that may develop from a primary vessel.

complex carbohydrates A term used to describe foods high in starch (bread, cereals, fruits, and vegetables) as contrasted with simple carbohydrates such as table sugar.

conduction In relation to body temperature, the transfer of heat from one substance to another by direct contact.

congenital heart disease Certain heart defects that are present at birth.

convection In relation to body temperature, the transfer of heat via currents in either the air or water.

copper A reddish metallic element essential to human nutrition; it functions with iron in the formation of hemoglobin and cytochromes.

core temperature The temperature of the deep tissues of the body, usually measured orally or rectally.

coronary arteries The arteries that supply blood to the heart muscle.

coronary artery disease A narrowing of the coronary arteries. *See also* arteriosclerosis and atherosclerosis.

coronary heart disease *See* CHD.

coronary occlusion A blockage of blood supply in a coronary artery.

coronary risk factors The behaviors (smoking) or body properties (cholesterol levels) that may predispose an individual to coronary heart disease.

coronary thrombosis A clot in a coronary artery that may lead to a coronary occlusion.

creeping obesity A gradual accumulation of body fat, possibly over several years, that leads to obesity. *See also* adult-onset obesity.

curl-up An abdominal exercise similar to a sit-up, but the individual sits up only part way, about 30 degrees from the floor.

cyanocobalamin Vitamin B_{12}.

dehydration A reduction of the body water to below the normal level of hydration; water output exceeds water intake.

delayed muscle soreness Muscle soreness or pain that develops a day or two after a severe exercise bout and usually involves eccentric muscle contractions.

diabetes mellitus A disorder of carbohydrate metabolism due to inadequate production of insulin; results in high blood glucose levels and loss of sugar in the urine.

diastolic blood pressure The blood pressure in the arteries when the heart is at rest between beats.

diet The food consumed to obtain essential nutrients. A balanced diet will provide adequate nutrition. Adjectives may be used to describe specific diets, e.g., low-Calorie diet, diabetic diet, etc.

dietary fiber Fiber in plant foods that cannot be hydrolyzed by the digestive enzymes.

disuse phenomena The degeneration that may occur in various body tissues or systems when they are not used; lack of exercise may result in certain pathological effects in some body tissues.

DNA Deoxyribonucleic acid; a complex protein, found in chromosomes, that is the carrier of genetic information and the basis of heredity.

duration concept One of the major concepts of aerobic exercise; duration refers to the amount of time spent exercising during each bout.

dynamic flexibility Flexibility exercises that involve rapid, bouncing movements to stretch a particular muscle group.

dysmenorrhea Painful cramps during the menstrual flow period.

early-onset obesity Obesity that develops early in life, as early as the first year of life or even at puberty. May often be a hyperplasia-type obesity.

eccentric muscle contraction A lengthening muscle contraction in which the muscle is trying to shorten, but the outside force is greater, causing the muscle to lengthen.

ECG The electrocardiogram, a measure of the electrical activity of the heart.

electrolytes A solution that contains ions and can conduct electricity; often the ions of salts such as sodium and chloride are called electrolytes. *See also* ions.

embolus A blood clot that travels freely in the bloodstream.

EMR Exercise metabolic rate; an increased metabolic rate due to the need for increased energy production during exercise; the BMR may be increased more than twenty-fold.

endorphins Naturally occurring chemicals produced in the brain that resemble narcotic drugs and may help reduce pain.

energy The ability to do work; energy exists in various forms, notably mechanical, heat, and chemical forms in the human body.

energy balance The concept that weight control is a measure of energy, or caloric, balance. *See also* positive and negative energy balance.

enzyme A complex protein in the body that serves as a catalyst, facilitating reactions between various substances without being changed itself.

epidemiology A science that investigates the relationship between various factors and the prevalence of a disease or other physiological condition in a given population.

essential amino acids Those amino acids that must be obtained in the diet and cannot be synthesized in the body.

essential fat Fat in the body that is an essential part of the tissues, such as cell membrane structure, nerve coverings, and the brain. *See also* storage fat.

essential fatty acid The unsaturated fatty acid that may not be synthesized in the body and must be obtained in the diet; linoleic fatty acid.

essential nutrients Those nutrients found to be essential to human life and optimal functioning.

estrogen The female sex hormones responsible for the development of secondary sexual characteristics and the various phases of the menstrual cycle.

ethanol Alcohol; ethyl alcohol.

ethyl alcohol Alcohol; ethanol.

evaporation The conversion of a liquid to a vapor that consumes energy; evaporation of sweat cools the body by using body heat as the energy source.

exercise ECG stress test An exercise test usually administered on a treadmill. The ECG is recorded to determine if any pathological condition is present in the heart, to derive information for an exercise prescription, and to determine present fitness level.

exercise frequency In an aerobic exercise program, the number of times per week that an individual exercises.

exercise intensity The tempo, speed, or resistance of an exercise. Intensity can be increased by working faster, doing more work in a given amount of time.

exercise metabolic rate *See* EMR.

fasting Starvation; abstinence from eating that may be partial or complete.

fast-twitch fibers Muscle fibers characterized by high contractile speed.

fatigue A generalized or specific feeling of tiredness that may have a multitude of causes; may be mental or physical.

fats Triglycerides; a combination, or ester, of three fatty acids and glycerol.

fatty acids Any one of a number of aliphatic acids containing only carbon, oxygen, and hydrogen; they may be saturated or unsaturated.

feeding center A collection of nerve cells in the hypothalamus that are involved in the control of feeding reflexes.

FFA Free fatty acids; formed by the hydrolysis of triglycerides.

fiber In general, the indigestible carbohydrate in plants that forms the structural network. *See also* cellulose.

fibrin A protein, formed in the blood, that is involved in the blood clotting process.

flexibility A measure of the range of motion of a given joint in the body; usually a measure of the flexibility or elasticity of the soft tissues such as muscles and tendons.

fluoride A salt of hydrofluoric acid; a compound of fluorine that may be helpful in the prevention of dental decay.

folacin Folic acid.

folic acid A water-soluble vitamin that appears to be essential in preventing certain types of anemia.

food additives *See* additives.

Food Exchange Lists A grouping of foods into six different exchange lists; foods in each list are similar in caloric value and carbohydrate, fat, and protein content.

free fatty acids *See* FFA.

fructose A monosaccharide known also as levulose or fruit sugar; found in all sweet fruits.

genetics The science or study of heredity and the differences or similarities among organisms.

glucose A monosaccharide; a thick, sweet, syrupy liquid.

glucose intolerance An inability to metabolize glucose properly; usually determined by a glucose tolerance test.

glycogen A polysaccharide that is the chief storage form of carbohydrate in animals; it is stored primarily in the liver and muscles.

glycogen sparing effect The theory that certain dietary techniques, such as the utilization of caffeine, may facilitate the oxidation of fatty acids for energy and thus spare the utilization of glycogen.

glycolysis The degradation of sugars into smaller compounds; the main quantitative anaerobic energy process in the muscle tissue.

hamstrings The three muscles in the posterior portion of the thigh.

HDL cholesterol High density lipoprotein cholesterol; one mechanism whereby cholesterol is transported in the blood. (High HDL levels are somewhat protective against CHD.)

heat cramps Painful muscular cramps or tetanus following prolonged exercise in a hot environment without water or salt replacement.

heat exhaustion Weakness or dizziness from overexertion in a hot environment.

heat stroke Elevated body temperature of 106°F or greater caused by exposure to excessive heat gains or production and diminished heat loss.

heat syncope Fainting caused by excessive heat exposure.

height-weight charts Charts that use combinations of height and weight to determine if an individual is overweight or underweight.

hemoglobin The protein-iron pigment in the red blood cells that transports oxygen.

hernia The protrusion of some body tissue through a weakened wall of the cavity within which it is normally contained.

high blood pressure *See* hypertension.

high density lipoprotein A protein-lipid complex in the blood that facilitates the transport of triglycerides, cholesterol, and phospholipids. *See* HDL cholesterol.

hip flexion Bending over at the waist or raising the thigh forward.

histidine An essential amino acid for children.

homeostasis A term used to describe a condition of normalcy in the internal body environment.

hormones A chemical substance produced by specific body cells, secreted into the blood, and then acting on some specific target tissues.

HR max The normal maximal heart rate of an individual during exercise.

hunger A basic physiological desire to eat that is normally caused by a lack of food; may be accompanied by stomach contractions.

hydrogenated fats Fats to which hydrogen has been added, usually causing them to be saturated.

hypercholesteremia Elevated blood cholesterol levels.

hyperglycemia Elevated blood glucose levels.

hyperplasia An increased number of cells.

hyperplasia-type obesity Obesity that is caused by an increased number of fat cells.

hypertension A condition with various causes whereby the blood pressure is higher than normal.

hypertriglyceridemia Elevated blood levels of triglycerides.

hypertrophy An enlargement of cells.

hypertrophy-type obesity Obesity that is caused by an increased size of fat cells.

hypoglycemia A low blood sugar level.

hypohydration Dehydration; a state of decreased water content in the body.

hypothalamus A part of the brain involved in the control of involuntary activity in the body; contains many centers for neural control such as temperature, hunger, appetite, and thirst.

imagery A relaxation technique whereby a relaxing image is created in the mind to help reduce stress.

insensible perspiration Perspiration on the skin that is not detectable by ordinary senses.

insulin A hormone secreted by the pancreas involved in carbohydrate metabolism.

insulin-dependent diabetes Diabetes in which insulin is required to help control it. Most common in juvenile-onset diabetes.

insulin response Blood insulin levels rise following the ingestion of sugar and the resultant hyperglycemia; the insulin causes the sugar to be taken up by the muscles and liver, possibly creating a reactive hypoglycemia.

International Unit *See* IU.

interval training A form of training that involves repeated bouts of exercise with intervals of rest between each repetition.

inverted-U hypothesis The hypothesis that both too much and too little anxiety will lead to inferior performance levels.

iodine A nonmetallic element that is necessary for the proper development and functioning of the thyroid gland.

ions Particles with an electrical charge; anions are negative and cations are positive.

iron A metallic element essential for the development of several chemical compounds in the body, notably hemoglobin.

iron deficiency anemia Anemia caused by an inadequate intake or absorption of iron, resulting in impaired hemoglobin formation.

isokinetic Meaning same speed, or a muscle contraction in which the speed of movement is controlled.

isoleucine An essential amino acid.

isometric Meaning same length, or a muscle contraction in which very little or no movement occurs.

isotonic Meaning same tension, or a muscle contraction in which the same tension is developed through a range of motion.

IU International Unit; a method of expressing the quantity of some substance (such as vitamins) that is an internationally developed and accepted standard.

jogging A term used to designate slow running; although the distinction between running and jogging is relative to the individual involved, a common value used for jogging is a 9 minute mile or slower.

juvenile-onset diabetes Diabetes that occurs at a young age; now known as insulin-dependent diabetes.

KC Kilocalorie or KCAL. *See* Calorie.

key nutrient concept The concept that if certain key nutrients are adequately supplied by the diet, the other essential nutrients will also be present in adequate amounts.

kilocalorie A large Calorie. *See* Calorie.

kilogram A unit of mass in the metric system; in ordinary terms, 1 kilogram is the equivalent of 2.2 pounds.

Krebs cycle The main oxidative reaction sequence in the body that removes hydrogen ions in order to generate ATP; also known as the citric acid or tricarboxylic acid cycle.

lactic acid The anaerobic end product of glycolysis; it has been implicated as a causative factor in the etiology of fatigue.

lactic acid system The energy system that produces ATP anaerobically by the breakdown of glycogen to lactic acid; used primarily in events of maximal effort for one to two minutes.

lactovegetarian A vegetarian who includes milk products in the diet as a form of high-quality protein.

LDL cholesterol Low density lipoprotein cholesterol; a mechanism whereby cholesterol is transported in the blood. (High blood levels are associated with increased incidence of CHD.)

lean body mass The body weight minus the body fat; composed primarily of muscle, bone, and other nonfat tissue.

legume The fruit or pod of vegetables including soybeans, kidney beans, lima beans, garden peas, black-eyed peas, and lentils; high in protein.

leucine An essential amino acid.

life expectancy The number of years of life expected from birth for a given individual in the population. The median for men in the United States is 68 years, for women, 75 years.

life span The biological limit to the length of life; the potential median life span age is 85.

lipids A group of fats or fatlike substances, including triglycerides, phospholipids, and cholesterol.

lipoprotein A combination of lipid and protein, possessing the general properties of proteins. Practically all the lipids of the plasma are present in this form.

lipostatic theory The theory that hunger and satiety are controlled by the lipid level in the blood.

liquid protein diets Protein in a liquid form; a common form consists of predigested protein into simple amino acids.

local muscular endurance The ability of a small muscle group to perform prolonged exercise, such as sit-ups that focus on the abdominal muscles.

long-haul concept Relative to weight control, the idea that weight loss via exercise should be gradual and the individual should not expect to lose large amounts of weight in a short period of time.

low back pain syndrome Pain (usually of the dull, aching type) that persistently occurs in the lumbar region of the lower back.

low density lipoprotein A protein-lipid complex in the blood that facilitates the transport of triglycerides, cholesterol, and phospholipids. *See also* LDL cholesterol.

lumbar lordosis An increased forward curve in the lower (lumbar) region of the back.

lysine An essential amino acid.

magnesium A white metallic mineral element essential in human nutrition.

major minerals Those minerals essential to human nutrition with an RDA in excess of 100 mg/day: calcium, magnesium, phosphorus, sodium, potassium, chloride.

malnutrition Poor nutrition that may be due to inadequate amounts of essential nutrients or due to too many Calories leading to obesity.

mantra A secret word or phrase that is used as part of the relaxation technique in Transcendental Meditation (TM).

maturity-onset diabetes Diabetes that occurs later in life, usually after age forty. It is usually the noninsulin-dependent type.

maximal heart rate *See* HR max.

maximal heart rate reserve The difference between the maximal HR and resting HR. A percentage of this reserve, usually 60–90 percent, is added to the resting HR to get the target HR for aerobic training programs.

maximal oxygen uptake *See* $\dot{V}O_2$ max.

metabolic aftereffects of exercise The theory that the aftereffects of exercise will cause the metabolic rate to be elevated for a period of time, thus expending Calories and contributing to weight loss.

metabolic disorders Diseases of human metabolism; a common one is diabetes.

metabolic rate The energy expended in order to maintain all physical and chemical changes occurring in the body.

metabolic water The water that is a by-product of the oxidation of carbohydrate, fat, and protein in the body.

metabolism The sum total of all physical and chemical processes occurring in the body.

methionine An essential amino acid.

METS A measurement unit of energy expenditure; one MET equals approximately 3.5 ml O_2/kg body weight per minute.

mineral An inorganic element occurring in nature.

mitochondria Structures within the cells that serve as the location for the aerobic production of ATP.

mode of exercise The means by which a person exercises, such as running, swimming, or bicycling.

molybdenum A hard, heavy, silvery-white metallic element.

monosaccharides Simple sugars (glucose, fructose, and galactose) that cannot be broken down by hydrolysis.

muscle fiber A muscle cell. A common method of classifying muscle fibers is by their speed of contraction (either fast twitch or slow twitch).

muscle fiber splitting A theory that muscle cells can increase in number by splitting and forming two cells from one.

muscle glycogen The form in which carbohydrate is stored in the muscle.

muscular hypertrophy An increase in the size of a muscle.

mutagens Compounds or agents that cause genetic mutations, including such agents as chemicals or ultraviolet rays.

myocardial infarct Death of part of the heart muscle, the myocardium.

myofibrils A protein substructure in the muscle fiber. Many myofibrils make up a single muscle fiber.

myoglobin An iron-containing compound, similar to hemoglobin, found in the muscle tissues; myoglobin binds oxygen in the muscle cells.

natural, organic foods Foods that are stated to be grown without the use of man-made chemicals such as pesticides and artificial fertilizers.

Nautilus® A brand of exercise equipment designed for strength training programs; uses a principle to provide optimal resistance throughout the full range of motion.

negative addiction A term coined by Dr. William Morgan to indicate the excessive devotion some individuals have to running, to the extent that they disregard other important facets of their lives such as family and job.

negative energy balance A condition whereby the caloric output exceeds the caloric intake, thus contributing to a weight loss.

niacin Nicotinamide; nicotinic acid; part of the B complex and an important part of several coenzymes involved in aerobic energy processes in the cells.

nicotinamide An amide of nicotinic acid; niacin.

nicotine A poisonous compound found in the tobacco plant, primarily in the leaves.

nicotinic acid Niacin.

nitrogen A colorless, tasteless, odorless gas comprising about 80 percent of the atmospheric gas; an essential component of protein that is formed in plants during their developmental process.

nonessential amino acids Amino acids that are formed in the body and thus need not be obtained in the diet. *See also* essential amino acids.

noninsulin-dependent diabetes Diabetes that may be controlled by diet, exercise, and possibly other medication besides insulin; usually associated with the adult-onset diabetes.

nulliparity Having never given birth to a child.

nutrient density The degree of concentration of nutrients in a given food.

nutritional labeling A listing of selected key nutrients and Calories on the label of commercially prepared food products.

obesity An excessive accumulation of body fat; usually reserved for individuals who are 20–30 percent or more above the average weight for their size.

oligomenorrhea Infrequent or scanty blood flow.

osteoarthritis A chronic disease of the joints characterized by destruction of articular cartilage and decreased function.

osteoporosis Increased porosity or softening of the bone.

overload principle The major concept of physical training whereby the individual imposes a stress greater than that normally imposed upon a particular body system.

overweight Body weight greater than that which is considered normal. *See also* obesity.

ovolactovegetarian A vegetarian who also consumes eggs and milk products as a source of high-quality animal protein.

ovovegetarian A vegetarian who includes eggs in the diet to obtain adequate amounts of protein.

oxygen A gas essential for human cell metabolism and the production of energy in the body.

oxygen consumption The total amount of oxygen utilized in the body for the production of energy; it is directly related to the metabolic rate.

oxygen system The energy system that produces ATP via the oxidation of various foodstuffs, primarily fats and carbohydrates.

pancreas A gland that produces many hormones (including insulin) associated with digestion and metabolism.

pantothenic acid A vitamin of the B complex.

parasympathetic nervous system A part of the autonomic nervous system that helps maintain homeostasis.

PC Phosphocreatine; a high energy phosphate compound found in the body cells; part of the ATP-PC energy system.

pelvic tilt A movement of the pelvic girdle in an anterior, posterior, or lateral direction. An anterior tilt will increase lumbar lordosis while a backward tilt will decrease it.

peripheral circulation The vessels that carry blood to and from the various body tissues. (Compare to central circulation.)

peripheral vascular disease Arteriosclerosis in the peripheral blood vessels other than the coronary and cerebral arteries.

peripheral vascular resistance The resistance to blood flow that is provided by the peripheral blood vessels.

phenylalanine An essential amino acid.

phospholipids A lipid-containing phosphorus that, in hydrolysis, yields fatty acids, glycerin, and a nitrogenous compound. Lecithin is an example.

phosphorus A nonmetallic element essential to human nutrition.

phosphorus-calcium ratio The ratio of calcium to phosphorus intake in the diet; the normal ratio is 1:1.

photosynthesis The process whereby nature harnesses the energy from the sun to produce plant food.

phylloquinone Vitamin K; essential in the blood-clotting process.

physical fitness A general term to denote the ability to do certain activities that are characteristic of specific types of fitness.

phytates Salts of phytic acid; produced in the body during the digestion of certain grain products; can combine with some minerals, such as iron, and possibly decrease their absorption.

pituitary gland An endocrine gland located in the brain that produces a wide variety of hormones that may eventually affect almost all tissues in the body. Often called the master gland.

plaque The material that forms in the inner layer of the artery and contributes to atherosclerosis. It contains cholesterol, lipids, and other debris.

polyunsaturated fatty acids Fats that contain two or more double bonds and thus are open to hydrogenation.

positive energy balance A condition whereby caloric intake exceeds caloric output; the resultant effect is a weight gain.

Positive Health Life-style A life-style characterized by health behaviors that are designed to promote health and longevity by helping to prevent many of the chronic diseases afflicting modern society.

potassium A metallic element essential in human nutrition; it is the principal cation present in the intracellular fluids.

power Work divided by time; the ability to produce work in a given period of time.

power-endurance continuum In relation to strength training, the concept that power or strength is developed by high resistance and few repetitions, while endurance is developed by low resistance and many repetitions.

PRE Progressive resistive exercise.

preventive medicine The concept that certain health behaviors may be able to prevent chronic diseases such as coronary heart disease.

principle of recuperation   The principle in exercise training that rest is essential between workouts in order for the muscle tissue to develop properly.

principle of specificity   The principle that training should be specific to the energy system and the activity that the individual desires to improve.

principle of use   The principle that if a body system is not used, it will lose its potential to perform optimally.

Pritikin program   A dietary program developed by Nathan Pritikin that severely restricts the intake of certain foods (like fats and cholesterol) and greatly increases the consumption of complex carbohydrates.

progressive relaxation   A form of relaxation training in which various muscle groups are contracted and then consciously relaxed, progressively covering all major muscle groups in the body.

progressive resistance principle   A training technique, primarily with weights, in which resistance is increased as the individual develops increased strength levels.

progressive resistive exercise (PRE)   The concept that as one gets stronger through a weight training program, then the resistance needs to be increased progressively in order to continue to gain strength.

protein   Any one of a group of complex organic compounds containing nitrogen; formed from various combinations of amino acids.

protein complementarity   The practice among vegetarians of eating foods from two or more different food groups together (usually legumes, nuts, or beans with grain products), in order to ensure a balanced intake of essential amino acids.

protein sparing effect   An adequate intake of energy Calories, as from carbohydrates, will decrease somewhat the rate of protein catabolism in the body and hence spare protein.

prudent health behavior   Although many of the health behaviors of the Positive Health Life-style have not been proven to increase longevity, they are prudent health behaviors because there is a very strong possibility they can increase longevity by prevention of many chronic diseases.

psoas major   One of the main muscles involved in hip flexion, but it may also increase lumbar lordosis in the lower spine when a sit-up is done improperly.

pyridoxine   A component of the vitamin B complex, vitamin B_6.

radiation   Electromagnetic waves given off by an object; the body radiates heat to a cool environment.

ratings of perceived exertion   See RPE.

RDA   Recommended dietary allowances; the levels of intake of essential nutrients considered to be adequate to meet the known nutritional needs of practically all healthy persons.

recommended dietary allowances   See RDA.

recommended dietary goals   Dietary goals for Americans that have been established by a United States Senate subcommittee on nutrition; goals stress dietary reduction of fat, cholesterol, salt, and sugar and stress an increase in complex carbohydrates.

rectangular society   The concept used to explain the fact that the life expectancy is approaching the life span, so that the longevity curve becomes more rectangular in shape.

rectus abdominis   One of the main muscles involved in doing a curl-up. Strength of this muscle is important in prevention of low back pain.

rectus femoris   One of the main muscles for hip flexion and knee extension; may be involved in creating lumbar lordosis in some improperly performed exercises.

relative humidity   The percentage of moisture in the air compared with the amount of moisture needed to cause saturation (which is taken as 100).

repetition maximum In weight training, the amount of weight that can be lifted for a specific number of repetitions.

repetitions In relation to weight training or interval training, the number of times that an exercise is done.

resistance In weight training, it is the amount of weight to be lifted.

resting metabolic rate *See* RMR.

retinol Vitamin A.

rheumatoid arthritis A form of arthritis characterized by joint inflammation, swelling, stiffness, and pain.

RHR Resting heart rate.

riboflavin Vitamin B_2, a member of the B complex.

risk factor A health behavior or condition that predisposes an individual to a disease that has been statistically related to that behavior or condition.

RMR Resting metabolic rate; the energy required to drive all physiological processes while in a state of rest. *See also* BMR and EMR.

RNA Ribonucleic acid; a cellular component involved in the formation of cell proteins.

round shoulders A postural condition in which the shoulders are inclined forward and inward.

routine In weight training, a number of different types of exercises constitutes a routine.

RPE A subjective rating, on a numerical scale, used to express the perceived difficulty of a given work task.

running Although the distinction between running and jogging is relative to the individual involved, a common value used for running is 9 minutes/mile or faster.

sacroiliac The immovable joint in the lower back region where the sacrum of the spine meets the ilium which is part of the hip bone.

satiety center A group of nerve cells in the hypothalamus that responds to certain stimuli in the blood and provides a sensation of satiety.

saturated fatty acids Fats that have all chemical bonds filled.

SDA Specific dynamic action; often used to represent the increased energy cost observed during the metabolism of protein in the body.

secondary amenorrhea A cessation of normal menstrual flow after it has once been established at puberty, as contrasted with primary amenorrhea, in which menstruation never appears in the first place.

selenium A nonmetallic element resembling sulfur; poisonous to some animals.

self-actualization One of the highest levels in Maslow's hierarchy of development in which the individual exhibits characteristics of a well-adjusted personality.

self-concept The feelings individuals have about their worth or value as an individual; their self-esteem.

serum cholesterol The level of cholesterol in the blood serum.

serum lipid level The concentration of lipids in the blood serum.

set In weight training, a certain number of repetitions constitutes a set; for example, a lifter may do three sets of six repetitions in each set.

shin splints A painful condition in the shin area of the lower leg that often develops in joggers or runners who run on hard surfaces such as concrete.

silicon A nonmetallic element.

simple carbohydrates Usually refers to table sugar, or sucrose (a disaccharide); may also refer to other disaccharides and the monosaccharides.

skinfold technique A technique used to compute an individual's percentage of body fat; various skinfolds are measured and a regression formula is used to compute the body fat.

slow-twitch fibers Red muscle fibers that have a slow contraction speed; designed for aerobic activity.

sodium A soft metallic element; combines with chloride to form salt; the major extracellular cation in the human body.

soft tissues In relation to flexibility, the muscles and tendons that can be stretched due to their content of elastic fibers.

somatotype A classification system for body types; for example, endomorphs are round and fat, mesomorphs are muscular, and ectomorphs are thin.

spinal flexion A forward, bending movement of the spine.

sports anemia A temporary condition of low hemoglobin levels often observed in athletes during the early stages of training.

spot reducing The theory that exercising a specific body part, such as the thighs, will facilitate the loss of body fat from that spot.

standardized exercise An exercise task that conforms to a specific standardized protocol.

state anxiety A transient period of anxiety caused by a temporary stressor; state anxiety disappears when the stressor is removed.

static flexibility Flexibility as measured by a slow, steady movement to the limit of the range of motion. Static flexibility exercises are done slowly. (Compare with dynamic flexibility.)

steady state A level of metabolism, usually during exercise, when the oxygen consumption satisfies the energy expenditure and the individual is performing in an aerobic state.

steady-state threshold The intensity level of exercise in which the production of energy appears to shift rapidly to anaerobic mechanism, such as a rapid rise in lactic acid. The oxygen system will still supply a major portion of the energy, but the lactic acid system begins to contribute an increasing share.

stimulus period In exercise programs, the time period over which the stimulus is applied, such as an HR of 150 for 15 minutes.

storage fat Fat that accumulates and is stored in the adipose tissue. *See also* essential fat.

strength The ability of a muscle to exert maximal force during one contraction.

stress The physiological response the body makes to any stressor. *See also* stress response.

stress management Procedures or treatments that are designed to decrease the potential harmful effects of stress on the individual.

stress response The characteristic physiological responses that the human body makes when confronted by a stressor.

stressor Anything that will elicit a stress response in a given individual.

stroke Common term used to describe the results of a cerebral vascular accident or a ruptured blood vessel in the brain.

stroke volume The amount of blood pumped by the heart during each beat.

substance abuse Excessive reliance on drugs, such as alcohol or tobacco, to cope with society.

sucrose Table sugar, a disaccharide; yields glucose and fructose upon hydrolysis.

sulfur A pale yellow nonmetallic element essential in human nutrition; a component of the sulfur-containing amino acids.

synovial fluid The fluid in the joint capsule that aids in lubrication and decreases friction during movement.

systolic blood pressure The blood pressure in the arteries when the heart is contracting and pumping blood.

target heart rate In an aerobic exercise program, the heart rate level that will provide the stimulus for a beneficial training effect.

target heart rate range (target HR) The range of heart rate response during exercise that is necessary to achieve a beneficial training effect from the exercise.

tendon The connective tissue in the muscle that merges with and connects the muscle to the bone.

testosterone The male sex hormone produced by the testes.

thiamin Vitamin B_1.

threonine An essential amino acid.

threshold stimulus In exercise, the intensity level necessary to elicit a beneficial training effect, such as a target heart rate.

thrombus A blood clot that does not move.

tocopherol Generic name for an alcohol that has the activity of vitamin E.

total body fat The sum total of the body's storage and essential fat stores.

trace elements Those minerals essential to human nutrition that have an RDA less than 100 mg daily.

trait anxiety A more enduring anxiety level that appears to be characteristic of a given individual. (Compare to state anxiety.)

Transcendental Meditation (TM) A passive relaxation technique characterized by quiet meditation.

triglycerides One of the many fats formed by the union of glycerol and fatty acids.

tryptophan An essential amino acid.

type A personality A personality trait of an individual characterized by constant anxiety or time urgency.

underwater weighing A technique for measuring the percentage of body fat in humans.

United States recommended daily allowances See U.S. RDA.

Universal Gym® A brand name for exercise equipment, particularly weights, for strength development.

unsaturated fatty acids Fatty acids that contain double or triple bonds and hence can add hydrogen atoms.

U.S. RDA The United States recommended daily allowances; the RDA figures used on labels representing the percentage of the RDA for a given nutrient contained in a serving of the food.

validity The degree to which a test accurately measures what it is designed to measure.

valine An essential amino acid.

Valsalva phenomena A condition in which a forceful exhalation is attempted against a closed epiglottis so no air escapes; such a straining may cause the person to faint or black out due to an eventual lack of blood to the brain.

vegan An extreme vegetarian who eats no animal protein.

vegetarian An individual whose food is of vegetable or plant origin. See also lacto-vegetarian, ovovegetarian, ovolactovegetarian, and vegan.

veins The blood vessels that carry blood back to the heart.

very low density lipoprotein See VLDL.

vitamin, natural Often referred to as a vitamin derived from natural sources; i.e., foods in nature. (Contrast with vitamin, synthetic.)

vitamin, synthetic A man-made vitamin commercially produced from the separate components of the vitamin.

vitamin A An unsaturated aliphatic alcohol that is fat soluble.

vitamin B_1 Thiamin; the antineuritic vitamin.

vitamin B_2 Riboflavin.

vitamin B_6 Pyridoxine and related compounds.

vitamin B$_{12}$ Cyanocobalamin.

vitamin B$_{15}$ Not a vitamin but marketed as one; usual composition is calcium gluconate and dimethylglycine (DMG).

vitamin C   Ascorbic acid; the antiscorbutic vitamin.

vitamin D   Any one of related sterols that have antirachitic properties; it is fat soluble.

vitamin deficiency   Subnormal body vitamin levels due to inadequate intake or absorption; specific disorders occur, depending on the deficient vitamin.

vitamin E   Alpha-tocopherol (one of three tocopherols); it is fat soluble.

vitamin K   The antihemorrhagic (or clotting) vitamin; it is fat soluble.

vitamins   A general term for a number of substances deemed essential for the normal metabolic functioning of the body.

VLDL   Very low density lipoproteins; a protein-lipid complex in the blood that transports triglycerides, cholesterol, and phospholipids and has a very low density. *See also* HDL and LDL cholesterol.

V̇O$_2$ max   Maximal oxygen uptake; measured during exercise, the maximal amount of oxygen consumed reflects the body's ability to utilize oxygen as an energy source; equals the maximal cardiac output times the maximal arterio-venous oxygen difference.

warm-down   A gradually tapering period after the stimulus period of an exercise bout in which the individual exercises mildly. Also known as a cool-down period after exercise.

warm-up   Low level exercises used to increase the muscle temperature and/or stretch the muscles before a strenuous exercise bout.

water   A tasteless, colorless, odorless fluid essential to life; composed of two parts hydrogen and one part oxygen (H_2O).

water depletion heat exhaustion
Weakness caused by excessive loss of body fluids such as through exercise-induced dehydration in a hot or warm environment.

weight lifting   A competitive sport; the two most common lifts are the clean-and-jerk and the snatch.

weight training   A conditioning method with heavy weights designed to increase strength, power, and muscle size.

wellness clinics   Educational seminars designed to help individuals develop health behaviors characteristic of a Positive Health Life-style.

work   Effort expended to accomplish something; in terms of physics, force times distance.

zinc   A blue-white crystalline metallic element essential to human nutrition.

Index